G. P. Krestin · G. M. Glazer (Eds.)

Advances in CT IV

Springer

Berlin
Heidelberg
New York
Barcelona
Budapest
Hong Kong
London
Milan
Paris
Santa Clara
Singapore
Tokyo

G. P. Krestin · G. M. Glazer (Eds.)

Advances in CT IV

4th International Scientific User Conference SOMATOM PLUS CT Rotterdam, March 1998

With 115 Figures, some in Color, and 23 Tables

Springer

Gabriel P. Krestin, M. D., Ph. D.
Professor and Chairman
Dept. of Radiology
University Hospital Rotterdam
Erasmus University
Dr. Molewaterplein 40
3015 GD Rotterdam
The Netherlands

Gary M. Glazer, M. D.
Professor and Chairman
Dept. of Radiology
Stanford University
Stanford, CA 94305-5488
USA

ISBN 3-540-64348-6 Springer-Verlag Berlin Heidelberg New York

Die Deutsche Bibliothek – CIP-Einheitsaufnahme
Advances in CT IV / 4th International Scientific User Conference
SOMATOM Plus, CT, Rotterdam, March 1998. G. P. Krestin ; G. M. Glazer (ed.). – Berlin ; Heidelberg ; New York ; Barcelona ; Budapest ; Hong Kong ; London ; Milan ; Paris ; Santa Clara ; Singapore ;
ISBN 3-540-64348-6

CIP data applied for

Production: PRO EDIT GmbH, D-69126 Heidelberg
Cover Design: design & production GmbH, D-69121 Heidelberg
Typesetting: Zechnersche Buchdruckerei, D-67346 Speyer

SPIN: 10673245 18/3137-5 4 3 2 1 0 – Printed on acid-free paper

Preface

We are in the midst of major advances in medical imaging, converting static presentation of anatomic information into near real-time interactive imaging and displays capable of depicting both structure and function. This will have profound impact on diagnosis and image-guided therapies.

These advances have been most notable in the modalities of computed tomography and magnetic resonance. These technologies have become capable of acquiring volumetric images in short periods of time. Speed gains in MRI were very significant in the early 1990s with the development of clinically usable pulse sequences for gradient-recalled and echo-planar imaging. It appears that further speed gains in MRI will be difficult to achieve.

The development of spiral CT has ushered in an era in which major speed gains in CT are also possible. This has enabled creation of new types of applications such as CT angiography, which has already come to replace catheter angiography at many medical centers throughout the world. We are very pleased that the results from industrial and academic laboratories have been transferred to the bedside to improve patient care at a speed that may be faster than in any other area of medicine.

Concurrent with advances in CT technology there have been dramatic strides in the performance characteristics and costs of computer hardware and software. The combination of volumetric high-speed CT and enhanced computer graphics permits developments of novel applications such as virtual CT colonoscopy and virtual CT bronchoscopy. The general theme of these applications is to develop CT-based techniques that will screen patients so that only those who will benefit will proceed to the "real" invasive procedures. The potential importance of this work is very major, since a large number of patients undergoing colonoscopy or bronchoscopy present no abnormal findings.

Furthermore, advances in the use of genetic screening to identify subsets of patients who are at high risk for developing cancers will result in a greater need for anatomic localization of malignant disease using non-invasive methods. Finally, we are aware of developments using multiple rows of detectors which will further improve volumetric CT data acquisition.

There have been no national boundaries in the creation of these advances, and therefore the 4th International Somatom Plus CT Scientific User Conference, held in Rotterdam on 6–7 March 1998, assembled a distinguished international faculty. Recognizing further the international flavor of the meeting, we expanded the hosting of the conference to include two universities, Erasmus and Stanford, which are separated geographically but linked by a spirit of discovery, innovation and education.

We are happy to present the proceedings of this conference and are grateful to Siemens Medical Systems for their continuing support as well as to Springer-Verlag for the prompt and professional publication. We very much look forward to the next Somatom Plus User Conference to hear of the improved patient care resulting from continued technological innovation and clinical development.

Rotterdam, The Netherlands, April 1998 GABRIEL P. KRESTIN, M.D., Ph.D.
Stanford, USA, April 1998 GARY M. GLAZER, M.D.

Contributors

S. Achenbach
Institute of Medical Physics
University of Erlangen-Nürnberg
Krankenhausstrasse 12
91054 Erlangen
Germany

K. H. Allmann
Department of Diagnostic Radiology
University Hospital Freiburg
Hugstetterstrasse 55,
79106 Freiburg
Germany

M. E. Baker
Section Abdominal Imaging
Division of Radiology
Cleveland Clinic Foundation
9500 Euclid Ave, Ste HB-6
Cleveland OH 44195
USA

G. Battaglia
Department of Radiology
University of Brescia
Policlinico Satellite,
25123 Brescia
Italy

W. A. Bautz
Institutes of Diagnostic Radiology
and Medical Physics
University of Erlangen-Nürnberg
Krankenhausstrasse 12
91054 Erlangen
Germany

M. Bohnert
Institute for Legal Medicine
University Hospital Freiburg
Hugstetterstrasse 55
79106 Freiburg
Germany

A. H. H. Bongaerts
Department of Radiology
Daniel den Hoed Cancer Center
University Hospital Rotterdam
The Netherlands

H. Bosmans
Department of Radiology
University Hospitals KU Leuven
Herestraat 49
3000 Leuven
Belgium

C. H. Buitrago-Téllez
Department of Diagnostic Radiology
University Hospital Freiburg
Hugstetterstrasse 55
79106 Freiburg
Germany

A. Chiesa
Department of Radiology
University of Brescia
Policlinico Satellite,
25123 Brescia
Italy

C. Claussen
Department of Radiology
University of Tübingen
Hoppe-Seyler-Str. 3
72076 Tübingen
Germany

F. Codazzi
Department of Radiology
University of Brescia
Policlinico Satellite,
25123 Brescia
Italy

P. Costello
Department of Radiology
Queen Elizabeth Hospital, and
University of Adelaide
28 Woodville Road
Woodville South
South Australia 5011

R. A. Coulden
Department of Radiology
Papworth Hospital
Papworth Everard
Cambridge CB3 8RE
UK

J. J. Cross
Department of Radiology
Addenbrooke's Hospital, and
University of Cambridge
Cambridge CB2 2QQ
UK

W. J. Davros
Division of Radiology
Cleveland Clinic Foundation
9500 Euclid Ave, Ste HB-6
Cleveland, OH 44195
USA

J. de Mey
Akademisch Ziekenhuis
Vrije universiteit Brussel
Laarbeeklaan 101
1090 Brussels
Belgium

A. K. Dixon
Department of Radiology
Addenbrooke's Hospital, and
University of Cambridge
Cambridge CB2 2QQ
UK

C. Engelke
Department of Diagnostic Radiology
Medical School Hannover
Carl-Neuberg-Str. 1
30625 Hannover
Germany

D. Farina
Department of Radiology
University of Brescia
Policlinico Satellite
25123 Brescia
Italy

E. K. Fishman
Johns Hopkins University
School of Medicine
601 North Wolfe St.
Baltimore, MD 21205
USA

C. D. R. Flower
Department of Radiology
Addenbrooke's Hospital, and
University of Cambridge
Cambridge CB2 2QQ
UK

J. J. Froelich
Department of Radiology
Hospital of the Philipps University
Baldingerstrasse
35043 Marburg
Germany

M. Galanski
Department of Diagnostic Radiology I
Medical School Hannover
Carl-Neuberg-Str. 1
30625 Hannover
Germany

M. Gies
Institute of Medical Physics
University of Erlangen-Nürnberg
Krankenhausstrasse 12
91054 Erlangen
Germany

H. Greess
Institutes of Diagnostic Radiology
and Medical Physics
University of Erlangen-Nürnberg
Krankenhausstrasse 12
91054 Erlangen
Germany

D. Hahn
Department of Diagnostic Radiology
Julius-Maximilians-University
Josef-Schneider-Str. 2
97080 Würzburg
Germany

K. Hashi
Department of Neurosurgery
Sapporo Medical University School
of Medicine
South-1, West-16, Chuo-ku
Sapporo, 060-8543
Japan

M. P. Hayball
Department of Radiology
Papworth Hospital
Papworth Everard
Cambridge CB3 8RE
UK

L. Heuser
Department of Radiology
and Nuclear Medicine
Knappschaft Hospital Langendreer
Hospital of the Ruhr University Bochum
In der Schornau 23–25
44892 Bochum
Germany

P. Hilfiker
Department of Radiology
University Hospital Zurich
Zurich
Switzerland

R. Hupke
Siemens Medical Engineering
CT Department
Siemensstrasse 1
91301 Forchheim
Germany

P. Huppert
Department of Radiology
University of Tübingen
Hoppe-Seyler-Str. 3
72076 Tübingen
Germany

Y. Ibayashi
Department of Neurosurgery
Sapporo Medical University School
of Medicine, South-1, West-16
Chuo-ku, Sapporo, 060-8543
Japan

R. B. Jeffrey
Stanford University, School of Medicine
Dept. of Radiology
300 Pasteur Drive
Stanford, CA 94305
USA

M. Kachelriess
Institute of Medical Physics
University of Erlangen-Nürnberg
Krankenhausstrasse 12
91054 Erlangen
Germany

W. A. Kalender
Institutes of Diagnostic Radiology
and Medical Physics
University of Erlangen-Nürnberg
Krankenhausstrasse 12
91054 Erlangen
Germany

M. Karakaya
Institute of Medical Physics
University of Erlangen-Nürnberg
Krankenhausstrasse 12
91054 Erlangen
Germany

E. W. Khoo
Department of Radiology
Queen Elizabeth Hospital
and University of Adelaide
Woodville South
South Australia 5011

M. Kimmig
Department of Diagnostic Radiology
University Hospital Freiburg
Hugstetterstrasse 55
79106 Freiburg
Germany

K. Klingenbeck-Regn
Siemens Medical Engineering
CT Department
Siemensstrasse 1
91301 Forchheim
Germany

K. J. Klose
Department of Radiology
Hospital of the Philipps University
Baldingerstrasse
35043 Marburg
Germany

E. Klotz
Siemens Medical Engineering
CT Group
Siemensstrasse 1
91301 Forchheim
Germany

M. König
Department of Radiology
and Nuclear Medicine
Knappschaft Hospital Langendreer
Hospital of the Ruhr University Bochum
In der Schornau 23–25
44892 Bochum
Germany

M. Langer
Department of Diagnostic Radiology
University Hospital Freiburg
Hugstetterstrasse 55
79106 Freiburg
Germany

P. Maculotti
Department of Radiology
University of Brescia
Policlinico Satellite,
25123 Brescia
Italy

G. Marchal
Department of Radiology
University Hospitals KU Leuven
Herestraat 49
3000 Leuven
Belgium

R. Maroldi
Department of Radiology
University of Brescia
Policlinico Satellite
25123 Brescia
Italy

F. Mehnert
Department of Radiology
University of Tübingen
Hoppe-Seyler-Str. 3
72076 Tübingen
Germany

M.T. Modic
Division of Radiology
Cleveland Clinic Foundation
9500 Euclid Ave, Ste HB-6
Cleveland, OH 44195
USA

W. Moshage
Institute of Medical Physics
University of Erlangen-Nürnberg
Krankenhausstrasse 12
91054 Erlangen
Germany

J. Nossen
Institute of Medical Physics
University of Erlangen-Nürnberg
Krankenhausstrasse 12
91054 Erlangen
Germany

M. Ohtaki
Department of Neurosurgery
Sapporo Medical University School
of Medicine, South-1, West-16, Chuo-ku
Sapporo
060-8543 Japan

B. Op de Beeck
Akademisch Ziekenhuis
Vrije universiteit Brussel
Laarbeeklaan 101
1090 Brussels
Belgium

M. Osteaux
Academic Hospital
Free University Brussels
Laarbeeklaan 101
1090 Brussels
Belgium

M. Oudkerk
Department of Radiology
Daniel den Hoed Cancer Center
University Hospital
Groene Hilledijk 301
3075 EA Rotterdam
The Netherlands

P. Pelkonen
Department of Radiology
University Hospital Zurich
Zurich
Switzerland

P. Pereira
Department of Radiology
University of Tübingen
Hoppe-Seyler-Str. 3
72076 Tübingen
Germany

M. Prokop
University of Vienna
Dept. of Radiology
Währinger Gürtel 18–20
1090 Vienna
Austria

G. D. Rubin
Stanford University, School of Medicine
Dept. of Radiology
300 Pasteur Drive
Stanford, CA 94305
USA

C. M. Schaefer-Prokop
University of Vienna
Dept. of Radiology
Währinger Gürtel 18–20
1090 Vienna
Austria

G. Schultz
Department of Diagnostic Radiology
Julius-Maximilians-University
Josef-Schneider-Str. 2
97080 Würzburg
Germany

M. J. Siegel
Mallinckrodt Inst. Radiology
Dept. of Radiology
510 S Kingshighway Blvd.
St. Louis, MO 63110-1076
USA

C. Steiner
Division of Radiology
Cleveland Clinic Foundation
9500 Euclid Ave, Ste HB-6
Cleveland, OH 44195
USA

C. Suess
Institute of Medical Physics
University of Erlangen-Nürnberg
Krankenhausstrasse 12
91054 Erlangen
Germany

S. Tanabe
Department of Neurosurgery
Sapporo Medical University School
of Medicine, South-1, West-16, Chuo-ku
Sapporo
060-8543 Japan

T. Uede
Department of Neurosurgery
Sapporo Medical University School
of Medicine, South-1, West-16, Chuo-ku
Sapporo
060-8543 Japan

E. J. R. van Beek
Department of Radiology
Academic Medical Center
Amsterdam
The Netherlands

S. van de Straete
Department of Radiology
University Hospitals KU Leuven
Herestraat 49
3000 Leuven
Belgium

L. van Hoe
Department of Radiology
University Hospitals KU Leuven
Herestraat 49
3000 Leuven
Belgium

G. Verhoek
Department of Radiology
Queen Elizabeth Hospital, and
University of Adelaide
28 Woodville Road
Woodville South
South Australia 5011

T. von der Haar
Siemens Medical Engineering
CT Department
Siemensstrasse 1
91301 Forchheim
Germany

H. Wolf
Institutes of Diagnostic Radiology
and Medical Physics
University of Erlangen-Nürnberg
Krankenhausstrasse 12
91054 Erlangen
Germany

Contents

Part I
Dose Reduction

1 Relationships Between Time, Dose, and Quality in Helical CT 3
L. van Hoe, S. van de Straete, H. Bosmans, G. Marchal

2 Improvement of CT Performance by UFC Detector Technology 9
T. von der Haar, K. Klingenbeck-Regn, R. Hupke

3 Dose Reduction vs. Image Quality in Spiral CT:
How Far Down Can We Go in Clinical Practice? 16
M. Prokop, C. M. Schaefer-Prokop, M. Galanski

4 Dose Reduction in CT by Anatomically Adapted Tube Current
Modulation: Principles and First Results 27
W. A. Kalender, H. Wolf, C. Suess, M. Gies, H. Greess, W. A. Bautz

5 Dose Reduction in CT by Anatomically Adapted Tube Current
Modulation: First Patient Studies 35
H. Greess, H. Wolf, W. A. Kalender, W. A. Bautz

Part II
Neuro, Head and Neck

6 Spiral CT and its Use in Neuroradiology: A Review of Spiral
CT Techniques, Real Time Volume Rendering, and Real Time
Neuro-Navigation 43
W. J. Davros, C. Steiner, M. T. Modic

7 Determination of Regional Brain Perfusion by Functional CT 49
M. König, L. Heuser, E. Klotz

8 The Diagnostic Accuracy and the Role of Three-Dimensional
CT Angiography for the Diagnosis of Cerebral Aneurysms 59
S. Tanabe, M. Ohtaki, T. Uede, Y. Ibayashi, K. Hashi

9 Spiral CT vs. Subsecond Conventional CT in Head and Neck Malignancies 70
R. Maroldi, G. Battaglia, P. Maculotti, D. Farina, F. Codazzi, A. Chiesa

10 Spiral CT in Maxillofacial Trauma 76
C. H. Buitrago-Téllez, M. Bohnert, M. Kimmig, K. H. Allmann, M. Langer

Part III
Chest

11 Optimizing CT Angiography of the Chest 85
C. M. Schaefer-Prokop, M. Prokop, C. Engelke, M. Galanski

12 The Diagnostic Impact of Spiral CT for Pulmonary Embolism 98
A. K. Dixon, J. J. Cross, C. D. Flower

13 Cost-Effectiveness Analysis of Diagnostic Management of Pulmonary Embolism 106
M. Oudkerk, E. J. R. van Beek, A. H. H. Bongaerts

14 Helical CT in the Pediatric Chest 115
M. J. Siegel

15 Cardiac CT with Prospective Cardiac Gating 126
R. A. Coulden, M. P. Hayball

16 Imaging of the Heart by ECG-Oriented Reconstruction from Subsecond Spiral CT Scans 137
M. Kachelriess, W. A. Kalender, M. Karakaya, S. Achenbach, J. Nossen, W. Moshage, W. A. Bautz

17 CT-Guided Diagnostic Punctures of the Chest 144
D. Hahn

Part IV
Abdomen, Musculoskeletal

18 Three-Dimensional Imaging and Virtual Reality Applications of Spiral CT 149
R.B. Jeffrey

19 Automatic Bolus Traking for Spiral CT of the Liver 154
C. Claussen, F. Mehnert, P. Pereira, P. Huppert

20 Dual-Phase Spiral CT of Pancreatic Neoplasms 165
R.B. Jeffrey

21 Contribution of Fast and Spiral CT to Diagnostic Punctures of Abdominal Lesions 171
J. de Mey, B. Op de Beeck, M. Osteaux

22 Spiral CT of the Musculoskeletal System 175
E. K. Fishman

Part V
Technical Developments, Postprocessing

23 Spiral CT: How New Technology Has Improved Scanner Utilization and Productivity 189
M. E. Baker

24 Volumetric Analysis of Spiral CT Data 196
G. D. Rubin

25 Impact of Real-Time Three-Dimensional Rendering of CT Data on Diagnostic Performance 207
G. P. Krestin, P. Hilfiker, P. Pelkonen, G. Verhoek

26 Interactive Three-Dimensional Volume Rendering – Vascular Applications 212
P. Costello, E. W. Khoo

27 Guidance of Nonvascular Interventional Procedures with Real-Time CT-Fluoroscopy: Early Clinical Experience with C.A.R.E. Vision CT 225
J. J. Froelich, K. J. Klose

Subject Index 235

Part I
Dose Reduction

Moderators: R. B. Jeffrey, P. Vock

1 Relationships Between Time, Dose, and Quality in Helical CT

L. Van Hoe, S. Van de Straete, H. Bosmans, G. Marchal

1.1 Introduction

Helical computed tomography (CT) constitutes an evolution of conventional (incremental) CT and offers marked advantages with respect to image quality and speed. In physical terms, image quality can be described by the spatial resolution, the low contrast visibility, and the signal-to-noise ratio. In clinical practice, the degree of confidence in detecting or excluding disease is more generally used to set up specific procedures. Any optimization, however, should take account of the ALARA principle, and the relationship between image quality, acquisition time, and dose therefore needs to be carefully studied.

A series of parameters have an influence on the image quality of a helical CT image, including the total acquisition time, the scanned volume and the number of scans per volume, the table feed/collimation (or pitch), the filtration of the X-ray spectrum, the efficiency of the detector and its configuration, the resolution of the monitor for image display, and the selection of look-up tables for printing. The quality of post-processed images (e.g., three-dimensional renderings) depends on many parameters, such as the image reconstruction interval, appropriate selection of threshold, and appropriate automated or manual image editing.

Short examination times allow for breath-hold scanning (thus eliminating data gaps caused by respiratory misregistration) and for an optimal use of intravenous contrast media. Short examination times can be obtained by using a short rotation time (e.g., 0.75 s), by selecting a large collimation and table feed, or by reducing the volume covered. Since the volume to be examined is usually fixed and determined by the clinical question, tradeoffs exist between longitudinal spatial resolution and in-plane contrast resolution on the one hand and imaging time on the other.

The selection of the ratio of table feed to collimation (i.e., pitch) should be optimized in order to keep the degree of SSP broadening as low as possible and to avoid rotation- or stair-step artifacts specific for helical CT. On the other hand, higher pitches significantly reduce the total dose per scan.

A practical issue that should be discussed is the need to adapt acquisition protocols to the expected patterns of contrast uptake of organs and lesions (e.g., necessity of dual- or multiphase contrast-enhanced scanning). Again, a tradeoff exists between the maximum number of scans per volume and per time unit on the one hand and resolution on the other.

The purpose of this study was twofold. First, in a physical study, we used a low contrast phantom (Siemens, Erlangen, Germany) to analyze the influence of radiation dose reduction on low contrast visibility. Second, in a clinical study, we attempted to develop a flow chart for radiation dose reduction in abdominal helical CT based on measurement of the abdominal perimeter.

1.2 Materials and Methods

1.2.1 Experimental Study

The low contrast phantom was scanned using a Siemens Somatom Plus 4 helical CT scanner. The parameters studied were the voltage (140 vs. 120 kV), the rotation time (0.75, 1.5 s), and the mA value (360, 240, 171, 111, 60, and 43 mA). The influence of these parameters on object conspicuity was determined.

1.2.2 Clinical Study

The clinical study was performed in 120 randomly chosen patients referred for an upper abdominal helical CT study. Before the acquisition, the abdominal perimeter was measured at the level of the umbilicus. The patients were divided into four groups (I–IV). In each group, different tube currents were used: 240, 171, 111, and 60 mA. A tube current of 240 mA used to be the routine value in our department.

Further parameters were voltage (140 kV), rotation time (0.75 s), slice thickness and table feed (8 mm/12 mm), window setting (enhanced scans: window width 350 HU, window level 50 HU; unenhanced scans: window width 350 HU, window level 0 HU).

Four images per patient were selected for further evaluation at the level of the hepatic veins, the portal vein, the pancreatic body, and the renal hilum. Images were scored independently by five radiologists using the following subjective gradings for image quality, delineation of contours and conspicuity of focal structures or lesions: 1, unsatisfactory; 2, satisfactory; 3, good; 4, optimal results. The five scores per patient and per slice were added, and an average score was calculated from the scores assigned to each of the four separate images. In this way, the final total score ranges between 5 and 20. This score was analyzed as a function of the dose and the patient's perimeter.

1.3 Results

1.3.1 Experimental Study

The experimental study showed no surprising results. As could be predicted [1, 2], there was a nonlinear relationship between object size, dose, and conspicuity. All objects were visible with the following parameters: rotation time 0.75 s, 140 kV, and 360 mA. Using 240 mA and with unchanged values of the other parameters, the 3-mm objects became nearly invisible; at 111 mA, 4-mm objects became invisible (see Fig. 1.1).

1.3.2 Clinical Study

Surprisingly, we found no statistically significant influence of the patient's perimeter. The mean scores as a function of the mA value used are given in Fig. 1.2. Even the image quality in the third group (using only 111 mA) was scored as "good." There were no statistically significant differences between the scores of group I and group II (*p* value, 0.147). Statistically significant differences were seen between the scores of patients scanned at 240 and at 171 mA on the one hand and at 111 and 60 mA on the other hand.

1.4 **Conclusion**

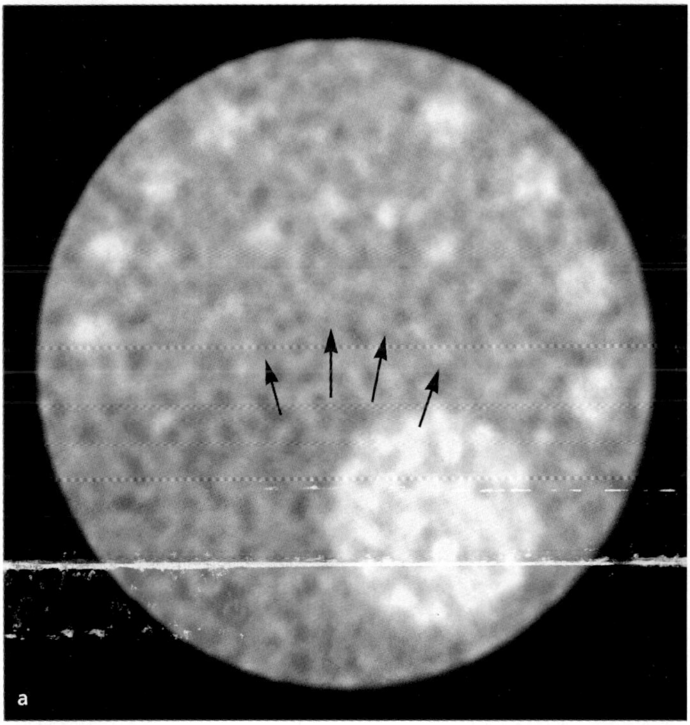

Fig. 1.1a–d. Low-contrast phantom scanned with four different mA values: **a** 360, **b** 240, **c** 171, and **d** 111 mA. Even at the high mA setting, the smallest objects are rather unsharp (*arrows*)

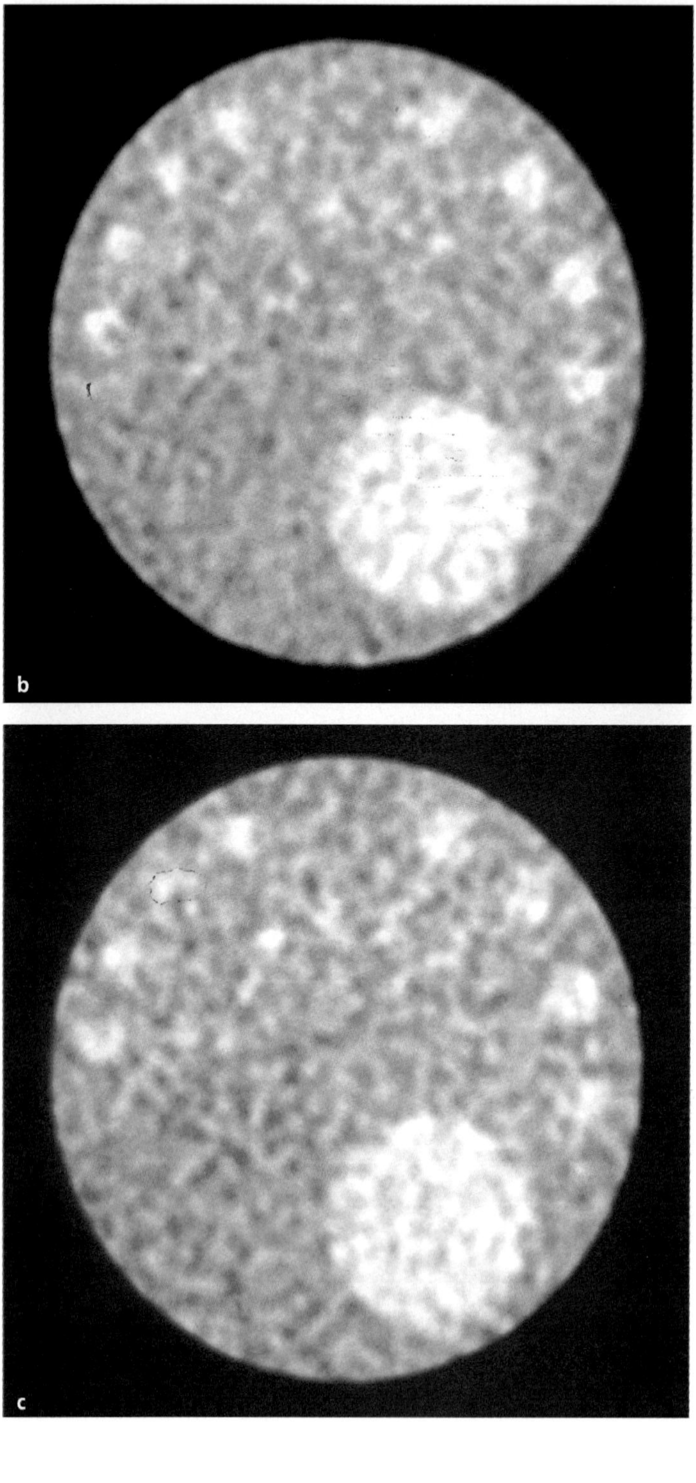

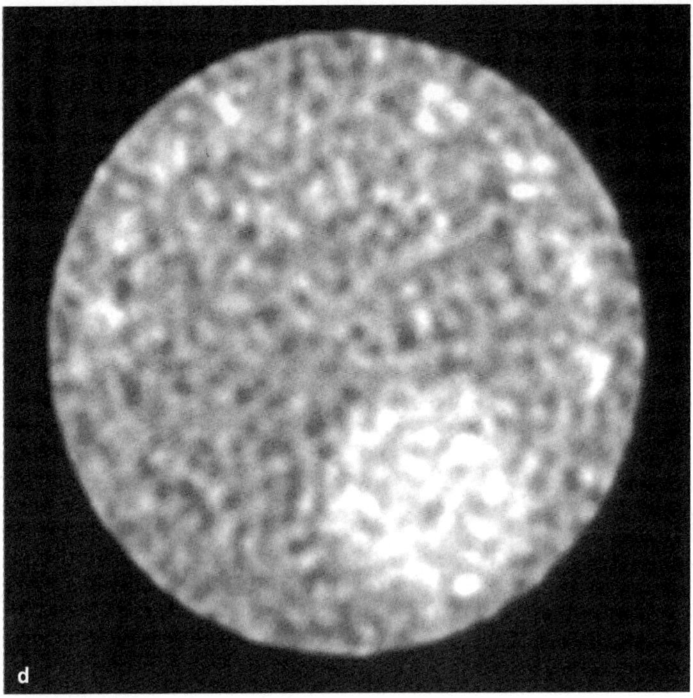

Fig. 1.1b–d. Low-contrast phantom scanned with four different mA values: **b** 240, **c** 171, and **d** 111 mA. Even at the high mA setting, the smallest objects are rather unsharp

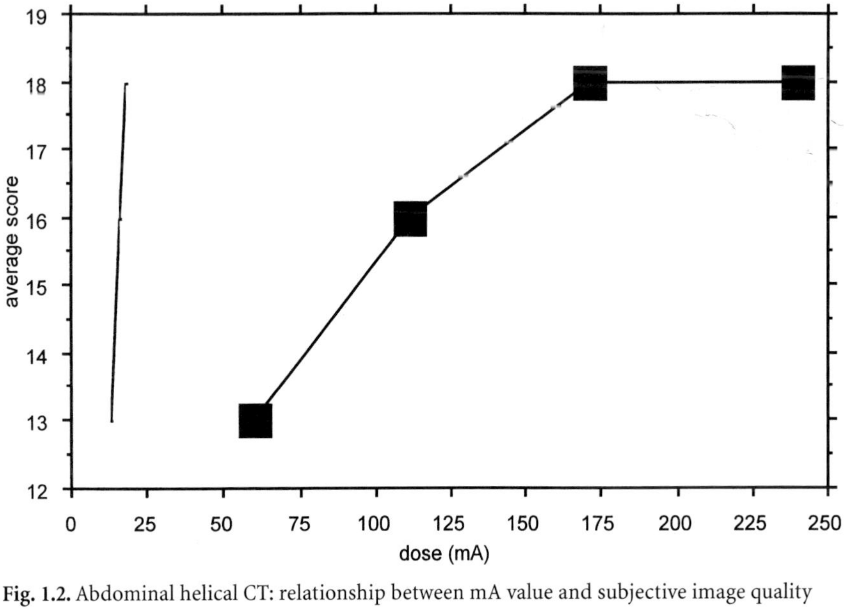

Fig. 1.2. Abdominal helical CT: relationship between mA value and subjective image quality

Many parameters affect image quality in helical CT. We tried to reduce the radiation dose in abdominal helical CT by calculating the optimal dose as a function of the patient's perimeter. Unfortunately, no such method could be developed because the patient's perimeter was not an important determinant of image quality at a given dose.

A second conclusion from this study was that even a remarkable reduction of radiation doses (e.g., 111 mA vs. 240 mA, 46% of the original value) still gave rise to a "good" (subjective) image quality. This result suggests that mAs values could be significantly reduced in a clinical setting.

The phantom study, however, enabled us to put these results into perspective. The tests illustrate that too much noise is detrimental for the signal-to-noise ratio and low contrast visibility. The reduction of radiation dose led to a dramatic decrease in conspicuity of small, low-contrast lesions. It could therefore be argued that the low mA setting should be used for screening studies only, and not for dedicated studies of the liver or pancreas, for instance.

References

1. Martin JE, Schlesinger AE, Niklason LT, Guire KE (1994) Radiation dose reduction in CT of the pediatric pelvis. Radiology 190:683–687
2. Haaga JR, Miraldi F, MacIntyre W, LiPuma JP, Bryan PJ, Wiesen E (1981) The effect of mAs variation upon computed tomography image quality as evaluated in in vivo and in vitro studies. Radiology 138:449–454

2 Improvement of CT Performance by UFC Detector Technology

T. von der Haar, K. Klingenbeck-Regn, R. Hupke

2.1 Introduction

Since the early days of computed tomography (CT), solid state detectors have been used to detect the X-ray radiation transmitted through the patient's body. These detectors have been based on the combination of classical scintillators with photodetectors, e.g., NaI with photomultipliers or CsI ($CdWO_4$) with photodiodes. Early CT scanners were of the rotate–rotate type with pulsed radiation and change of the direction of rotation from scan to scan.

With the advent of slip-ring technology, continuous radiation, and spiral imaging [1], these classical scintillators became obsolete, mainly due to their slow temporal response, afterglow, and radiation drift. Xenon detectors were the ideal alternative as they combine fast response and high X-ray absorption. Optimized Xenon detectors (high gas pressure and deep chambers) allow spiral imaging at high spatial resolution(high sampling density, fast response) and excellent low contrast resolution (high X-ray efficiency) without artifacts due to insufficient detector response. The first subsecond (750 ms) scanner – the Siemens Somatom Plus 4, introduced in 1994 – also relied on Xenon detectors due to the advantages mentioned above.

The challenge for the next generation of solid state detectors was to overcome the limitations of the known scintillators and at the same time to realize advantages over Xenon detectors for improved clinical performance in subsecond spiral imaging. This goal has been achieved by a comprehensive material research which resulted in the development of a scintillating ceramics, the ultrafast ceramics (UFC) scintillator.

2.2 UFC Detectors: Design Goal

The clinical demands for modern CT scanners are their ability to perform long spirals or multispirals in rapid succession without interruptions due to tube cooling and with excellent image quality. Dose savings without compromising image noise are an important requirement in view of recent discussions on dose recommendations which are under development in several countries of the European Union. On the other hand, the CT system must offer an ample dose to obtain a reliable diagnosis in obese patients. Yet another requirement is the scanning of anatomical volumes with narrow slice collimation for the detection of small lesions and for the identification of small structures in three-dimensional representations.

A core component to achieve such demands is the efficiency of the detection system, including low noise readout electronics. The dose efficiency of the CT scanner determines the amount of radiation necessary to achieve a certain noise level in the CT image. Closely related to image noise is the low contrast detectability: the contrast of a lesion needed for its detection in a noisy image is directly proportional to noise. The overwhelming majority of diagnostic medical applications of CT requires optimum low contrast detectability for a certain applied dose. The most important design criterion is therefore dose efficiency, which we will discuss first.

2.2.1 Dose Efficiency

The most obvious factor contributing to dose efficiency is the geometric efficiency of the detector. The geometric efficiency is defined as the ratio of the active area to the total area of a single element of the detector array. This ratio is smaller than 1 due to dead spaces between elements needed for (optical) separation and antiscatter collimators. It is important to realize that the geometric efficiency is determined by the "fine art" of mechanics. For state-of-the-art designs, a geometric efficiency of about 80% is standard.

The second most obvious factor contributing to dose efficiency is the X-ray absorption efficiency. From solid state physics, we can conclude that once a scintillator of sufficiently high atomic number is employed, an absorption efficiency of well above 90% will be achieved (for the X-ray energies used in CT).

The question that naturally arises in this context concerns the differentiating elements of the UFC detector. The most important answers to this question are: The UFC material features an extremely high light output per absorbed X-ray photon. The efficient optical coupling to photodiodes converts the scintillation light into electrical signals with minimum losses. These signals are directly converted into image information, as no further noise-enhancing correction procedures need to be applied; this is because the UFC has the fastest decay and virtually no afterglow compared to other scintillators used in CT scanners, no radiation drift is present (at least at the exposure levels of CT), and scattered radiation is practically eliminated. Finally, due to the minimum dead time of the readout electronics, virtually all absorbed X-ray photons are used for image formation.

Summarizing the above discussion, the UFC achieves its outstanding efficiency by optimizing the whole chain of information transfer from X-ray absorption to the final clinical image. Highest signal-to-noise ratio is maintained by carefully balancing the chemistry of the scintillator and by avoiding any signal losses and any noise-enhancing signal corrections.

The excellent dose efficiency which is thereby achieved is demonstrated by measurements of the noise in a 20-cm water phantom. Figure 2.1 compares the image noise as a function of dose for the same scanner equipped with a Xenon detector and a UFC detector, respectively. The quality factor used for the comparison in Fig. 2.1 is defined as the product of image noise with the square root of

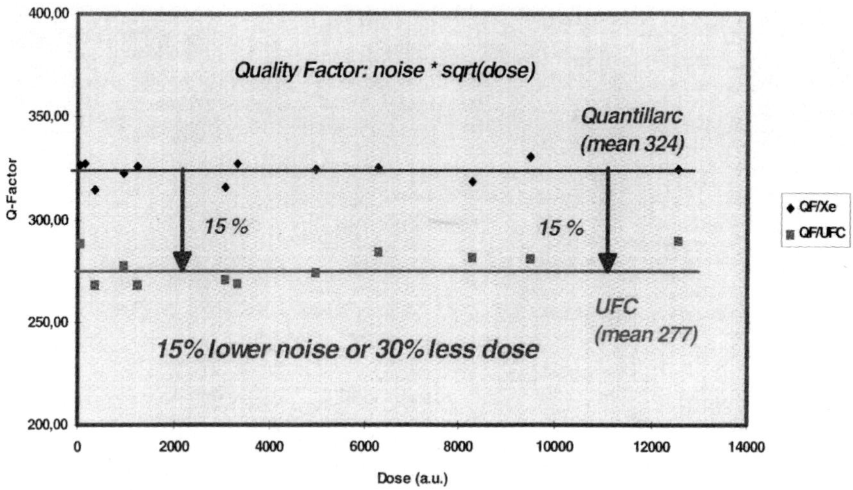

Fig. 2.1. Quality factor as a function of dose for a scanner with a Xenon and with a UFC detector, respectively. (Data by courtesy of Professor W. Kalender, Erlangen, Germany)

the applied dose. Obviously, over a wide range of dose values, this quality factor is independent of dose, indicating that image noise is solely determined by quantum noise. This finding is important to prove that there are no other sources of system noise to detoriate image quality.

Using the UFC detector, an average decrease of noise of about 15% is observed for the same dose, which amounts to a dose saving of about 30% for equal image noise. Corresponding improvements of low contrast detectability and spiral performance are discussed in Sect. 2.3 below.

2.2.2 High Contrast Resolution

Figure 2.2 demonstrates the spatial resolution capabilities of the UFC system. The limiting resolution for the case of negligible noise is illustrated by the graph of the modulation transfer function (MTF) in Fig. 2.2a from measurements with a thin wire phantom in air. The (unmeasurable) cutoff frequency of 18.6 lp/cm is determined by the aperture of the detector elements and by the geometry of the scanner. The usual measure of the spatial resolution, the frequency for the 2% MTF value, is seen in Fig. 2a to be about 17 lp/cm. According to the Rayleigh criterion, the spatial resolution related to this frequency is about 0.29 mm. A more intuitive illustration of spatial resolution is given in Fig. 2b: an image of the high contrast resolution section of the Catphan (commercial phantom; Phantom Laboratory, POB 511, Salem, New York, USA, 12865–0511). The bar pattern for 16 lp/cm is clearly resolved, and the pattern for the limiting resolution is significantly corrupted by noise.

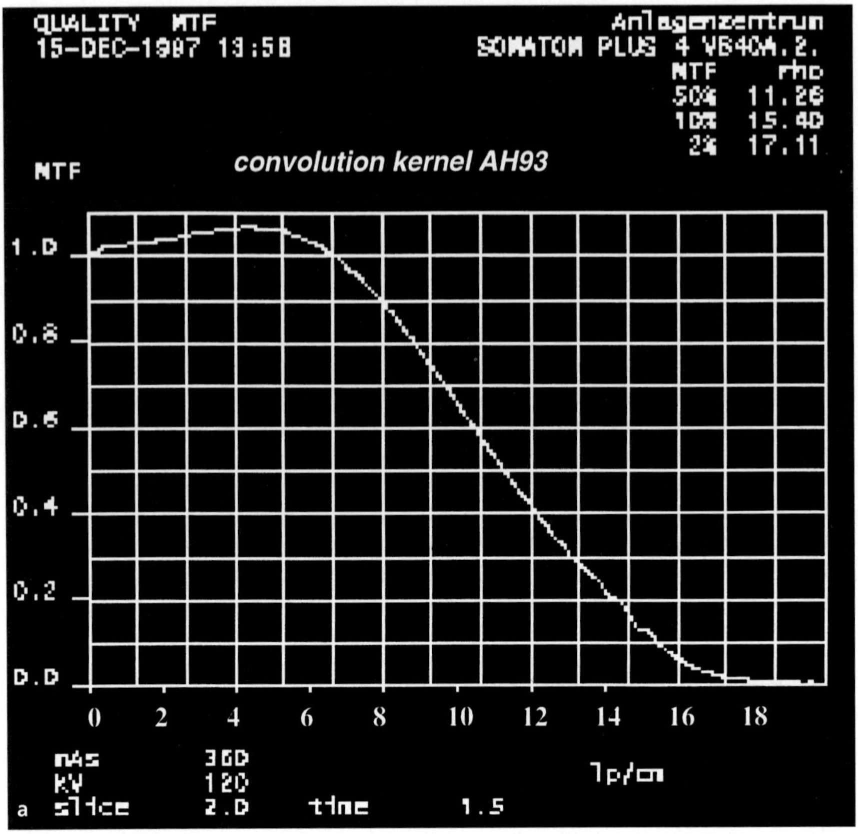

Fig. 2.2. a The modulation transfer function (MTF) of a Somatom Plus 4, UFC, for the high resolution kernel AH93

2.2.3 CT Number Stability

An important feature of high-performance spiral scanners is the stability of the CT numbers in long spirals or in multispirals. Due to practically no radiation drift and to extremely low afterglow, the UFC detectors guarantee this stability even under extreme conditions. Repeated test series with continuous serial imaging at high X-ray power over 100 s proved the extraordinary stability. CT numbers of the first and last image (20-cm water phantom) of multiple 100-s series differ by a fraction of 1 HU, only which is well within the statistical uncertainties.

2.3 Practical Considerations

The improved dose efficiency of the UFC system as compared to Xenon systems can be employed in two different ways in practice

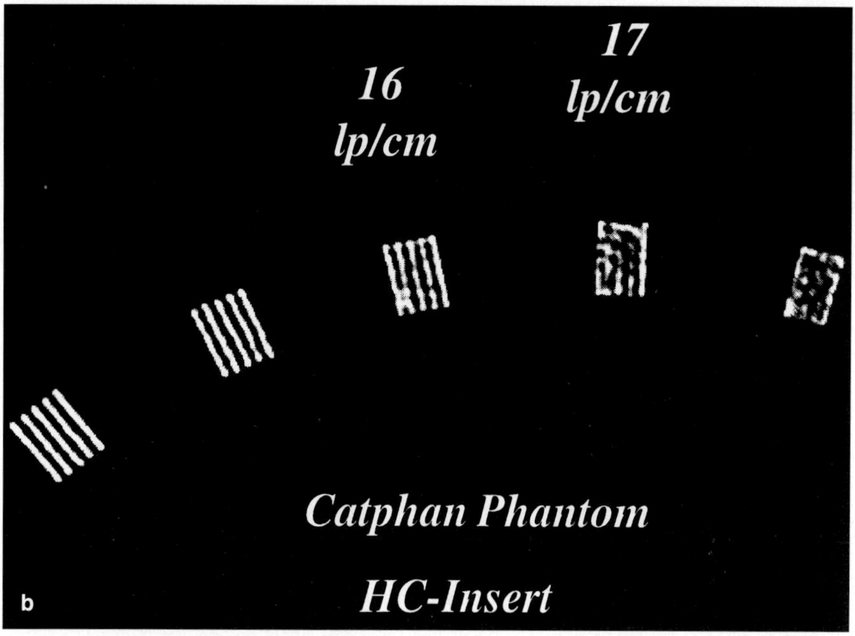

Fig. 2.2. b Image of the high contrast resolution insert of the Catphan (Somatom Plus 4, UFC, AH93)

1. For the same patient dose, a significant reduction of image noise and a correspondingly improved low contrast detectability can be achieved.
2. For a comparable image quality, the patient dose can be significantly decreased, thereby also reducing the tube load and increasing the tube life. Since the tube load decreases nonlinearly with decreasing tube current, the spiral performance in terms of demanding protocols in rapid succession is improved considerably.

In the following, we shall illustrate these issues by means of some examples. The specifications of the low contrast detectability of Somatom Plus 4 systems are shown in Fig. 2.3 compared to those of another scanner equipped with ceramic scintillation detectors. For the same size (5 mm) and the same contrast (3 HU) of the object (low contrast insert of the Catphan, 20 cm diameter; Phantom Laboratory, Salem, USA), the UFC system obviously allows for a remarkably low dose of only 20 mGy.

The dose values quoted in Fig. 2.3 are taken from measurements with a pencil ionization chamber (length, 100 mm) positioned on top of the Catphan phantom. For the same low contrast detectability, the Quantillarc system needs about 30% more dose, reflecting the results of Fig. 2.1 on noise reduction due to the dose efficiency of the UFC. The other scanner also equipped with solid state detectors needs 45% more dose.

These facts underline the comments made on dose efficiency in the preceding section. To beat the efficiency of optimized Xenon systems by solid state detector systems, a careful design and tuning of the various steps involved in converting absorbed X-rays into image information is required. The X-ray power needed for the specified dose (also given in Fig. 2.3) is determined by additional factors such as the scanner's geometry.

The dose efficiency also limits the image quality of long volume scans. This is illustrated in Fig. 2.4 for the same CT systems as in Fig. 2.3. The graphs in Fig. 2.4

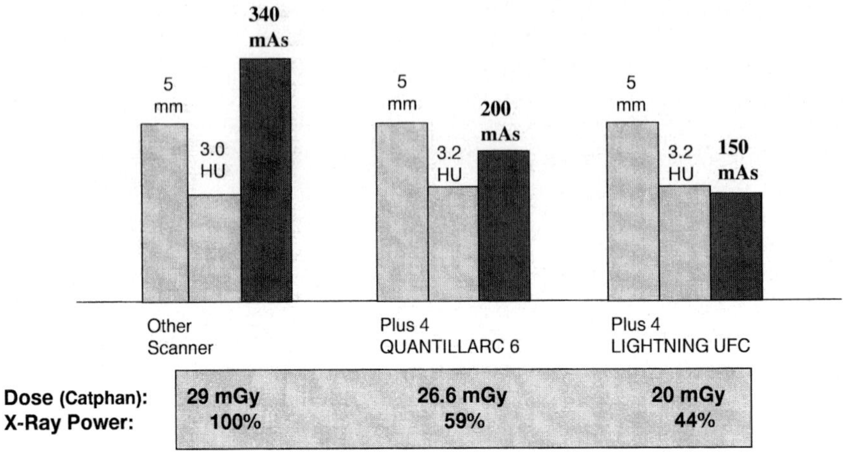

Fig. 2.3. Specifications of low contrast detectability

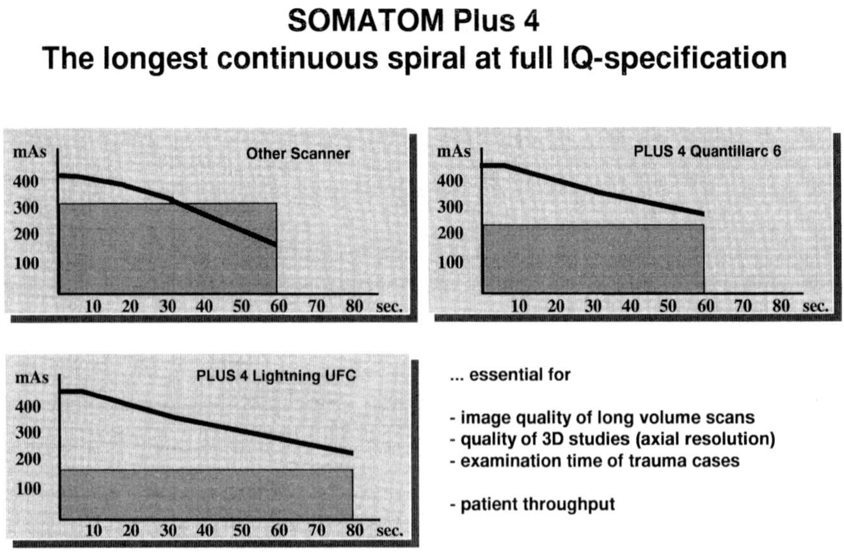

Fig. 2.4. Spiral scan times and maximum possible mAs settings. See text for further details

show the maximum possible mAs values as a function of the total scan time. Spiral imaging at the specified low contrast detectability requires mAs settings above the gray hatched area of Fig. 2.4. Obviously, the UFC system is capable of scanning demanding spiral protocols at the specified image quality.

2.4 Conclusions

It has been shown that the UFC detector technology has made an important contribution to significantly increase the dose efficiency of modern CT scanners. In clinical practice this outstanding efficiency can be employed in two ways:

Without compromising image quality dose savings of about 30% can be realized. The resulting lower tube current facilitates longer spiral runs, minimizes tube cooling times and increases tube life.

On the other hand, the image quality, especially the low contrast detectability, can be significantly improved by keeping the patient dose constant. Furthermore the axial resolution may be enhanced by using narrower slice widths.

The UFC detectors fully support subsecond scanning; in combination with the flying focal spot technique, the limits for high contrast resolution could be extended significantly. Finally, the UFC material is completely nontoxic, adding to environmental safety and to the protection of future detector technologies based on UFC.

In the context of dose savings, it should be mentioned that a dose modulation, adapted to the individual patient's geometry, provides another significant potential to reduce patient dose by as much as 40% [2] (see also Chap. 2, this volume). Combining both technologies, an overall dose reduction by a factor of 2 is well within the realm of modern CT technologies.

References

1. Kalender WA, Seissler W, Klotz E, Vock P (1990) Spiral volumetric CT with single-breath-hold technique, continuous transport and continuous scanner rotation. Radiology 176:181–183
2. Kalender WA, Wolf H, Suess C, Hentschel D, Bautz W (1997) Dose reduction in CT by anatomically adapted tube current modulation: experimental results and first patient studies. Radiology 205 (P) [Suppl]:471

3 Dose Reduction Versus Image Quality in Spiral CT: How Far Down Can We Go in Clinical Practice?

M. Prokop, C. M. Schaefer-Prokop, M. Galanski

Abstract

Computed tomography significantly contributes to the radiation exposure of the population of western countries. As compared to conventional radiography, an increase in dose by factors of up to 100 has been reported. With respect to spiral CT, the discussion focuses on a potential dose increase by bi- or triphasic examinations and the tendency to use smaller slice collimation. This chapter will give an outline how a conscientious choice of scanning protocols may dramatically reduce the radiation exposure to the patient (even with the standard Xenon detector) without having to sacrifice diagnostic accuracy. This can be achieved by individualizing mAs settings dependent on patient diameter, by choosing a pitch factor >1.5, and by considering the influence of the raw data interpolation and image reconstruction on spatial resolution and image noise. Concerning the trade-off between spatial resolution and dose requirements, a little less sharpness will in many cases mean a lot less dose to the patients' algorithms.

3.1 Introduction

CT significantly contributes to the radiation exposure of the population of Western countries. In Great Britain, CT accounted for only 2% of the total number of X-ray examinations but was responsible for 20% of the radiation exposure due to diagnostic medial examinations [13, 14]. As compared to conventional radiography, an increase in dose by factors of up to 100 has been reported [16]. Dependent on the scan parameters, a chest CT will cause an organ dose to the breasts of up to 20 mSv. This dose exceeds the radiation exposure due to a single mammogram by a factor of 10 [15].

With respect to spiral CT, there is a fear that the increased use of bi- or triphasic examinations [9] and the tendency to use smaller slice collimation will lead to a marked further increase in radiation exposure.

Thus there is a strong need for a conscientious choice of scan parameters in order not to cause an unnecessary radiation hazard to patients. It is therefore important to know how the various scan parameters influence the two major criteria of image quality, image noise and spatial resolution.

3.2
Material and Methods

In order to quantify the influence of scan parameters on image noise and spatial resolution, we performed various phantom experiments on the Somatom Plus 4 A (Xenon detector) and correlated our results with a brief patient study.

3.2.1
CTDI Measurements

In order to be able to compare the exposure with varying slice thickness and kVp settings, we performed CTDI measurements (in air) using an pencil ionization chamber of 14 cm in length (PTW, Freiburg), positioned at the center of the gantry, and we repeated each measurement five times. Dose measurements were performed at three different mAs settings for each slice collimation. Measurements were repeated for 80kVp, 120 kVp, and 140 kVp.

3.2.2
Phantom Experiments

Noise Measurements. For the measurement of the influence of slice collimation, raw data interpolation, pitch factor, and reconstruction algorithm, we performed measurements using circular water phantoms of 10 cm, 20 cm, and 30 cm in diameter.

Our standard parameter set was as follows: 120kVp, 3-mm slice collimation, pitch 1, 1 s tube rotation, an AB50 filter kernel, and "slim2" raw data interpolation. A 30-cm phantom was used if not mentioned otherwise. Depending on the experiment, various scan parameters were altered.

Since the 360°LI interpolation includes data from two rotations for calculating one image, we reconstructed images every second rotation in order to gain independent data sets for noise measurements. For each set of scan parameters, five images were reconstructed.

Image noise is not distributed homogeneously over the cross-sectional area of the phantom [12]. Thus we measured noise in two regions of interest (ROIs at opposing sides of the phantom) close to the periphery and two ROIs close to the center of the phantom and averaged the values for each pair of ROIs.

Spatial Resolution Measurements. The spatial resolution was determined using a small lead bead (diameter, <0.2 mm) as a delta impulse (e.g., [1]). CT number profiles through the center of the bead yield the point spread function in all three spatial dimensions. After signal normalization, this point spread function directly converts into the slice sensitivity profile for the z-direction, while its Fourier transform in the x-direction yields the MTF (within the scan plane).

Spiral scans were performed with a slice collimation of 1, 2, 3, 5, 7, and 10 mm and a pitch of 1. For 3-mm collimation, the pitch factor was varied from 1 to 3, and all available raw data interpolation algorithms were employed. The reconstruction interval was chosen as at least one tenth of the table feed (0.1–0.3 mm).

3.2.3 Patient Studies

A total of 25 patients with various imaging studies of the chest and abdomen were selected arbitrarily. From each spiral study, single images at the following levels were selected for noise measurements: shoulders, mediastinum at the pulmonary hila, center of the diaphragm, liver hilum, abdomen just above the pelvic bones, and small pelvis. The images were chosen so that no artifacts from breathing, pulsation, or contrast application were visible.

At each level, noise measurements were performed in multiple homogenous ROI of at least 1 cm^2 that were placed as close as possible to the center of the patient. The median number was determined for each level.

These test images were printed on laser film (43 × 35 cm, 12 on each) in random order. Four staff radiologists with more than 5 years of experience in CT evaluation were asked to rate each image on a 5-point scale (1 = excellent to 5 = diagnostically inadequate) with respect to the image noise, definition/sharpness of contours, and image contrast.

3.2.4 Display Noise

In order to test the hypothesis that the window width is a major contributing factor to the subjective perception of image noise, even at soft tissue window settings, we normalized the pixel noise σ (standard deviation of CT numbers) to the window width W and called this number display noise σ^*. It was calculated according to the following equation:

$$\sigma^* = \sigma \times 100/W$$

and corresponds to the visually perceived noise level (given as a percentage of the ratio between maximum to minimum available gray level on the image display).

Noise ratings from the patient study were correlated to the pixel noise and to this display noise. Ratings were also compared between observers and between the various criteria for image quality.

3.3 **Results**

3.3.1 CTDI Measurements

Figure 3.1 demonstrates that the CTDI increases linearly with mAs ($r > 0.9999$). While there are only minor differences between collimations of 2 mm or above, the CTDI for 1-mm slices increases by a factor of (approximately) 2.

For the same mAs settings, the $CTDI_{air}$ increased by a factor of 1.4 if 140 kVp was used instead of 120 kVp, while the $CTDI_{air}$ fell by a factor of 4 when 80 kVp was employed.

3.3.2 Individualizing mAs Setting

Image noise increases exponentially with increasing phantom diameter (Fig. 3.2). From the slope of the curve, the half layer (for noise) can be determined. Depending on the kVp, the values vary between 5.8 and 7.1 cm at 3-mm slice collimation. The numbers decrease with lower mAs, lower kVp, and narrower slice collimation. When all measurements were taken into account (variation of mAs settings, collimation, phantom diameter, and kVp), half layers between 6 and 7.5 cm were found for the clinically relevant choices of scan parameters.

3.3.3 Slice Collimation

As can be expected from theory, image noise decreased with increasing slice collimation (SC) (Fig. 3.3). This relationship could be described using the following equation:

$$\sigma = a \times SC^{-b}$$

In this equation, the exponent *b* should be equal to 0.5 if only quantum noise contributes to the measured pixel noise. Dependent on the phantom size, we found numbers that varied between 0.46 and 0.53 for 120 kVp, suggesting that other components due to electronic noise of the CT equipment are less important for the chosen mAs.

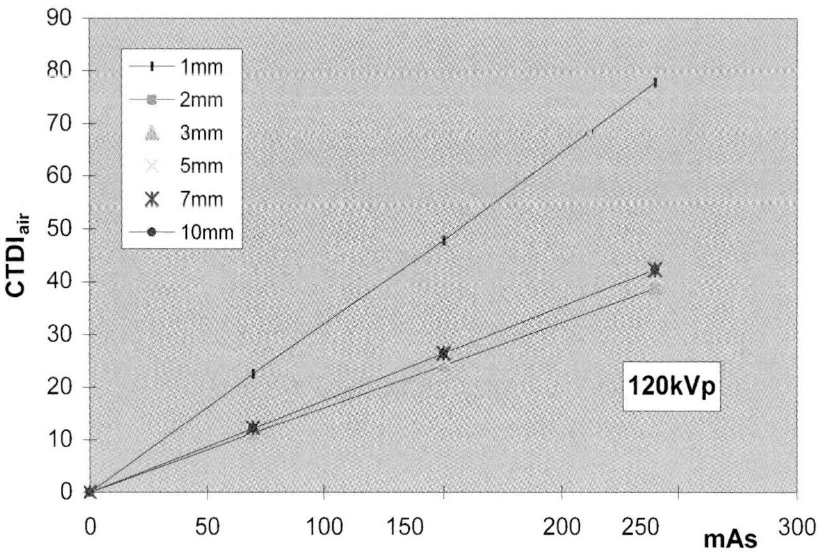

Fig. 3.1. CTDI measurements in air (dosimeter length, 14 cm) for 120 kVp and various slice collimations: the numbers for 1 mm increase by a factor of 2 over all other collimations

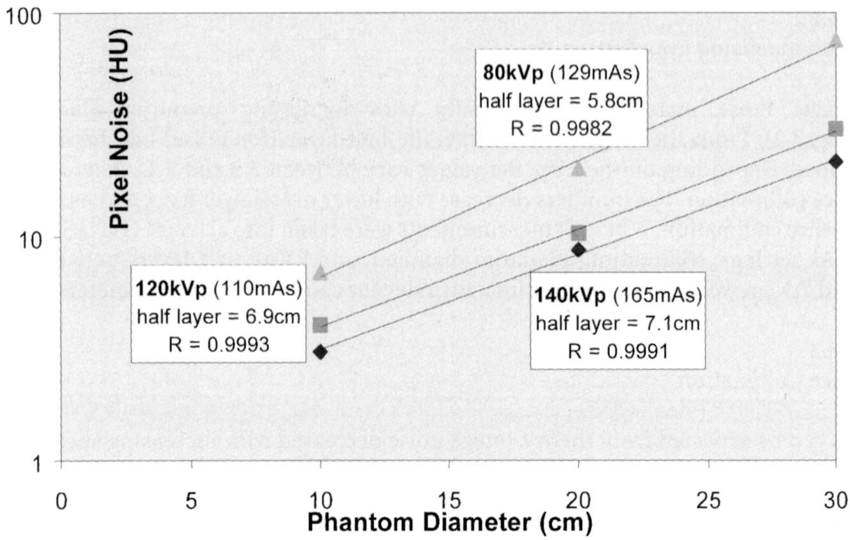

Fig. 3.2. Image noise increases exponentially with increasing phantom diameter: half layers for 80 kVp, 120 kVp, and 140 kVp differ substantially

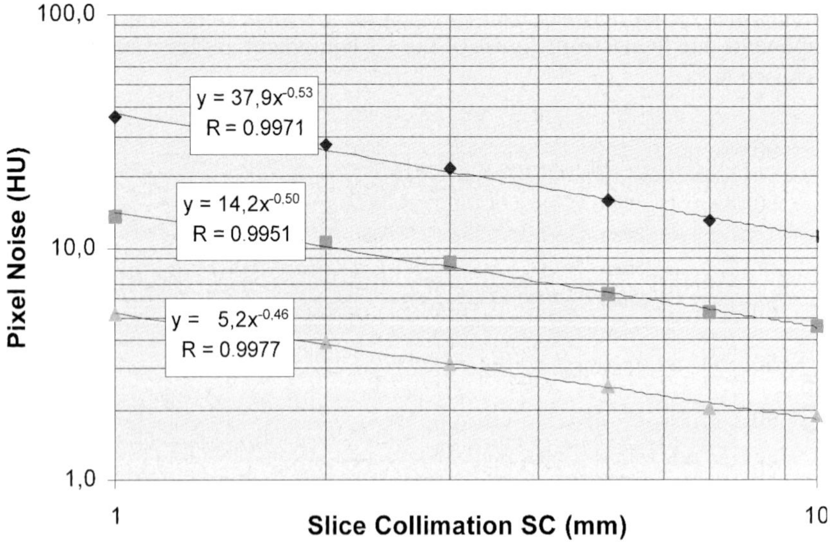

Fig. 3.3. Image noise decreases with increasing slice collimation

In clinical practice, this simple finding should have the following consequences: For an identical image quality in terms of image noise, the mAs would have to be increased with smaller slice collimation and could be decreased when larger collimation is used.

Although trivial, this does not seem to have influenced the choice of mAs settings in most institutions. A survey of all recent papers published in *Radiology* and *Röfo* during the years 1996/1997 demonstrates that there is almost no correlation between slice collimation and choice of mAs values (Fig. 3.4). While some dedicated low-dose protocols use 50 mAs, some standard protocols apply as much as 350 mAs to the chest. These findings have to be seen as an indicator that the choice of exposure parameters in CT is still largely intuitive.

The detector dose is proportional both to the slice collimation and the mAs settings ($I \times t$). If one assumes the noise level at a certain slice collimation SC_0 acceptable (e.g., for high-resolution CT of the lung, 350 mAs at 2 mm), one can calculate the required mAs settings for a different slice collimation using the following equation:

$$(I \times t) = SC_0 \times (I \times t)_0 / SC$$

Using this equation, one can calculate that only a fifth of the dose (70 mAs) would be required for 10-mm slice collimation in the chest if the same noise level is considered acceptable as with 2 mm and 350 mAs.

3.3.4 Pitch Factor

At a given slice collimation (here, 3 mm), the pixel noise remained constant independent of pitch factor and raw data interpolation (slim, slim2, wide). Thus, if a

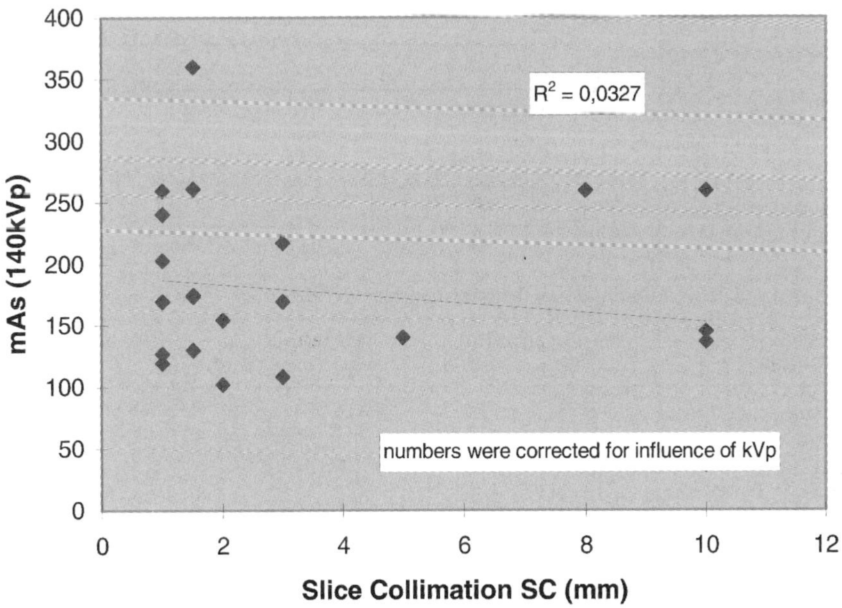

Fig. 3.4. Current status in chest CT (survey of all recent papers in *Radiology* and *Röfo* during the years 1996/1997): no correlation between slice collimation and choice of mAs values

higher pitch factor is chosen, the patient dose falls proportionally to the pitch without leading to an increased image noise (although the effective slice thickness increases slightly).

3.3.5 Raw Data Interpolation Algorithm

When the image noise was compared with the various raw data interpolation algorithms, there was no significant influence of other factors such as slice collimation, pitch, or phantom diameter. The relative contribution of image noise due to the interpolation is given in Table 3.1.

Since we measured only 89% of the noise of standard CT slices with the new slim2 raw data interpolation, it allows for marked dose reduction as compared to 113% with the older slim algorithm: noise is reduced by 21%. This corresponds to potential dose savings of 38%. At the same time, there was no significant deterioration of the slice sensitivity profile, and the effective slice thickness remained constant.

3.3.6 Image Reconstruction Algorithm (Filter Kernel)

Image noise is heavily dependent on the image reconstruction algorithm (filter kernel). Table 3.2 provides the relative contribution of various reconstruction algorithms to image noise and demonstrates that marked differences occur. If these

Table 3.1. Relative contribution of various interpolation algorithms to image noise

Interpolation	Relative noise (%)
Standard CT	100
VAR	69
Wide (360°LI)	82
Slim2 (180°LI)	89
Slim (180°WI)	113

Table 3.2. Relative contribution of various reconstruction algorithms to image noise

Reconstruction algorithm	Relative noise (%)	Relative dose requirements (%)[a]	Spatial resolution[b]
AB10	56	32	4.1
AB20	71	50	4.7
AB30	78	60	5.0
AB40	85	72	5.2
AB50	100	100	5.8
AB60	117	137	6.2
AB70	136	184	6.6
AB82	281	789	7.6
AB91	280	786	7.7

[a] Measured close to the center of 30 cm water phantom; AB50 = 100%.
[b] Spatial resolution is given as MTF at 20% level (measured by metal bead).

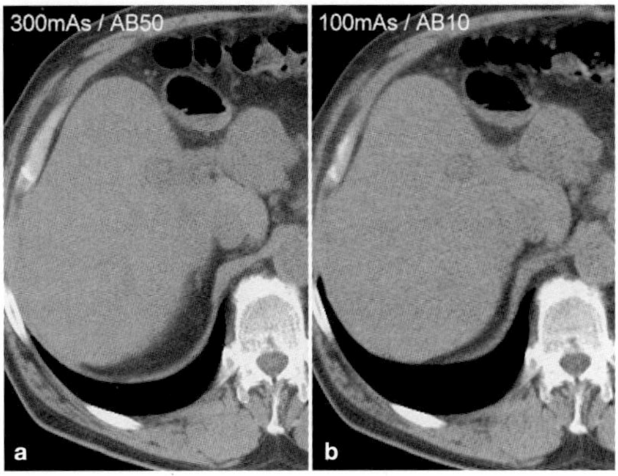

Fig. 3.5a,b. For CT of the liver, a dose reduction by a factor of 3 is possible if an AB10 (**b**) reconstruction kernel is employed instead of AB50 (**a**). As a tradeoff, contours are less sharply demarcated and there is a an increased coarseness of noise

differences are compensated by variations in mAs settings, the potential for dose savings and the need for dose increase become clear.

As one moves from an AB50 standard kernel to AB30, the noise level decreases to approximately 78% (potential dose savings, 40%). If AB10 is acceptable (with respect to spatial resolution), the noise level will decrease to 56% (dose savings of more than factor 3; see Fig. 3.5).

On the other hand, an AB70 kernel requires 1.8 times more dose than AB50 for identical image noise, and AB82 or AB91 require seven to eight times more dose if the noise level is to be maintained.

3.3.7 Window Width

As was demonstrated with the use of high resolution reconstruction algorithms, a noise level similar to that of soft tissue imaging can no longer be maintained, since dose increases would have to be excessive. Nevertheless, image noise hardly plays a role for most of the high-resolution applications. The reason for this is that high-resolution algorithms are employed mainly for high-contrast objects such as the lungs or skeletal structures.

It is well known that window settings influence our perception of image noise. In general, however, this has had little impact on the choice of parameters for most common CT applications. Figure 3.6 demonstrates that we found almost no correlation between pixel noise (standard deviation of CT numbers) and subjective perception of image noise, while there was satisfactory correlation between noise perception and display noise. This display noise is inversely proportional to the window width. The good correlation suggests that this noise definition is superior to describe the subjective effect of noise on image quality.

As a consequence, mAs settings may be reduced with larger window width: since window width influences noise directly (inversely proportional) while dose dependence is described by a square root function ($1/\sqrt{I \times t}$), even an increase in the window width from 300 to 350 HU allows for a reduction in the mAs settings of 26% if the perception of image noise is to remain constant.

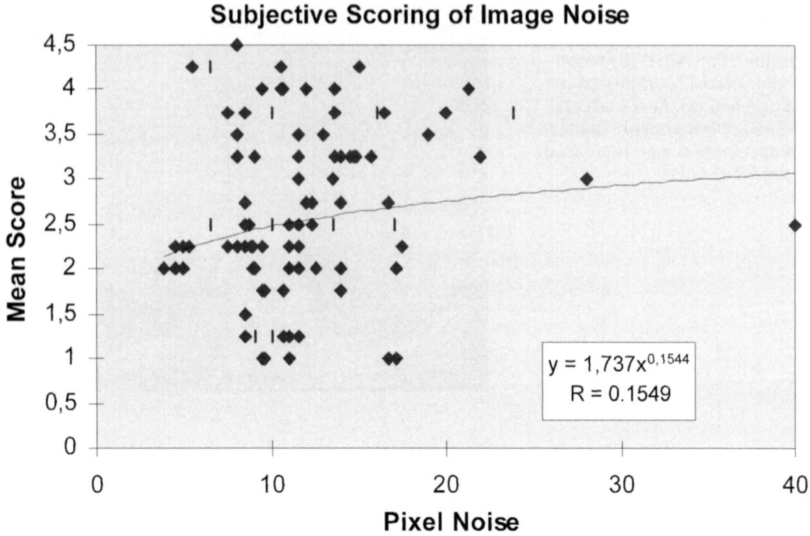

a

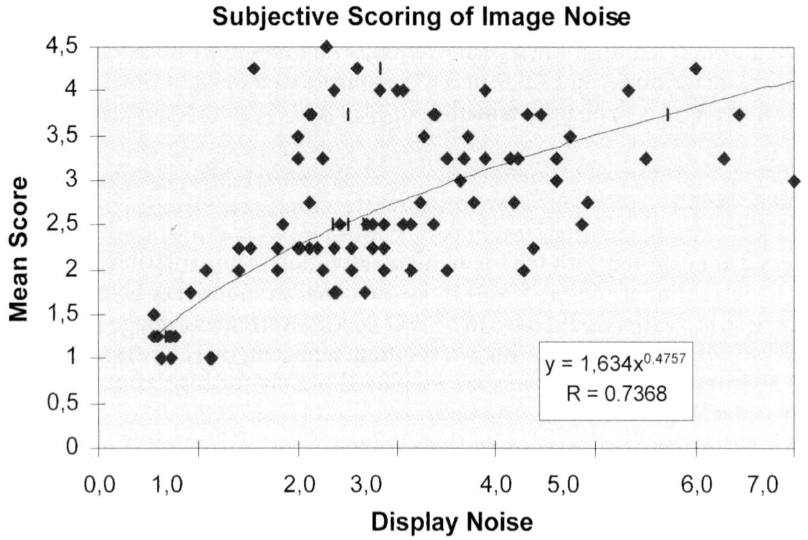

b

Fig. 3.6a,b. Subjective evaluation of image noise (5-point scale). Almost no correlation with standard deviation of CT numbers ("pixel noise," **a**), but satisfactory correlation with pixel noise normalized to window width ("display noise," **b**) 100/*W*

3.4 Discussion

In most clinical environments, the choice of mAs settings is largely intuitive and is determined by personal preferences and individual taste. Variations in patient exposure may be dramatic, as was shown for the example of chest CT: while some institutions applied up to 350 mAs, others reduced the settings to 50 mAs. A reduction in mAs settings with larger-slice collimation appears feasible in most clinical applications. Given the above-mentioned adaptation of mAs to slice collimation, a dose reduction by approximately a factor of 3 appears feasible as compared to the most commonly suggested standard parameters for the chest (10 mm, 200 mAs). Since there is marked dependence on patient diameter, however, the mAs settings have to be increased in patients with more adipose tissue.

As can be demonstrated by comparing the increase of image noise due to a high-resolution kernel (with AB82, noise is higher by a factor of 2.5–2.7 than with AB50) and the decrease of perceived image noise (display noise) when moving from a mediastinal window (width, 300–500 HU) to a lung window (width, 1000–2000 HU; i.e., decrease in image noise by a factor of 3–4), the choice of HR kernels is compensated by the increased window if one accepts a similar display noise. This implicitly requires that soft tissues and lungs have to be reconstructed using different kernels.

As is shown in Table 3.2, spatial resolution can be traded in for image noise. Since most diagnostically relevant structures, e.g., in the abdomen, are relatively large (approximately 1 mm), spatial resolution plays a minor role. This can be used to further reduce the required exposure dose. If an AB30 kernel is acceptable instead of AB50, mAs settings and thus patient dose can be reduced by 30%. Trading in an overly sharp definition of contours for a reduction of patient exposure may be well worthwhile.

A very important factor for potential dose savings is the choice of window width. This factor is usually neglected since it is merely considered to be a display parameter that does not influence the signal-to-noise ratio. In clinical practice, window width is a more or less preset parameter that is chosen depending on the displayed anatomic region. Only in very rare occasions is a more narrow window width used. It therefore makes sense to chose a certain "acceptable" display noise and chose the mAs settings accordingly. As a consequence, mAs reductions are not only possible for high-contrast structures, such as bones or lung parenchyma [2, 3, 5, 7, 8], but may also be feasible for soft tissue structures in the chest or abdomen.

Use of the new slim2 raw data interpolation should be recommended as the standard procedure, since it allows for either a dose reduction of more than 35% or a decrease in image noise of 23% as compared to the older standard, the slim (180°LI) raw data interpolation.

An important step towards minimizing patient exposure is to individualize mAs settings. It was shown that mAs settings can be cut in half if the patient is 3–4 cm thinner (slim individuals, children). Since measurements of patient diameters are cumbersome in clinical practice, one can often only estimate the dose requirements in an individual setting.

We are currently working on software that incorporates all dose-relevant scan parameters and allows for an individualized estimate of the mAs settings dependent on the chosen scan parameters, window settings, and reconstruction kernels. Initial results have shown that considerable dose savings are possible in slim patients, while image quality can be improved in individuals with more adipose tissue.

3.5 Conclusion

While adaptive exposure control and the use of new solid state detectors can dramatically reduce the dose requirements with the Somatom Plus 4, the conscientious choice of scan, reconstruction, and display parameters can already yield marked reductions in patent exposure that can be added to the new improvements in hardware and software. A little less sharpness will in many cases mean a lot less dose to the patient. It has to be noted, however, that the mAs settings have to be lowered in order to realize any of the mentioned dose saving.

References

1. Davros WJ, Herts BR, Walmsley JJ, Obuchowski NA (1995) Determination of spiral CT slice sensitivity profiles using a point response phantom. J Comp Assist Tomogr 19(5):838–843
2. Diederich S, Lenzen H, Puskas Z et al (1996) Niedrigdosis-Computertomographie des Thorax. Experimentelle und klinische Untersuchungen. Radiologe 36:475–482
3. Diederichs CG, Engelke WGH, Richter B, Hermann KP, Oestmann JW (1996) Must radiation dose for CT of the maxilla and mandible be higher than that for conventional panoramic radiography? AJNR 17:1758–1760
4. EUR 16262 (1997) Quality criteria for computed tomography. Working document by the European Commission's Study Group on Development of Quality Criteria for Computed Tomography
5. Felsenberg D, Kalender WA, Trinkwalter W, Wolf KJ (1990) CT-Untersuchungen mit reduzierter Strahlendosis. Röfo 153:516–521
6. Kalender WA (1995) Principles and performance of spiral CT. In: Goldman LW, Fowlkes JB (eds) Medical CT and ultrasound: current technology and applications. American Association of Physicists in Medicine, 379–410
7. Lenzen H, Roos N, Diederich S, Meier N (1996) Strahlenexposition bei der Niedrigdosiscomputertomographie des Thorax. Radiologe 36:483–488
8. Mayo JR, Hartman TE, Lee KS et al (1995) CT of the chest: minimal tube current required for good image quality with the least radiation dose. AJR 164:603–607
9. McNitt-Gray MF, Lu DS, Solberg TD, Cagnon C, Krasny RM, Kadell BM (1995) Two-phase and three-phase helical CT: dose measurements compared with conventional axial CT. Radiology 197(P):336
10. Polacin A, Kalender WA, Marchal G (1992) Evaluation of section sensitivity profiles and image noise in spiral CT. Radiology 185:29–35
11. Polacin A, Kalender WA (1994) Measurement of slice sensitivity profiles in spiral CT. Med Phys 21(1):133–140
12. Polacin A, Kalender WA (1995) Object adaptive section interpolation in spiral CT. Radiology 197(P):336
13. Shrimpton PC, Hart D, Hillier MC, Wall BF, Faulkner K (1991) Survey of CT practice in the UK. 1. Aspects of examination frequency and quality assurance. Chilton 1991, NRPB-R248. HMSO, London
14. Shrimpton PC, Jones DG, Hillier MC, Wall BF, Le Heron JC, Faulkner K (1991) Survey of CT practice in the UK. 2. Dosimetric aspects. Chilton 1991, NRPB-R248. HMSO, London
15. Stender HS, Saure D (1995) Qualitätskriterien in der diagnostischen Radiologie, Ziel und Realität. Akt Radiol 5:337–342
16. Zankl M, Panzer W, Drexler G (1991) The calculation of dose from external photon exposures using human reference phantoms and Monte Carlo methods. VI. Organ dose from computed tomographic examinations. GSF-Bericht 30/91. Gesellschaft für Strahlen- und Umweltforschung, Neuherberg

4 Dose Reduction in CT by Anatomically Adapted Tube Current Modulation: Principles and First Results

W. A. Kalender, H. Wolf, C. Suess, M. Gies, H. Greess, W. A. Bautz

4.1 Introduction

The performance of today's modern CT scanners is still improving, and the range of applications and the frequency of CT examinations show a continuous upward trend. This is contrary to many predictions in the late 1980s and early 1990s when a rapid decrease in the use of CT was expected. The introduction of spiral CT and the advent of faster and more powerful scanners specifically designed for volume CT scanning in spiral mode has led to a renaissance of CT.

Accompanying these positive technical and clinical trends has been an increasing awareness – sometimes even an irrational fear – of the dose associated with X-rays. This has been particularly strong in Europe, especially in Scandinavia, the United Kingdom, and Germany. A number of activities on European level are underway. In particular, the European Union has sponsored efforts aimed at limiting the dose and has demanded the establishment of reference dose levels for CT examinations [1]. This background has added to the motivation to limit the dose in CT or, better, to achieve the required level of image quality with minimum dose.

The purpose of this study was to investigate approaches and to develop technical means for dose reduction in CT which does not entail a loss of image quality. This means in particular that simple approaches, such as a general reduction in tube current (measured in milliampere, mA), are not a sufficient solution. mA reduction is available to any CT user at any time, but this results in increased pixel noise. We assume here that the optimal mA value and thereby the mAs product (tube current multiplied by scan time per 360° rotation) have been selected, i.e., noise is as high as tolerable and dose thereby chosen as low as acceptable for the given diagnostic task.

We sought to reduce total mAs without increasing pixel noise. The principal idea, as outlined below, is to redistribute the dose for a 360° rotation in accordance with the actual attenuation as a function of projection angle instead of maintaining the tube current constant, as is usually practiced today.

4.2 Methods and Materials

Noise in CT images varies proportional to the square root of the applied dose, i.e., proportional to the square root of the mAs product if the tube current is kept constant. However, noise in CT images is dominated by those projections in which attenuation is the highest. This is indicated in Fig. 4.1.

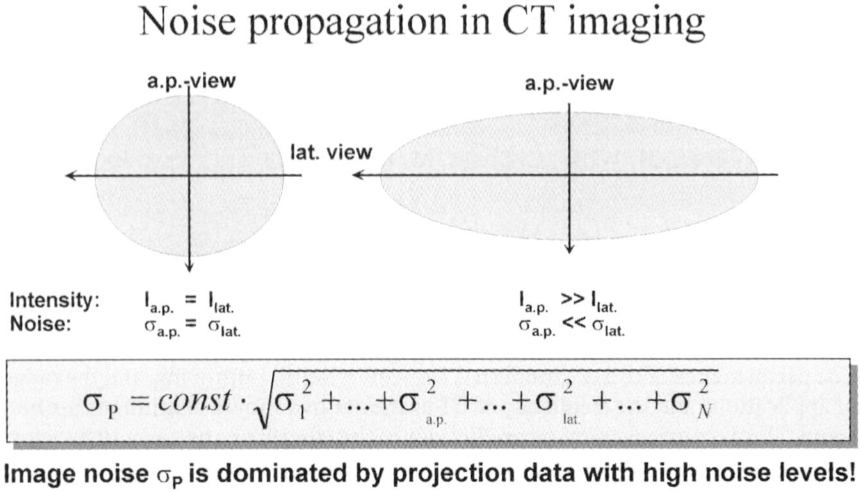

Fig. 4.1. Noise in the CT image is dominated by the noise of projection data with highest attenuation. Dose can be reduced in projections with low attenuation, here the a.p. projections, without significantly impairing image quality or increasing noise

For an object with circular cross-section, attenuation is constant over all projections, and all the measured values contribute equally. For a noncircular cross-section, however, attenuation varies strongly, sometimes by more than three orders of magnitude (Fig. 4.2). Noise in the data measured in high-attenuation projections, i.e., mostly in lateral direction, is decisive for the noise level in the CT image. This means that the dose for projections with relatively low attenuation, i.e., mostly in a.p. direction, can be reduced significantly without a measurable increase in image noise. The conclusion – and the basic consideration for our approach – is that tube current should be decreased as a function of rotation angle whenever attenuation is low. In consequence, we had to develop means for monitoring attenuation online and for variation of tube current as a function of projection angle.

The respective technical solution was implemented as a work-in-progress option on a Somatom PLUS 4 in cooperation with Siemens Medizinische Technik (Erlangen, Germany). Measured attenuation data were taken from the data acquisition system during scanning for further analysis. In this case the attenuation for the central channels of the detector system was determined as a function of projection angle. Various control functions can be derived from these data. We investigated trapezoidal, elliptical, sinusoidal, and anatomically adapted shapes by simulations and phantom measurements; both preprogrammed modulation functions and attenuation-based online control of the tube current were implemented. A circular, an elliptical, and two oval water phantoms with and without inserts were used. The respective phantoms, identical for simulations and physical measurements, and associated attenuation curves as a function of projection

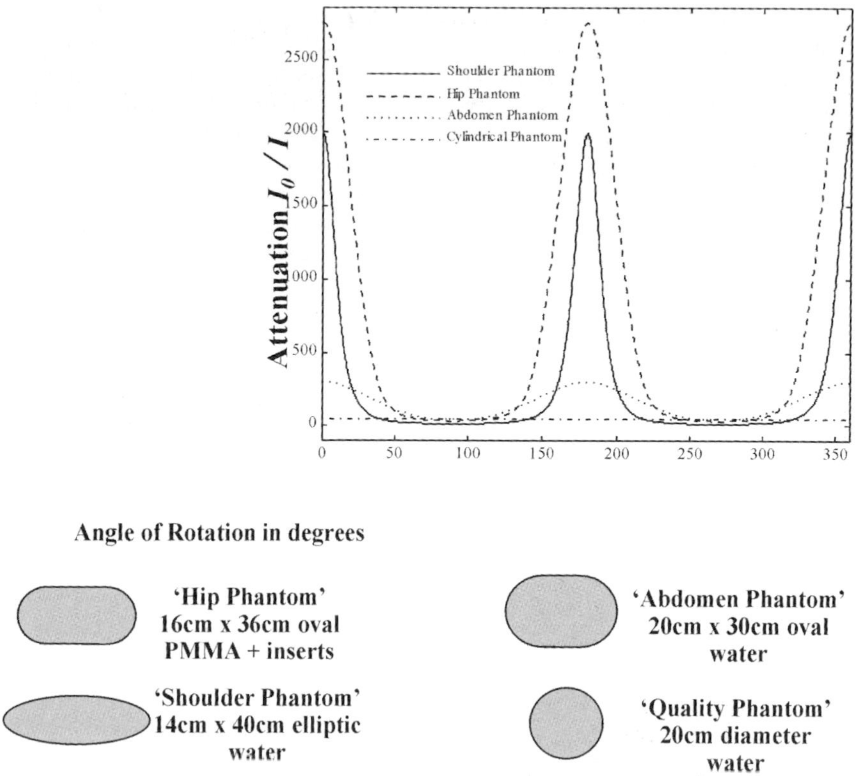

Fig. 4.2. Sketches of the phantoms used in simulations and physical measurements and associated attenuation values as a function of projection angle for the Somatom PLUS 4 at 120 kVp

angle are shown in Fig. 4.2. All relevant scan parameters were varied, including constraints such as the maximum modulation amplitude. The results of the simulations and phantom measurements were validated on six cadavers. First patient studies were also completed; they are the subject of a separate communication to this volume (see Chap. 5).

4.3 Results

The results of the simulation studies provided the basis for the decisions on optimization of our approach; the respective results are documented in a separate paper [2]. The most important findings were that tube current should be modulated as a function of the square root of measured attenuation and that the modulation amplitude available on a specific scanner is of great importance (Fig. 4.3). A modulation amplitude of at least 90% is desirable. This is available on our PLUS 4 for 2 s scanning; for 0.75 s scans we are presently limited to 60% modulation amplitude. This means that for very short scan times we fall significantly below the optimum for objects with large differences in attenuation (Fig. 4.3).

The results of our simulation studies were tested on various phantoms representing typical patient cross-sections. Agreement between simulations and measurements was very good (Table 4.1). As expected, no dose reduction was found in phantoms with circular cross-sections. However, dose reduction of up to 45% was found in phantoms with cross-sections mimicking the shoulder region (Fig. 4.4). Online attenuation-based control functions always yielded higher reductions in dose than fixed control functions, in this case a sinusoidal curve. A more detailed evaluation was given in a separate report [3].

Extensive studies on six human cadavers also yielded results which were in excellent agreement with the simulations and the phantom studies (Table 4.2). An example is presented in Fig. 4.5. It is noteworthy that the dose is reduced strongly not only in the shoulder region but also in most other body regions, with reduction values of more than 20%.

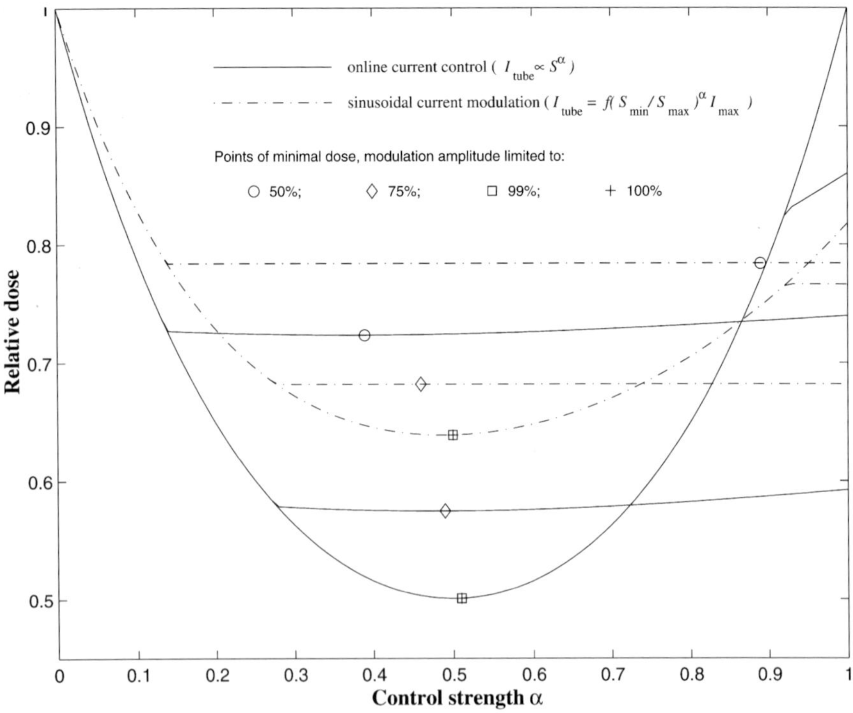

Fig. 4.3. Results of simulation studies for the shoulder phantom. Dose reduction is highest when tube current is modulated proportional to the square root of attenuation and when large modulation amplitudes are technically available

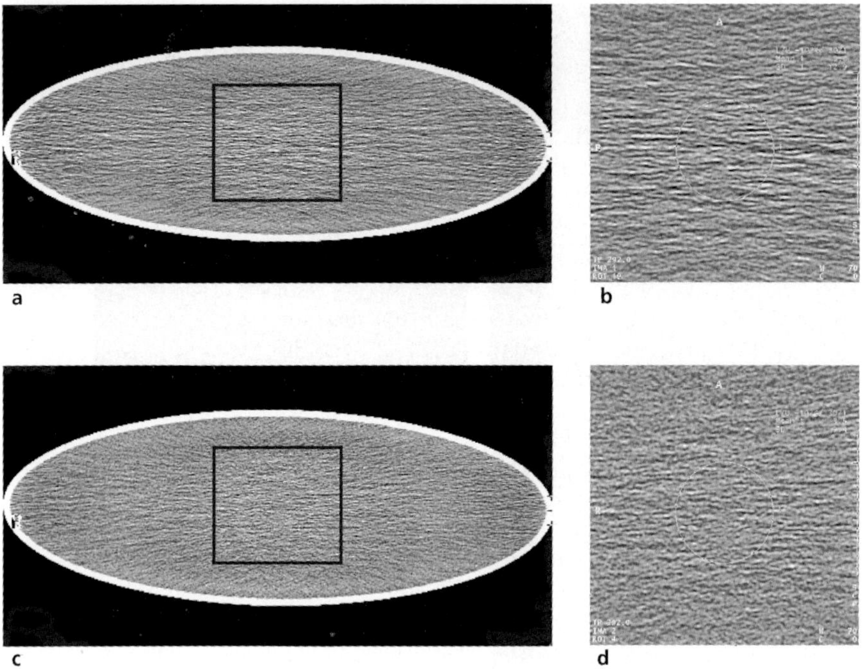

Fig. 4.4. Measurements on the shoulder phantom without (**a**, **b**) and with (**c**, **d**) tube current modulation. With online attenuation-based control the dose is reduced by 45% in this case

Table 4.1. Dose reduction in phantom scans determined by simulations and by measurements

Phantom	Modulation type	Simulated (%)	Measured (%)
Quality phantom	Sinusoidal	0	1
	Online control	0	0
Hip phantom	Sinusoidal	31	37
	Online control	37	41
Abdomen phantom	Sinusoidal	9	5
	Online control	10	10
Shoulder phantom	Sinusoidal	34	35
	Online control	45	41

Table 4.2. Mean dose reduction values determined by measurements on six cadavers with pixel noise kept constant

Anatomic region	Tube current modulation function (%)	
	Sinusoidal	Online control
Head ($n=3$)	7	11
Shoulder ($n=5$)	28	40
Thorax ($n=5$)	17	27
Abdomen ($n=6$)	18	23
Pelvis ($n=6$)	27	34
Upper legs ($n=3$)	23	27

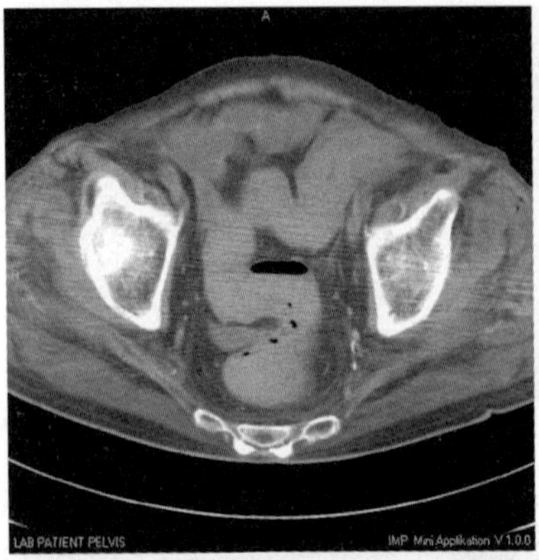

a

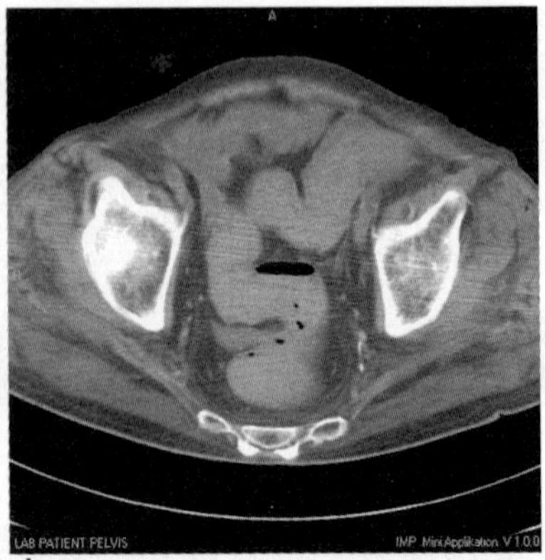

b

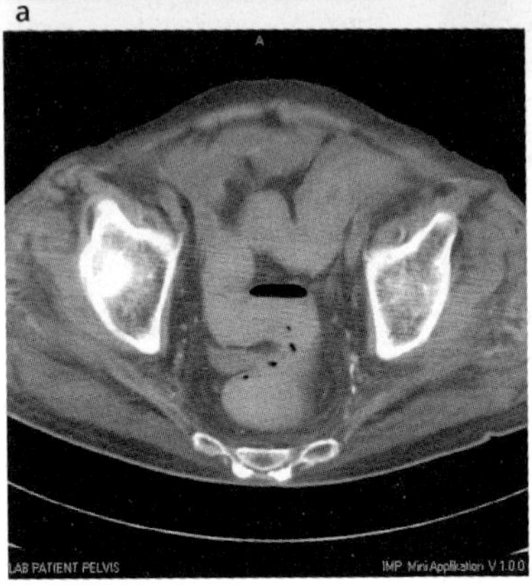

c

Fig. 4.5a–c. CT scans of a cadaver with different tube current modulation resulting in approximately equal noise levels, but significantly different dose values. **a** Standard scan with constant tube current: no dose reduction. **b** Scan with sinusoidal current modulation: 17% dose reduction. **c** Scan with attenuation-based online tube current modulation: 30% dose reduction

Very positive results were also achieved with a modification of our technique where the tube current was increased slightly (as compared to the standard scan mode) for lateral or other high-attenuation projections and decreased significantly in a.p. or other low-attenuation projections. This still resulted in a significant dose reduction but also yielded an increase in image quality. Clinical experience is still very preliminary in this case. A patient example for the shoulder region is presented in Fig. 4.6, with tube current increased by 25% for the highest attenuation values. However, a total dose reduction of 35% resulted in combination with a slight improvement in image quality, i.e., a reduction of structured noise in the areas indicated by arrows (Fig. 4.6).

4.4 Discussion and Conclusions

Since the beginning of CT imaging it has been a particular aim to use a minimal dose. This follows the ALARA principle which demands that dose should always be "**A**s **L**ow **A**s **R**easonably **A**chievable." In several respects CT technology can be

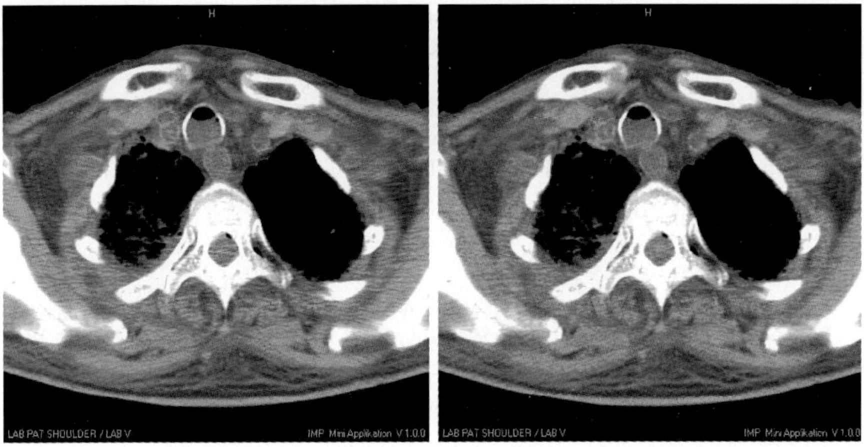

a b

Fig. 4.6a, b. A novel approach to improving image quality and reducing noise at the same time. A slight increase in tube current in lateral projections (+25%) combined with a significant decrease in low-attenuation projections (80% modulation amplitude) resulted in improved image quality and a dose reduction of 35%

considered mature; in particular, the available detector systems exhibit a very high dose efficiency. However, there is always room for improvement.

A novel technical approach to working with lower doses is to modulate the tube current during the 360° tube rotation. This idea was applied earlier by Kopka et al. [4] and Giacomuzzi et al. [5]. In their implementations, known as SmartScan, the modulation of current is based on attenuation measurements by two localizer radiographs and it is fixed over a complete anatomical range. Results presented in the literature so far are not convincing. Our approach goes beyond theirs in several respects: 1. no localizer radiographs (Topograms) are needed; 2. the current is modulated online with a delay of only half a rotation and is thus adapted from slice to slice and not fixed for a complete range; 3. our approach is strictly adapted to the actual course of attenuation and not to a geometric function, for example, a sinusoidal curve.

All these points add up to very favorable results. Cadaver studies which allowed free variation of all parameters and unambiguous evaluation and comparison of results yielded convincing data regarding the potential of our technique (Table 4.2). Dose reductions of 20%–30% appear realistic, and in some cases even higher reductions are possible.

We conclude that this technique should enter wide clinical use without delay. Online attenuation-based tube current modulation using the square root of attenuation as the control parameter appears to be the method of choice. The only deficiency at present is the amplitude of tube current modulation, which is still limited. The use of grid-controlled X-ray tubes which allow faster modulation of tube current would be a potential solution. In addition to the patients receiving less exposure, X-ray tubes will also profit from our approach since tube load is decreased to the same proportion as patient dose.

Acknowledgements. This study was supported in part by Siemens Medizinische Technik, Germany. We are grateful for valuable discussions with Drs. K. Klingenbeck and D. Hentschel, from Siemens CT R&D.

References

1. Bauer B, Bernhardt J, Stieve FE (eds) (1998) Reference doses and quality in medical imaging. Proceedings of the European Union Workshop held in Luxemburg, 23–25 October 1997. Radiat Protect Dosimetry [Suppl] (in press)
2. Gies M, Suess C, Wolf H, Kalender WA (1998) Dose reduction in CT by anatomically adapted tube current modulation. I. Simulation studies. Med Phys (submitted)
3. Wolf H, Kalender WA, Suess C, Gies M, Bautz WA (1998) Dose reduction in CT by anatomically adapted tube current modulation: experimental results and first patient studies. Med Phys (submitted)
4. Kopka L, Funke M, Breiter N, Hermann K-P, Vosshernrich R, Grabbe E (1995) Anatomisch adaptierte Variation des Röhrenstroms bei der CT. Fortschr Röntgenstr 163 (5):383–387
5. Giacomuzzi SM, Erckert B, Freund MC, Schöpf T, Dessl A, Jaschke W (1996) Dosisreduktion in der Computtomographie mit einem neuen Scan-Verfahren. Akt Radiol 6:110–113

5 Dose Reduction in CT by Anatomically Adapted Tube Current Modulation: First Patient Studies

H. Greess, H. Wolf, W.A. Kalender, W.A. Bautz

5.1 Introduction

The physical principles of dose reduction in computed tomography (CT) by anatomy-oriented attenuation-based tube current modulation, as discussed elsewhere in this volume (see Chap. 4), were tested in a first clinical patient study. Our aim was to reduce the dose applied in CT by current modulation and without a loss of image quality. Dose reduction was measured by the reduction of the mAs product, and image quality was assessed subjectively by experienced radiologists.

5.2 Methods and Materials

We used a Siemens Somatom PLUS 4 CT scanner for all our studies and clinical examinations; the physical principles and the work-in-progress adaptation of the apparatus for anatomy-oriented attenuation-based tube current modulation are described in detail in an accompanying report (see Chap. 4). We examined ten radiation therapy patients scheduled for CT as part of their routine work-up. For these patients four scan levels of the shoulder and upper thorax (the region where the greatest dose reduction was to be expected based on our prior experiments) were examined by single scans without and with tube current modulation. CT was performed without contrast medium to avoid ambiguities. All CT parameters were kept constant: 140 kVp, 5 mm slice thickness, 10 mm increment. Tube current was set to 206 mA without current modulation and to 274 mA maximum current for scans with current modulation. Scan times were either 1.0 s or 1.5 s depending on the cross section of the patient's body. The total mAs product was recorded to determine the respective dose reduction. Four experienced radiologists, blinded as to whether tube modulation was possible in the specific case, compared the two images for a given scan level and determined which was superior in terms of pixel noise, artifact behavior, contrast, and general impression.

5.3 Results

Dose Reduction. The mean difference in dose, measured by the difference in mAs product between scan without and with tube current modulation and expressed as a percentage of the mAs value without current modulation, was 38%,

Table 5.1. Dose reduction in the shoulder region, measured on ten patients and averaged over four levels

Pat. no.	Scan time (s)	mAs Off	mAs On	Dose reduction (%)
1	1	217	158.5	27
2	1.5	327	184.6	43
3	1	217	156.4	28
4	1	217	147.2	32
5	1	217	160.3	26
6	1.5	327	203.8	38
7	1.5	327	176.3	46
8	1.5	327	174.8	47
9	1.5	327	174.4	47
10	1.5	327	182.8	44
Mean				38

Tube current was set at 206 mA for constant current (off) and a peak value of 274 mA was used with current modulation (on).

ranging from 26% to 47% (Table 5.1). This result is quite impressive and is in very good agreement with measurements on cadavers, which yielded an average dose reduction of 40% for the shoulder region (Chap. 4). However, this does not necessarily mean that we have reached the optimum. The ratio of constant tube current to peak value for the modulated tube current was chosen based on simulations of an average shoulder and was only roughly adapted to the individual patient by choosing 1.0 s or 1.5 s scan time. This also means that we can expect that pixel noise is only roughly the same in both scans. Noise measurements are not practical in the highly restructured shoulder regions of patients; therefore noise was assessed subjectively.

Image Quality. The results of the subjective evaluation of pixel noise, contrast, artifact behavior and general impression are presented in Table 5.2.

Pixel Noise. Pixel noise impression was subjectively rated as better in 25% of the scans without current modulation, essentially the same in 58%, and improved in 17%, in spite of the significant dose reduction (Table 5.2). These balanced results are in agreement with expectations: we aimed for approximately unaltered noise levels, but noise reduction can also be achieved at the expense of increased peak mA value. An example of reduced pixel noise combined with significant dose reduction is demonstrated in Fig. 5.1. Improvement in the structure and amplitude

Table 5.2. Assessment of pixel noise, contrast resolution, artifact behavior and general impression: subjective ratings on 40 scan levels by four radiologists in a blinded fashion (relative values, in %)

	Better with current modulation	No significant difference	Better without current modulation
Pixel noise	17	58	25
Contrast resolution	21	30	49
Artifact behavior	48	21	31
General impression	29	42	29

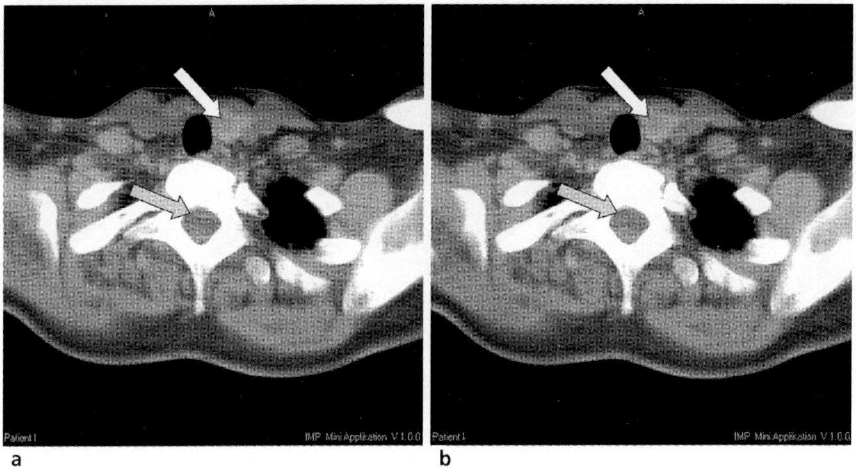

Fig. 5.1a, b. Scan of the shoulder region in patient 1. **a** Standard scan. **b** Scan with current modulation. The dose was reduced by 27% in the scan with current modulation, accompanied by improvement of noise structure (*arrows*)

of noise can be seen particularly well in the spinal canal (gray arrows) and in the left lobe of the thyroid gland (white arrows).

Contrast Resolution. The radiologists' assessment of contrast and of low-contrast resolution was not unambiguous. We expected that contrast of all structures would remain unchanged, but that contrast resolution would vary as a function of noise amplitude and pattern. Contrast resolution was assessed as unchanged in 30% of all ratings, better with current modulation in 21% and better without current modulation in 49% (Table 5.2). Figure 5.2 presents an example in which contrast resolution was rated inferior in the scan with current modulation. It is unclear, however, whether the deterioration was due to motion. The depiction of image content within the spinal canal is clearly better and not affected by structured noise in the case with current modulation.

Artifact Behavior. Assessment of artifact behavior did not yield a clear preference. Surprisingly, only a minority of scans were rated as not significantly different. It must be noted again that the judgement as to whether an artifact is present or not can be very subjective; it is also possible that in some cases the difference was due to other causes. The example shown in Fig. 5.3 was rated as inferior in the scan without current modulation due to an artifact, rated as a beam hardening effect, which was less pronounced in the image obtained with current modulation. The consensus regarding all scans generally was that there was no significant difference between the two scan modes.

General Impression. Ratings regarding general impression was more consistent and also conformed with expectations. In 42% of scans no significant difference

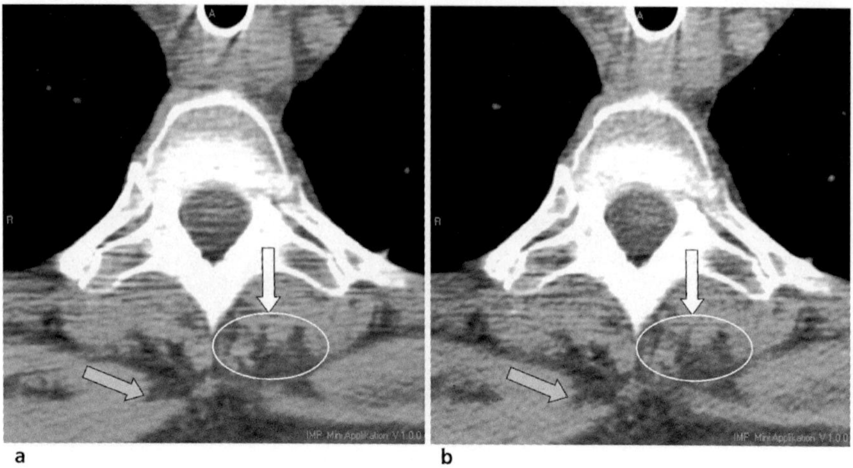

Fig. 5.2a, b. Scan of the shoulder region in patient 9. **a** Standard scan. **b** Scan with current modulation. The dose was reduced by 47% in the scan with current modulation. Low contrast resolution is better in the scan without current modulation (*arrows*). However, the spinal canal is depicted more clearly in the scan with current modulation

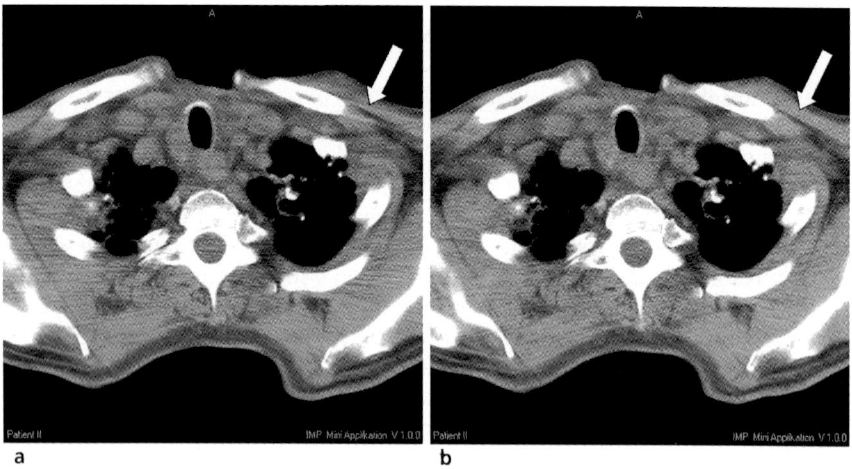

Fig. 5.3a, b. Scan of the shoulder region in patient 2. **a** Standard scan. **b** Scan with current modulation. The dose was reduced by 43% in the scan with current modulation. The bright zones lateral to the left clavicula was rated as a beam hardening artifact in the scan without current modulation, which did not appear in the same way in the scan with current modulation

was observed; equal numbers of the remaining scans were rated as better with and better without current modulation (Table 5.2, Fig. 5.4). This is in perfect agreement with our expectation, as the study was designed to maintain pixel noise and thereby image quality as approximately unaltered – the aim was to

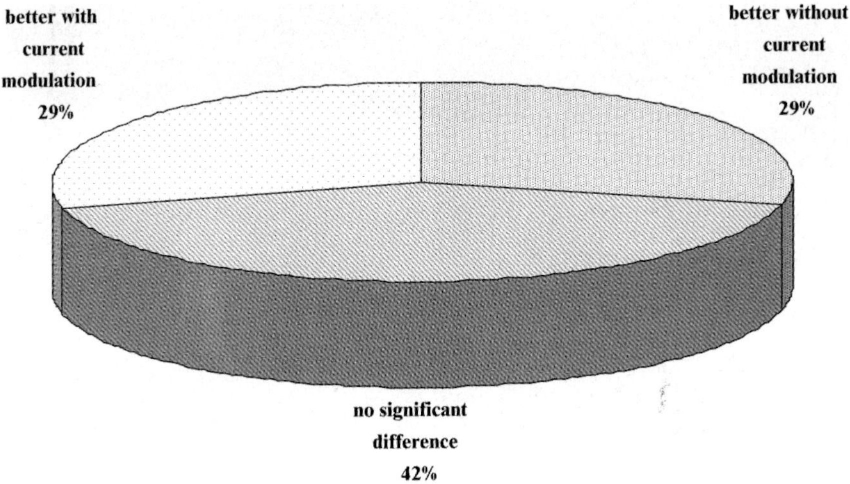

Fig. 5.4. Subjective assessment of image quality in general. There was no significant difference between the scans without and with current modulation. Ratings by four radiologists in a blinded fashion in favour of and against one type of scan were balanced

reduce dose. This was achieved convincingly by a mean dose reduction of 38% (Table 5.1).

5.4 Discussion and Conclusion

The first patient examinations with an anatomy-oriented attenuation-based tube current modulation demonstrated that a substantial dose reduction can be achieved in the shoulder region. A mean dose reduction of 38% was recorded, which is in good agreement with theoretical predictions [1] and phantom and cadaver studies (Chap. 4). It is difficult in a patient study to determine whether image quality differs in scans without and with tube current modulation. We tried to achieve this aim here by raising tube current slightly in lateral views of the shoulder and reducing it drastically in a.p. views. Subjective assessment of pixel noise by four radiologists blinded to whether tube current modulation was activated or not confirmed to a large extent that our initial goal was achieved. Pixel noise was rated as more or less unchanged and the general impression just the same (Table 5.2).

In spite of the significant reduction in dose, an improvement in the noise structure was observed, in particular a reduction of structured noise in the spinal canal. This is demonstrated by another example in Fig. 5.5.

Our results go beyond what has been reported in literature so far. For the use of a sinusoidal tube current modulation based on localizer radiographs (SmartScan), Giacomuzzi et al. [2] reported a dose reduction of maximally 18%; however, this was accompanied by an increase in pixel noise. Kopka et al. [3] and Leh-

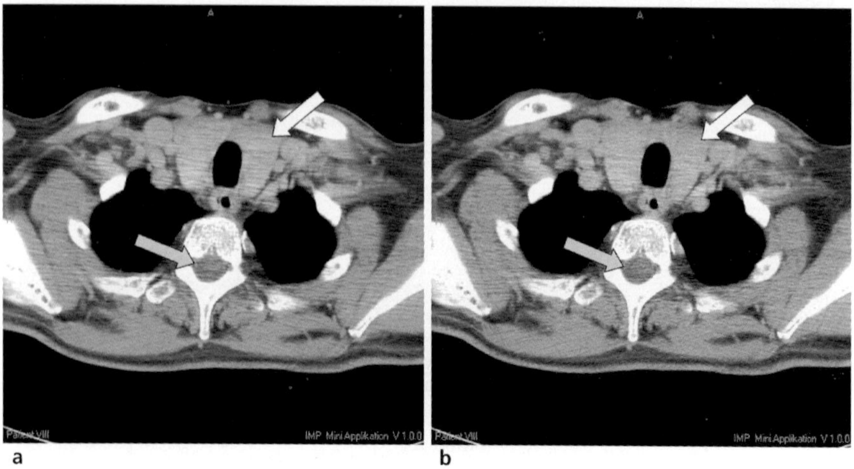

Fig. 5.5a, b. Scan of the shoulder region in patient 8. a Standard scan. b Scan with current modulation. The dose was reduced by 47% in the scan with current modulation. In addition, the improved noise patterns in the thyroid and the spinal canal (*arrows*) can be seen

mann et al. [4] reported a reduction of 11% with constant pixel noise. Our results are far more positive than this and confirmed by simulations, phantom and cadaver studies (Chap. 4). It appears that an online anatomy-oriented attenuation-based tube current control is much more efficient at simultaneously reducing dose and maintaining image quality. Therefore this new approach can play a significant role in efforts to reduce exposure. It must be taken as a standard for future CT systems. Extended clinical studies under well-defined and ethically approved protocols are on the way to evaluate this approach further for various other body regions.

References

1. Gies M, Suess C, Wolf H, Kalender WA (1998) Dose reduction in CT by anatomically adapted tube current modulation. I. Simulation studies. Med Phys (submitted for publication)
2. Giacomuzzi SM, Erckert B, Freund M. C, Schöpf T, Dessl A, Jaschke W (1996) Dosisreduktion in der Computertomographie mit einem neuen Scan-Verfahren. Akt Radiol 6:110–113
3. Kopka L, Funke M, Breiter N, Hermann K-P, Vosshernrich R, Grabbe E (1995) Anatomisch adaptierte Variation des Röhrenstroms bei der CT. Fortschr Röntgenstr 163 (5):383–387
4. Lehmann KJ, Wild M, Georgi M (1997) Klinischer Einsatz der softwaregesteuerten Röhrenstrommodulation "SmartScan" in der Spiral-CT. Akt Radiol 7:156–158

Part II
Neuro, Head and Neck

Moderators: L. Heuser, M. T. Modic

6 Spiral CT and Its Use in Neuroradiology: A Review of Spiral CT Techniques, Real-Time Volume Rendering, and Real Time Neuronavigation

W. J. Davros, C. Steiner, M. T. Modic

6.1 Introduction to Spiral CT

X-ray computed tomography (CT) became widely available in the early 1970s, and by the 1980s CT had reached a plateau that few thought could be improved; the technology had matured fully. However, in the early 1990s a new breed of CT scanner appeared: spiral CT. By the mid-1990s it was apparent that scan protocols would need to be entirely rewritten in order to harness the power and speed of spiral CT. We, as radiologists and referring physicians, would have to reevaluate the clinical potential of CT for locating disease. This chapter addresses a small part of this reevaluation: the role of spiral CT in neuroradiology and neurosurgery.

CT has evolved rapidly due to technological advances into a clinical modality that excels at portraying cross-sectional anatomy in stunning detail. CT has become faster at completing examinations as computer speed and memory have increased. Advances in X-ray tube technology have permitted longer and higher intensity exposures to be produced. Advances in detector materials have made more efficient use of X-rays. However, the single most important step in the evolution of CT has been the innovation of the slip ring gantry. The slip ring gantry permits an X-ray tube and detector bank assembly to rotate continuously about the gantry opening's axis of symmetry without the need to stop due to hard wiring limitations. The slip ring gantry is an electrical conduction path for data and power into and out of the X-ray tube-detector assembly. It works by means of spring loaded electrical contacts that ride on top of and slide over concentric conductive rings.

The clinical implications of this electrical arrangement have proven to have a profound effect on the way in which CT scanners can be used. Using spiral CT there is no need to stop the patient table from incrementally moving to the next position. Since the patient table does not have to be accelerated and decelerated at the beginning and end of each slice acquisition, the table can move a greater distance per unit time and at a constant velocity. In order to conceptually keep spiral scanning similar to conventional scanning, table travel per 360° gantry rotation was initially kept equal to the X-ray beam collimator setting (pitch = 1) early in the use of spiral CT. Later pitch factors greater than 1 were explored as a means of optimizing spiral CT protocols.

Pitch is a parameter for the distance that the table travels per 360° rotation of the gantry relative to the collimation setting. The following equation defines pitch: $P = d/c$, where d is the distance traveled (in millimeters) by the table per

360° rotation, and c is the collimator setting (in millimeters). Pitch is therefore a unitless quantity. Clinically pitches from 0.8 to 3.0 have been applied to varying degrees.

Also as a result of not having to stop the gantry rotation it became advantageous to collect data on a continuous basis as the patient in fed into the gantry opening at a constant velocity. The combination of constant velocity table travel and a continuously orbiting X-ray source form a spiral trajectory of X-rays about the patient's long axis, and hence the name spiral CT.

In conventional CT each rotation of the gantry produces a self-consistent set data of X-ray projections from which a single image is produced. In this scenario, each rotation of the gantry is intimately connected to a location on the patient and to a specific set of data from which an image of that unique location along the patient is made. Hence there is a one-to-one relationship between slice location as defined by the X-ray beam shining on the patient, the table position, and an image location. This one-to-one correspondence does not have meaning in spiral CT.

In spiral CT data are collected in a continuous fashion and form a spiral around the patient's long axis. After the projection data are collected, the user indicates to the reconstruction computer where along the spiral of raw data images are to be reconstructed. It is only then that the reconstruction computer selects the projections needed to reconstruct an image at each selected location. The selection of projections and their relative importance to the final image are chosen in such a way as to give added importance those projections that are nearest to the image location. This process is called z-axis interpolation.

In this implementation an image can be produced anywhere along the raw data stream so long as the mathematical constraints for sufficient projection data are met. This leaves open the possibility of producing overlapping images without using overlapping radiation fields. The concept of overlapping images will become apparent when 3D postprocessing and surgical neuronavigation are discussed.

Spiral CT permits shorter examination than conventional CT. There are two reasons. First, time is saved by not having to start and stop the table each time the X-ray tube is energized. In spiral scanning mode, once the table is moving, it is not stopped until the spiral acquisition is completed. Second, time is saved by not having to start and stop the gantry from rotating. Once the gantry is in motion about the table, it wants to stay in motion by virtue of its inertia. Because the gantry does not have to be rapidly accelerated and decelerated, it can be made to rotate at higher angular velocities. To date some scanners have angular velocities of 480° per second (one revolution in 0.75 s).

Spiral CT scanning has lead to increases in image quality. There are many reasons for this increase in quality. One reason is the suppression of motion artifacts from all sources. Patient motion is lessened because the scan is completed more quickly. Periodic motion such as cardiac motion and peristalsis are minimized because a complete set of projections is taken in less time due to increased gantry angular velocities. Partial volume averaging is also reduced by deemphasizing projections that are more distant from the image location.

Spiral CT has changed the way in which iodinated contrast media is used. Volume of injected media, injection rate, and delay between injection and the onset of scanning have been modified to optimize use of spiral techniques. One feature that stands out is the ability to track a bolus of contrast and scan a particular region when tissue contrast has reached its peak. Another key use of injectable contrast media has been improved spiral CT angiography. This is largely due to being able to scan through a region before the contrast media bolus has been diluted.

As described above, spiral CT scanning permits overlapping images to be reconstructed from projection data. When the image overlap reaches a point at which the distance between images is approximately one-third of the collimator setting, isotropic image volume elements (voxels) are produced. When this occurs, the usefulness of the image data set becomes much greater than that of the axial images by themselves. With isotropic resolution any arbitrary plane through the image data volume has the same spatial resolution, as do the original axial images. This point is important for advanced applications such as three-dimensional (3D) renderings and surgical navigation with real-time spiral CT image updating in any oblique plane.

6.2 Three Applications of Spiral CT in Neuroradiology

Visualization of intracranial pathology is not a new concept in CT. However, the use of spiral scanning protocols and application of high-speed computers for use in real-time three-dimensional modeling is a recent development. Spiral CT is ideally suited for use in intracranial imaging in that it allows rapid capture of a contrast bolus as is passes through the arterial structures of interest. When rapid, accurately timed scanning is combined with thin collimation and a high degree of image overlap, image data sets are produced that permit image postprocessing to be done.

Image postprocessing of intracranial and spinal pathology is useful for at least three broad applications. One is real 3D volume rendering, the second is real-time image updated intraoperative surgical navigation, and the third is 3D treatment planning for high dose radiosurgery (high-dose teletherapy).

6.3 Real-Time Three-Dimensional Volume Rendering

In real-time 3D volume rendering, overlapping images are loaded into a high-speed computer. This computer is optimized for performing 3D computations and display at real time rates. In the package that we are evaluating, the computer is a Silicon Graphics Incorporated ONYX workstation, and the software is 3D Virtuoso by Siemens Medical Systems. The software permits the user independently to include multiple anatomic objects in a rendering. This is done by selecting a range of Hounsfield units that best define the object. An example of this would be highly opacified arteries in the circle of Willis. For each object the user can also independently control the amount of object translucency. Additionally, structures that might obscure clinically relevant pathology can be excluded from view by positioning "exclusion or cut" planes. Lastly, the rendering can reviewed from any perspective simply by rotating the rendering on the display through the use of the computer mouse. Surgical planning of intracranial aneurysms is an example of where this technology is used. To date we have processed 15 cases in this fashion.

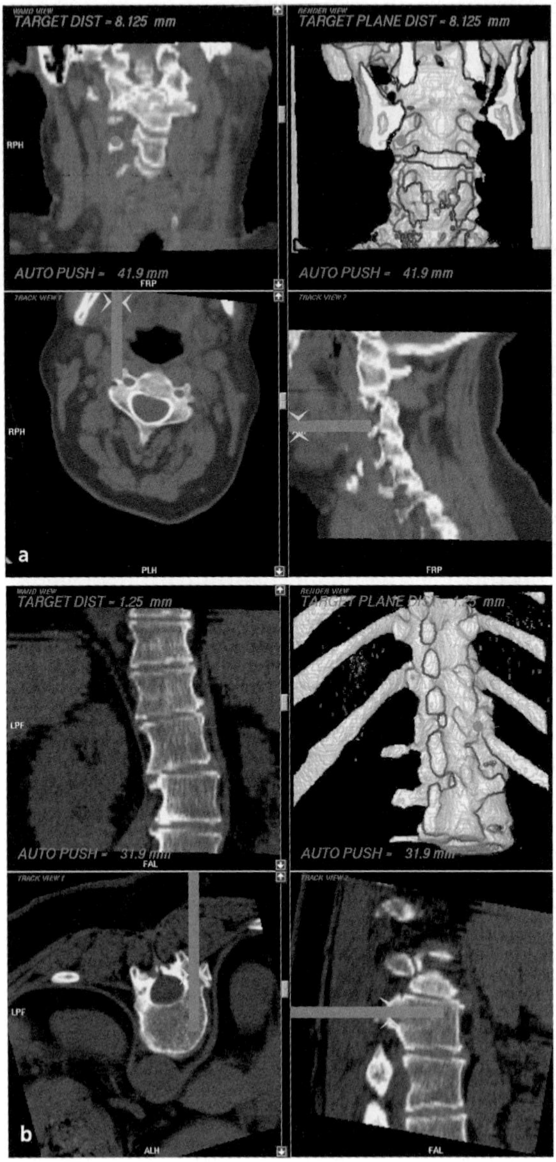

Fig. 6.1.

6.4
Real-Time Intraoperative Surgical Navigation

In real time intraoperative surgical navigation spiral CT image data is transferred to a computer that is optimized for high-speed 2D display. In this application a display has been designed that simultaneously displays axial, sagittal, and coronal slices that have a common point of intersection corresponding to a location in the surgical field (Fig. 6.1). The surgeon interacts with the computer through the use of a localizing stylus. This stylus is equipped with either optical or acoustic transmitters. The transmitted signals are received by a receiver array located

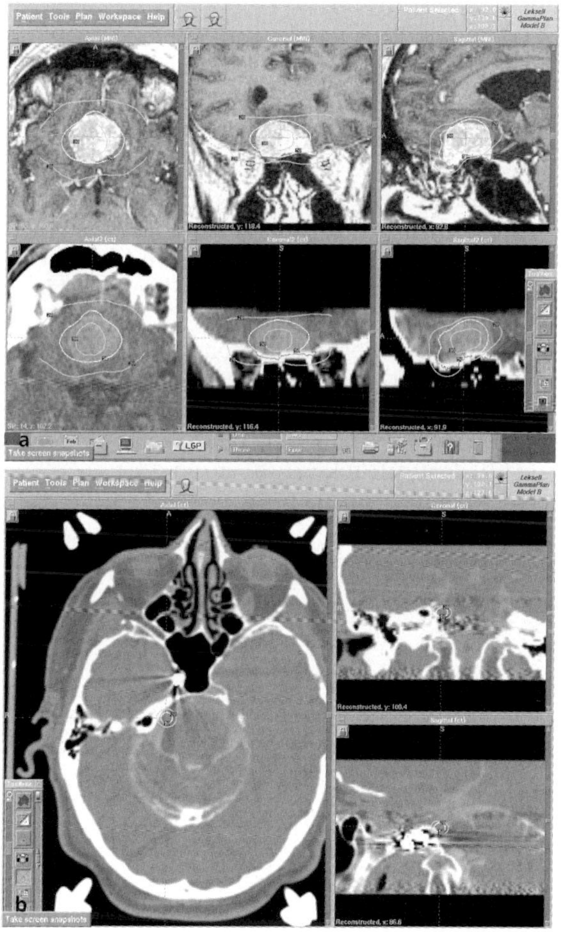

Fig. 6.2.

above the surgical field near the ceiling. The exact orientation of the stylus and its relationship to the pathology is initiated through a registration sequence. In this sequence the operator locates with the stylus fixed landmarks on the patient and in the image. The computer calculates the position of the stylus tip (x, y, z) and orientation angles (α, β, γ) of the stylus using an overdetermined data set. When the computer has registered a set of four to six landmarks each having unique (x, y, z) coordinates, an estimated positioning error is calculated. When that error is less than 1 mm, surgical navigation can commence. In 1997 the Division of Radiology performed 192 cervical spine spiral CT examinations and 379 lumbar spine spiral CT examinations. Of these approximately 400 were used in 1997 for spinal surgery navigation.

6.5 Three-Dimensional Radiosurgery Planning

The last spiral CT data sets are used in treatment planning for use with high-dose 3D radiosurgery such as the Gammaknife project. In this project thin section spiral CT data sets are made and fed into a treatment-planning computer. This computer then uses the spiral data set to calculate the 3D shape and location of one or more lesions in the brain (Fig. 6.2). The goal of this 3D planning is to deliver a dose of radiation to the lesions that is sufficient cause remission while sparing radiosensitive structures nearby. When performed correctly, 0.5-mm accuracy can be achieved. To date, spiral CT has been used in this capacity 251 times at the Cleveland Clinic Foundation.

Spiral acquisition at subsecond speeds, thin sections, the use of overlapping images, and high-speed computers have revolutionized CT. In the years to come, this technology will most likely grow to include cardiac gated CT, large-area detectors and possible intraoperative scanning. What is certain is that postprocessing will dominate future uses of spiral CT.

7 Determination of Regional Brain Perfusion by Functional CT

M. König, L. Heuser, E. Klotz

7.1 Introduction

Due to the increasing recognition that noninvasive measurements of cerebral blood flow (CBF) parameters may play a major role in the clinical management of patients with neurological disorders, a variety of functional imaging techniques have been developed in the past. Single photon emission computed tomography (SPECT) and xenon computed tomography (CT) have gained significant clinical acceptance, because these methods may be used as routine procedures for the investigation of chronic occlusive vascular disease. However, although accurate assessment of perfusion impairment has to be performed if modern therapeutic strategies are intended for acute stroke patients, only limited data are available concerning the application of these functional modalities within the first few hours of brain ischemia [1, 2]. Cerebral SPECT imaging using blood flow tracers provides useful information regarding the full three-dimensional extent of CBF impairment; however, it takes about 15–20 min for a complete examination to be performed. This causes substantial motion artifacts in many cases due to the limited compliance of the patients. Moreover, at present only a few community hospitals offer SPECT for 24 h a day as a routine measure. Xenon CT has not been widely applied in stroke patients within the acute phase due to the limited practicability of a measure that requires a face mask and inhalation of a narcotic gas to be accepted by the patient.

We used contrast enhanced dynamic computed tomography (CT) of the brain to calculate CBF parameters in acute stroke patients. The aim of this paper is to describe the principle of this new functional CT technique and to show its practicability and usefulness under clinical conditions.

7.2 Principle of Functional CT

Based on the indicator-dilution theory, the fundamentals of CBF measurements using dynamic CT scanning of the brain were developed by Axel in 1980 [3]. Rapid-sequence CT of a single section of the brain has been performed after intravenous bolus injection of iodine contrast material, which acts as a pure intravascular tracer as long as the blood–brain barrier is intact. During the first pass of the contrast bolus through the brain vasculature, local concentrations of iodine are simply reflected in changes of the attenuation values, as measured with CT. A set of parameters of cerebral bolus kinetics such as the area under the curve, the peak time, and the mean transit time of the local bolus passage may be derived from time–density curves for each pixel to calculate CBF and cerebral blood volume (CBV). However, additional gamma-variate fitting is necessary to avoid effects due to the recirculation of contrast material. For several reasons, this method has never reached a sufficient performance level to be acceptable as a clinical imaging technique, the most important of these reasons being the long cycle times and scan intervals of the older generations of CT scanners. Regarding the mean transit time, i.e., the time for a contrast bolus to pass through the normal human brain, of 3–5 s, more rapid scanning techniques with scan times of 1 s or less are required to obtain sufficient temporal resolution. For many years, dynamic CT played an important role for the investigation of the vascularity and perfusion characteristics of tumorous lesions of abdominal organs such as the liver and kidneys, because bolus transit times within these organs are substantially longer than within the brain. Fast and continuous data acquisition of slip-ring scanners now allows the detection of bolus kinetics within the cerebral vasculature even for calculating CBF and CBV. Due to the high spatial resolution of CT, this may be done on a pixel basis, leading to the generation of a set of functional maps of cerebral perfusion parameters.

7.2.1 Calculation of Cerebral Blood Flow

An alternative approach for the calculation of organ blood flow from CT data, which has been referred to as the "maximum slope model," was proposed by Miles et al. in 1991 [4]. Following this theory, organ blood flow expressed as flow *F* per unit volume *V* may be calculated as the relationship of the maximum slope of the tissue time–density curve divided by the maximum contrast enhancement within the supplying artery:

$$\frac{F}{V} = \frac{\text{maximum slope of tissue time density curve}}{\text{peak arterial enhancement}} \tag{1}$$

The model is based on a nuclear medicine technique using radiolabeled microspheres which are completely extracted from the circulation during the first pass of the tracer. Thus temporary retention of the substance within the organ to be investigated is a fundamental prerequisite. Application of this technique to CT perfusion measurements of abdominal organs (e.g., kidneys) has shown accurate results, because the prerequisite of tracer retention is sufficiently fulfilled even using iodine contrast material [4, 5]. However, to assess CBF using intravenous injection of contrast material, short transit times have to be taken into consideration. The lack of sufficient tracer retention may be an important limitation of the method, because as a result substantial overlap of the arterial inflow and venous outflow phase may occur, leading to the reduction of the upslope of the tissue time–density curve and subsequently to an underestimation of flow. In order to minimize this error, high rates of contrast injection have to be used to ensure that the arterial peak is reached before any contrast material leaves the brain via the venous route. This is equivalent to the requirement of keeping the arterial rise time as short as possible. However, in clinical practice, this may be counteracted by restrictions of the cardiac capacity of the patient, which may cause significant broadening of the time–density curve (Fig. 7.1). The theoretically expected dependence was clearly confirmed by measurements of CBF within cerebral gray matter and by determining the arterial rise time in our group of patients (Fig. 7.2). However, the results of flow measurements may be significantly distorted by an erroneous determination of the maximum enhancement within small arterial vessels due to partial volume effects. To correct for this, the peak enhancement is measured within the superior sagittal sinus, which usually has a large lumen within the chosen scan plane at the level of the basal ganglia. Due to

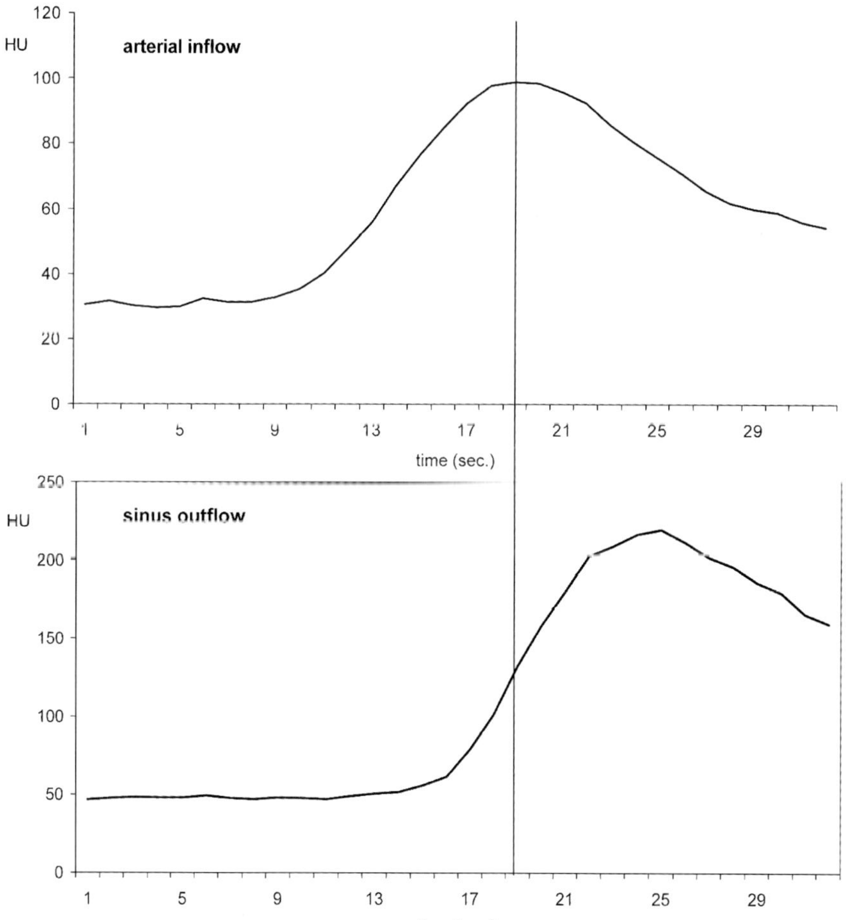

a

Fig. 7.1. a Due to cardiac insufficiency of the patient, the arterial bolus curve is flattened, causing overlap with the sinus outflow curve. Thus the condition of the maximum slope model is violated

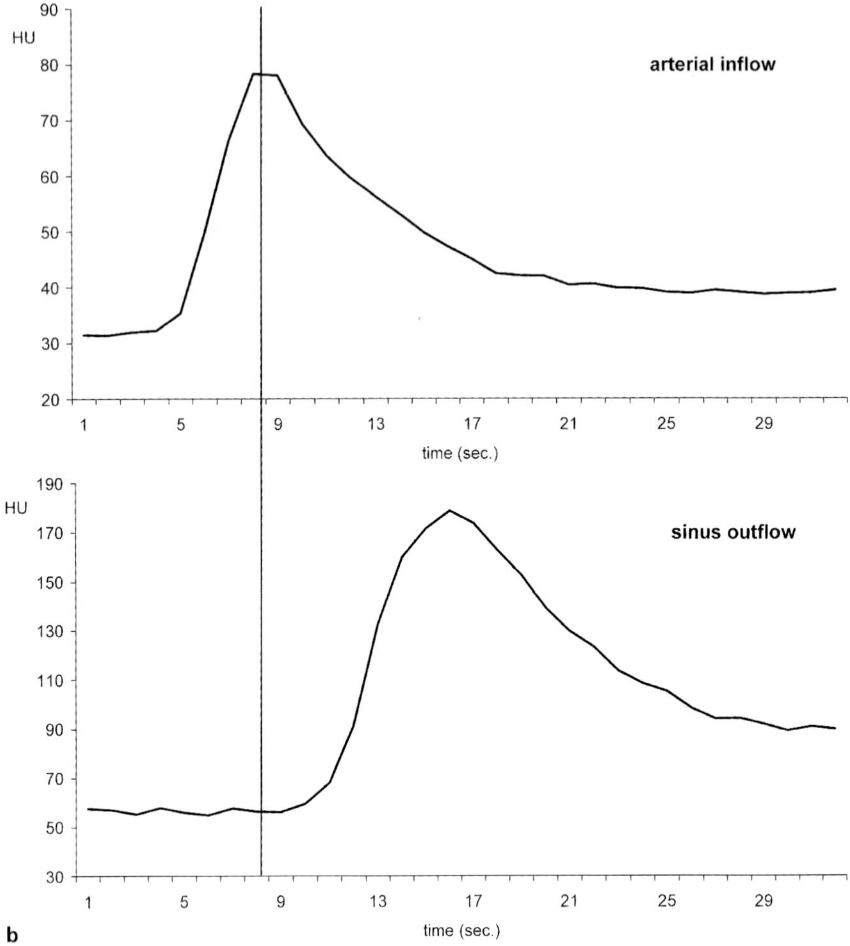

b

Fig. 7.1. b Very short arterial rise time following high rate of contrast injection in a patient with normal cardiac output

the short cerebral transit time, the difference of the peak enhancement values within the sinus and cerebral arteries with a large diameter may be expected to be relatively small. Nevertheless, it has to be borne in mind that the CBF values tend to be underestimated compared to the results of xenon CT studies [6, 7].

7.2.2 Calculation of Cerebral Blood Volume

Further analysis of the time-density curves in brain tissue and cerebral vessels allows the calculation of the fractional CBV according to the following simple equation:

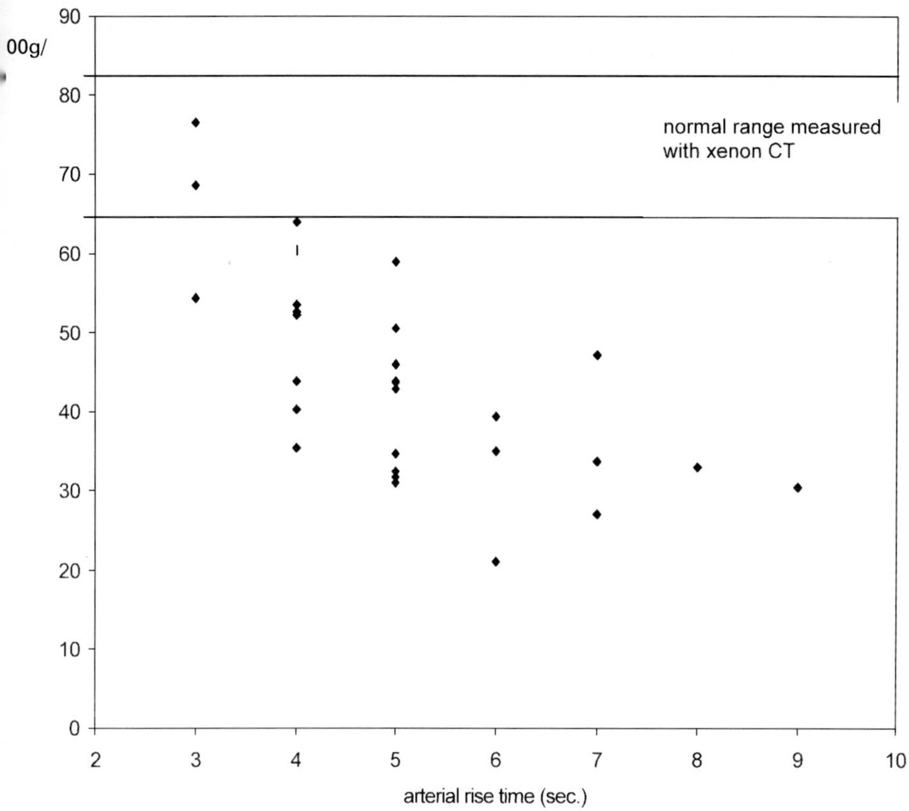

Fig. 7.2. Mean cerebral blood flow (CBF) values derived from the lentiform nucleus in the non-ischemic hemisphere of stroke patients showing a clear relationship to the rise time of the arterial time density curve

$$\mathrm{CBV} = \frac{\text{peak tissue enhancement}}{\text{peak enhancement in the superior sagittal sinus}} \tag{2}$$

The derivation of Eq. 2 has recently been published [8]. Like many others, our mathematical model for the calculation of blood flow is based on the assumption that the vasculature of the organ to be investigated may be described as a single compartment with one inlet and one outlet. Because this assumption only approximately holds true for the normal perfused brain and for vascular territories which are hypoperfused due to an embolic event, CBV cannot be accurately determined. However, the above equation provides a good estimate of CBV, yielding values that are quite similar to recently published results of photon emission tomography (PET) and SPECT studies, respectively [9–11].

7.3 Materials and Methods

7.3.1 Imaging Protocol

Functional CT was performed on a Somatom Plus S scanner using a standard imaging protocol with the following technical parameters: dynamic multiscan with an acquisition time of 32 s and a rotation time of 1 s; tube voltage, 120 kVp; tube current, 210 mA; and collimation, 10 mm. The position of the axial single slice was adjusted to the level of the basal ganglia to include most of the supratentorial vascular territories which are usually affected by ischemic stroke of the cerebrum. Because short arterial rise times are required to meet the condition of the underlying mathematical model, the use of an angiographic power injector is recommended to achieve high injection rates in the range of 15–20 ml/s. For each slice to be investigated, 50 ml high-density contrast material (Iopromide 370 mg/ml, Schering, Berlin) was injected via a large intravenous cannula (14 gauge) in the antecubital fossa.

7.3.2 Evaluation Procedure

Following image reconstruction using a time increment and reconstruction time of 1 s, images were transferred to an Intel PC-based workstation, where they were evaluated by means of the work-in-progress software "Perfusion CT" (Siemens, Erlangen, Germany).

To increase the speed of image processing, several preprocessing steps are carried out, including segmentation of the images. While exclusion of the skull bone is performed using contour finding, pixels representing cerebrospinal fluid (CSF) space are eliminated by setting appropriate thresholds. In addition, following reduction of the matrix size to 256, the images are subjected to a smoothing procedure to compensate for the limited signal-to-noise ratio of the images that results from the low contrast enhancement of the brain tissue. To avoid image blurring, this algorithm operates separately on brain tissue and vascular structures. Calculation of CBF and CBV is based on the generation of time–density curves of each pixel as well as the determination of the maximum enhancement within the superior sagittal sinus, as mentioned above. Parameters of the cerebral bolus kinetics such as the time to peak and the time to start may also be extracted from the curves and likewise shown as functional maps. Because thorough analysis of brain ischemia may be facilitated by comparison of corresponding regions within both hemispheres, several valuable tools are offered for further evaluation of the functional images. These include the use of mirrored regions of interest with any functional map as well as the graphical demonstration of the time–density curve of any part of the brain section. For better delineation of anatomic structures, a maximum-intensity projection (MIP) image of all consecutive images is included. Following expansion of the matrix to 512, each functional image may be printed on laser hard copies or displayed using an appropriate color scale. The time for a complete investigation typically amounts to 15 min, with the processing time being approximately 2 min. A striking advantage of the algorithm has been shown to be that, for calculation of the functional maps, data are extracted only from a very short period of time. Impairment of image quality due to patient motion is therefore not likely to occur.

To date, 48 patients with acute ischemic stroke have been included in a clinical study to apply perfusion CT within 6 h from symptom onset. Routine unenhanced CT scanning of the brain was performed as the initial method in all cases, followed by cerebral SPECT imaging using a blood flow tracer (99mTc-ECD) in 18 patients. For comparison of ischemic findings, the CBF image generated by functional CT and the appropriate slice of SPECT at the level of the basal ganglia were selected. Follow-up was performed with CT or magnetic resonance imaging (MRI).

7.4 Results

With regard to the results of the CBF maps, functional CT revealed areas of ischemic brain in 39 of 43 patients who showed definite cerebral infarcts on follow-up imaging studies. Thus the sensitivity was 90%. In four patients, no abnormality was detected by CT. In all these patients, the ischemic area was located outside the CT scan level. Based on their ischemic pattern, infarcts could be reliably classified as embolic ($n=34$), hemodynamic ($n=2$) (Fig. 7.3), or lacunar due to microangiopathy ($n=3$). The results of the CBF maps corresponded well to SPECT findings in 13 of 16 (81%) stroke patients, and two patients were shown to have a TIA. In many patients, functional CT revealed various degrees of perfusion impairment within the ischemic territory, thus giving rise to a very heterogeneous appearance. As a rule, the center of a lesion usually representing the core of ischemia showed marked reduction of blood flow, especially if the gray matter of the basal ganglia was affected. In these cases, CBV was also reduced and bolus arrival was not detectable on the time to peak image (Fig. 7.3). By contrast, at the outer margin of an ischemic area, the reduction of CBF and CBV was often less pronounced, indicating some residual flow via collaterals, as was confirmed by the bolus delay on the time to peak map.

7.5 Discussion

The standards of diagnostic imaging have changed considerably over the past few years as a result of modern treatment strategies for acute stroke patients.

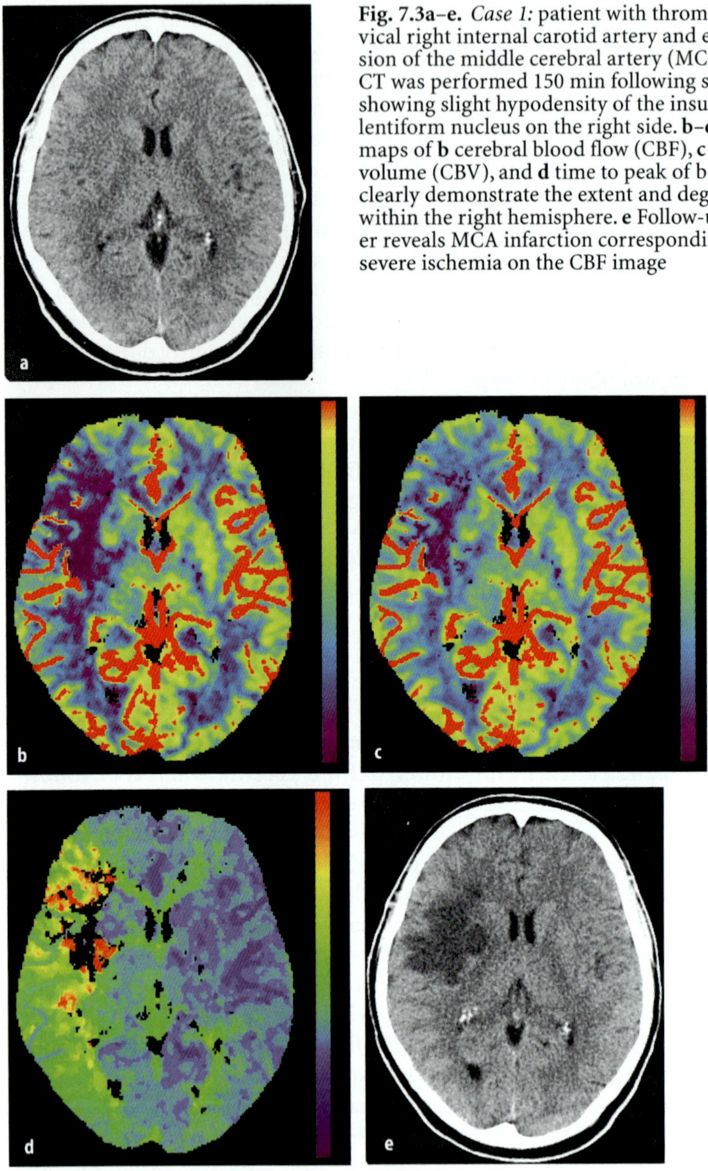

Fig. 7.3a–e. *Case 1:* patient with thrombosis of the cervical right internal carotid artery and embolic occlusion of the middle cerebral artery (MCA). **a** Standard CT was performed 150 min following symptom onset, showing slight hypodensity of the insular cortex and lentiform nucleus on the right side. **b–d** Functional maps of **b** cerebral blood flow (CBF), **c** cerebral blood volume (CBV), and **d** time to peak of bolus arrival clearly demonstrate the extent and degree of ischemia within the right hemisphere. **e** Follow-up CT 5 days later reveals MCA infarction corresponding well with the severe ischemia on the CBF image

There is now an increasing demand for new modalities which may provide functional information concerning the perfusion status of the ischemic brain within a few minutes. Functional CT of the brain based on the maximum slope model has proved to be a very fast and robust new imaging technique for the calculation of CBF, CBV, and certain time-dependent parameters of the cerebral bolus kinetics. Our data showed a clear relationship between CBF values measured using the

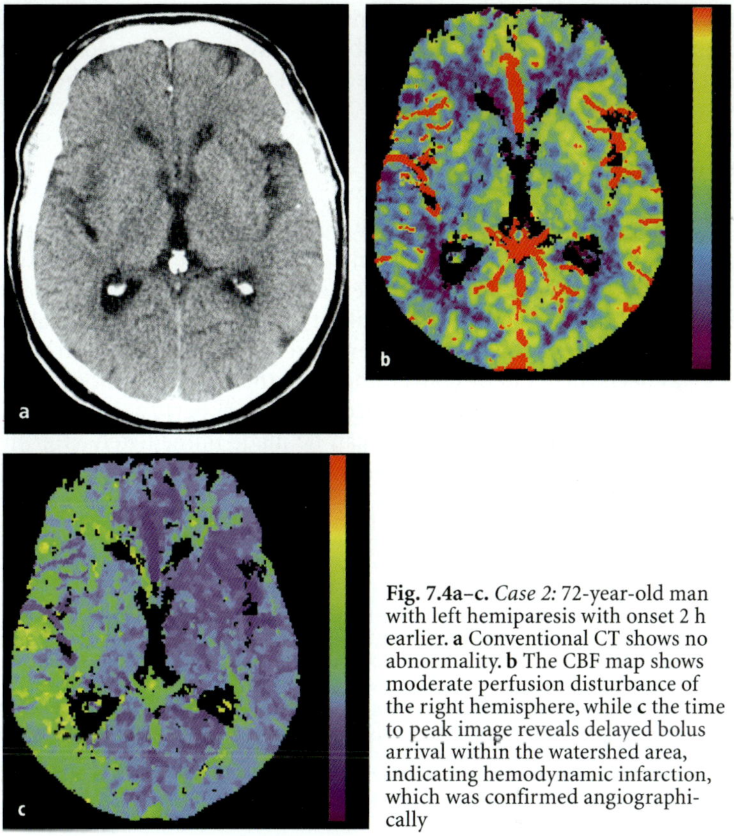

Fig. 7.4a–c. *Case 2:* 72-year-old man with left hemiparesis with onset 2 h earlier. **a** Conventional CT shows no abnormality. **b** The CBF map shows moderate perfusion disturbance of the right hemisphere, while **c** the time to peak image reveals delayed bolus arrival within the watershed area, indicating hemodynamic infarction, which was confirmed angiographically

perfusion CT technique and the rise time of the arterial input curve. Given an optimal contrast injection technique, CBF values may easily be calculated based on the maximum slope model. Although this modality does not provide accurate results for absolute values of CBF and CBV, the image quality is excellent in almost all patients, leading to a reliable assessment of cerebral perfusion impairments. The results of CBF images based on functional CT correspond well to the findings of SPECT, which has been shown to be a reliable technique for cerebral perfusion imaging over a period of many years. However, SPECT has the disadvantage of being more time-consuming than CT. Even using a single-slice examination, the sensitivity of the perfusion maps in our study was surprisingly high. In the case of a normal finding on the initial perfusion scan but clear evidence of cerebral ischemia due to clinical symptoms, the examination procedure can easily be repeated at a second level of the brain in order to depict the ischemic area or to obtain more information regarding the three-dimensional extent of the infarct. Thus the results might be even better than 90%. Imaging of the CBF is obviously the method of choice for the investigation of patients with acute stroke, because perfusion abnormalities can be demonstrated even in the very early phase when the pathological findings of conventional CT are very subtle. For better characterization of brain ischemia, it may be usefully complemented by details concerning CBV and information about the arrival time of a contrast bolus.

7.6 Conclusion

While in the near future functional imaging techniques should have a major impact on therapeutic decision-making in acute stroke patients, perfusion CT may be recommended even now for emergency applications in daily patient care due to its practicability and wide availability. With regards to optimal management, there is a major advantage for patients presenting with acute stroke: After bleeding has been ruled out by conventional CT, the same modality can be used to obtain information about the presence of regional perfusion abnormalities of the brain. Thus therapeutic decisions can be made immediately after the CT examination without moving the patient away to undergo another imaging method.

References

1. Imaizumi S, Sakurai Y (1995) Critical level of regional cerebral blood flow determined by xenon/computed tomography in acute cerebral infarction. In: Tomonaga M, Tanaka A, Yonas H (eds) Quantitative cerebral blood flow measurements using stable Xenon/CT: clinical applications. Futura, Armonk, pp 187–192
2. Sperling B, Overgaard K, Boysen G, Lassen NA (1993) The role of SPECT in acute stroke thrombolysis. In: del Zoppo GJ, Mori E, Hacke W (eds) Thrombolytic therapy in acute ischemic stroke II. Springer, Berlin Heidelberg New York, pp 206–211
3. Axel L (1980) Cerebral blood flow determination by rapid-sequence computed tomography: theoretical analysis. Radiology 137:679–686
4. Miles KA (1991) Measurement of tissue perfusion by dynamic computed tomography. Br J Radiol 64:409–412
5. Blomley MJ, Coulden R, Bufkin C, Lipton MJ, Dawson P (1993) Contrast bolus dynamic computed tomography for the measurement of solid organ perfusion. Invest Radiol 28 [Suppl 5]:72–77
6. Amano T, Meyer JS, Ikabe T et al (1982) Stable xenon CT cerebral blood flow measurements computed by a single compartment-double integration model in normal aging and dementia. J Comput Assist Tomogr 6:923–932
7. Segawa H (1985) Tomographic cerebral blood flow measurement using xenon inhalation and serial CT scanning: normal values and validity. Neurosurg Rev 8:27–33
8. König M, Klotz E, Luka B, Venderink DJ, Spittler JF, Heuser L. Perfusion CT of the brain: new diagnostic approach for early detection of ischemic stroke. Radiology (in press)
9. Phelps ME, Huang SC, Hoffmann EJ et al (1979) Validation of tomographic measurement of cerebral blood volume with C-11-labeled carboxyhemoglobin. J Nucl Med 20:328–334
10. Grubb RL, Raichle ME, Higgins CS et al (1978) Measurements of regional cerebral blood volume by emission tomography. Ann Neurol 4:322–328
11. Sakai F, Nakazawa K, Tazaki Y et al (1985) Regional cerebral blood volume and hematocrit measured in normal human volunteers by single-photon emission computed tomography. J Cereb Blood Flow Metab 5:207–213

8 The Diagnostic Accuracy and the Role of Three-Dimensional CT Angiography for the Diagnosis of Cerebral Aneurysms

S. Tanabe, M. Ohtaki, T. Uede, Y. Ibayashi, K. Hashi

8.1 Introduction

Digital subtraction angiography (DSA) has been considered as the gold standard for the diagnosis of cerebral aneurysms. However, this method is fairly invasive and requires an experienced and expert operator. Although magnetic resonance angiography (MRA) is less invasive, it has less spatial resolution than DSA. Recently developed three-dimensional computed tomography angiography (CTA) is a minimally invasive method and has higher spatial resolution than MRA. In this article, we report the usefulness of CTA in the diagnosis of cerebral aneurysms and its role in surgical planning.

8.2 Patients and Imaging Methods

Since 1992, we have performed CTA consecutively in cases with 111 unruptured cerebral aneurysms (73 patients), most of which were known or suspected by MRA and/or DSA, and 32 ruptured cerebral aneurysms (21 patients). The location of these aneurysms were as follows: anterior cerebral artery (ACA) ($n=27$), middle cerebral artery (MCA) ($n=31$), internal carotid artery (ICA) ($n=62$), basilar artery (BA) ($n=19$), and vertebral artery (VA) ($n=4$). With respect to the size of aneurysms, 44 aneurysms had a diameter of 1–3 mm, 72 aneurysms a diameter of 4–11 mm, 24 aneurysms a diameter of 12–40 mm; there were also three fusiform aneurysms.

CTA images were obtained using a Somatom Plus-S CT scanner with 120–140 kV, 180–210 mA, a slice thickness of 1 mm, a table increment of 1 mm/s, and an image interval of 1 mm. The three-dimensional images were reconstructed with the shaded surface reconstruction (SSR) method through a threshold of 120–180 HU and additionally 250–350 HU for detection of intracavernous ICA aneurysms. Maximum-intensity projection (MIP) and volume rendering modes were also employed. Nonionic iodinated contrast medium of 240–350 mgI/ml was administered at a rate of 4 ml/s using an automatic injector, and the total intravenous infusion volume was 150 ml. The scan was started 15–25 s after the initiation of the contrast medium injection.

In the present study, we adopted 4 key concepts to detect cerebral aneurysms at a higher rate:

1. A higher CT value of the target vessels by using large doses of the contrast medium is essential.

2. This method makes higher threshold image processing possible.
3. Target CTA with a 5- to 7-cm field of view is indispensable to investigate the target single vessel in detail.
4. The target images are reconstructed from all perspectives. In particular, the view from the opposite side should be investigated.

8.3 Diagnosis of Cerebral Aneurysms with CTA

8.3.1 Accuracy in Detection and Characterization

The results of our study indicate the distinct advantages of CTA in the diagnosis of cerebral aneurysms as compared to MRA and DSA, as described below. CTA was able to detect 140 of 143 aneurysms, i.e., had a high diagnostic rate of 97.9%, including two false-negative and one false-positive results. Concerning the size of aneurysms, CTA was able to demonstrate aneurysms with a diameter of more than 1 mm because of its higher spatial resolution (Fig. 8.1).

Three-dimensional image displays obtained by CTA are fundamentally different from the two-dimensional projection images of MRA and DSA. Thus CTA

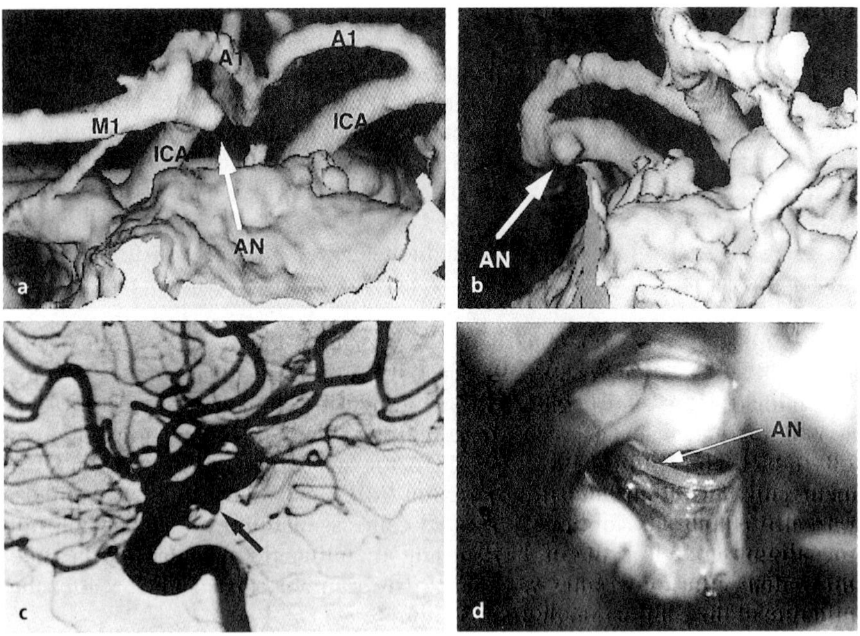

Fig. 8.1a–d. ICA anterior choroidal artery aneurysm (1.5 mm in diameter)
a CTA (posteroanterior view); **b** CTA (lateral view); **c**; **d** operative finding. For abbreviations in figure legends, refer to text

provides the useful anatomical presentation of the aneurysmal lesion, such as the shape of the neck and dome, the direction of aneurysmal growth, and adjacent arterial branches. In the present study, CTA was apparently superior to MRA in the diagnosis of any size of cerebral aneurysms (Fig. 8.2): small-sized (1–3 mm in diameter) in 25 of 26 aneurysms, medium-sized (4–11 mm) in 30 of 36 aneurysms, large-sized (12–40 mm) in 15 of 16 aneurysms (Table 8.1). Additionally, CTA was quite advantageous in the accurate detection of small-sized aneurysms as compared to DSA (18 out of 28 aneurysms detected). In most large-sized aneurysms, i.e., 12 of 18, CTA was considered more useful, particularly for surgical planning, because of detailed presentation of the aneurysmal neck and because it was independent of turbulent flow (Table 8.1, Fig. 8.3). MIP images were able to depict calcification within the arterial wall. This alerts the surgeon to possible intraoperative risk, especially while clipping the aneurysm.

In subarachnoid hemorrhage (SAH) resulting from ruptured cerebral aneurysms, excellent visualization of the intracranial vasculature was obtained by ordinal image processing. The CT number of acute subarachnoid clots did not usually exceed 90 HU; thus there was no difficulty in demonstrating contrast-filling arteries and aneurysms surrounded with blood clots by elevating thresholds up to 150 HU in SSR images (Fig. 8.4).

8.3.2 Disadvantages of CTA

CTA has several definite limitations to date. First, overlap with the skull base bone can constitute a major problem, especially in the detection of infraclinoidal aneu

Table 1. Comparison of diagnostic usefulness between CTA and DSA, MRA (94 cases, 143 aneurysms)

Diameter of aneurysm	Diagnostic usefulness		
1–3 mm (44 aneurysms)	CTA > MRA	25/26	
	CTA = MRA	1/26	
	CTA > DSA	18/28	
	CTA = DSA	8/28	(false positive)
	CTA < DSA	2/28	(false positive, false negative)
4–11 mm (72 aneurysms)	CTA > MRA	30/36	
	CTA = MRA	6/36	
	CTA > DSA	12/48	
	CTA = DSA	33/48	
	CTA < DSA	3/48	
12–40 mm (24 aneurysms)	CTA > MRA	15/16	
	CTA = MRA	1/16	
	CTA > DSA	12/18	
	CTA = DSA	6/18	
Fusiform (3 aneurysms)	CTA > MRA	2	
	CTA = DSA	1	

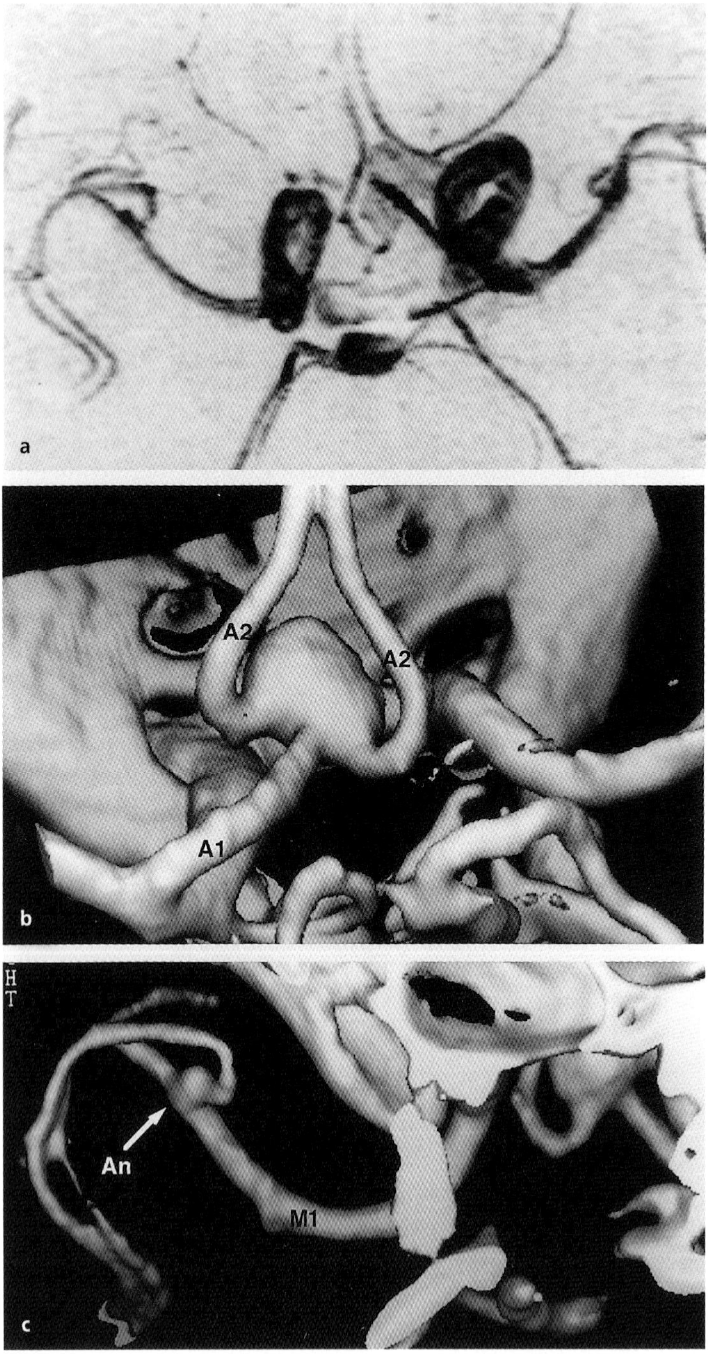

Fig. 8.2a–c. Multiple aneurysm [A com A (14 mm in diameter), MCA (2 mm in diameter)]. **a** MRA; **b** CTA (superoinferior view); **c** CTA (inferosuperior view)

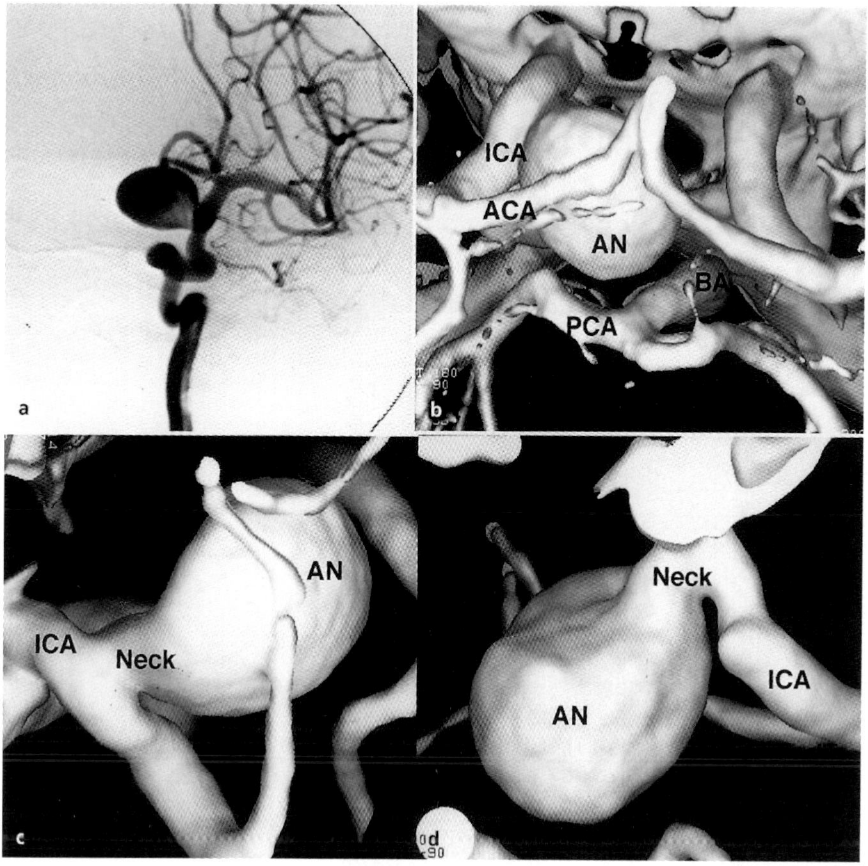

Fig. 8.3a–d. ICA ophthalmic artery aneurysm (17 mm in diameter).
a DSA; **b** CTA (superoinferior view); **c** target CTA (superoinferior view); **d** target CTA (inferosuperior view)

rysms. It is necessary during post-image processing to exclude the clinoidal processes, the lesser sphenoid wing, the clivus, and so on. These manipulations may be time-consuming. In such cases, however, CTA provides useful information concerning the anatomical relationship between the aneurysm and the bony structures, which can help surgical simulation for ICA and upper basilar trunk aneurysms. Early enhancement of the cavernous sinus can obscure the cavernous portion of the ICA, with the result that intracavernous aneurysms may be overlooked. As mentioned above, by means of both the large-dose infusion of contrast medium and elevation of the threshold over 250 HU in SSR images, aneurysms within or close to the cavernous sinus can be clearly visible (Fig. 8.5). Second, it is very hard to demonstrate the small vessels such as perforating arteries, hypoplastic posterior communicating arteries, and anterior choroidal arteries. Third, CTA

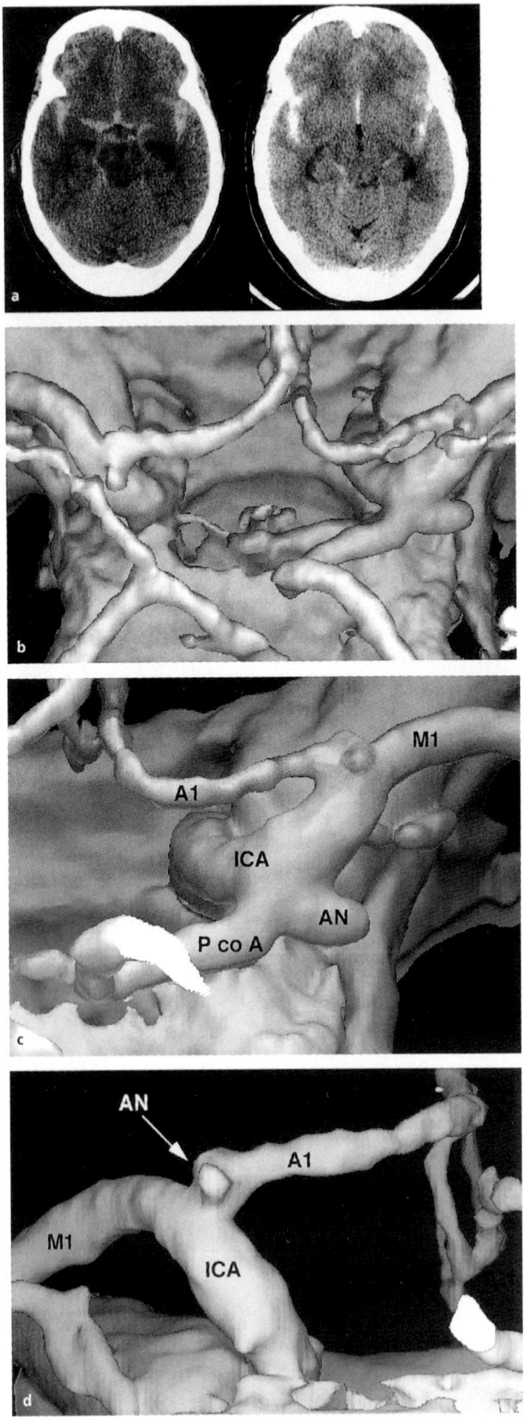

Fig. 8.4a–d. Multiple aneurysm [ruptured IC-CP (6 mm in diameter); unruptured ICA terminal (2 mm in diameter)]. **a** Plain CT; **b** CTA (superoinferior view); **c** target CTA (superoinferior view); **d** target CTA (posteroanterior view)

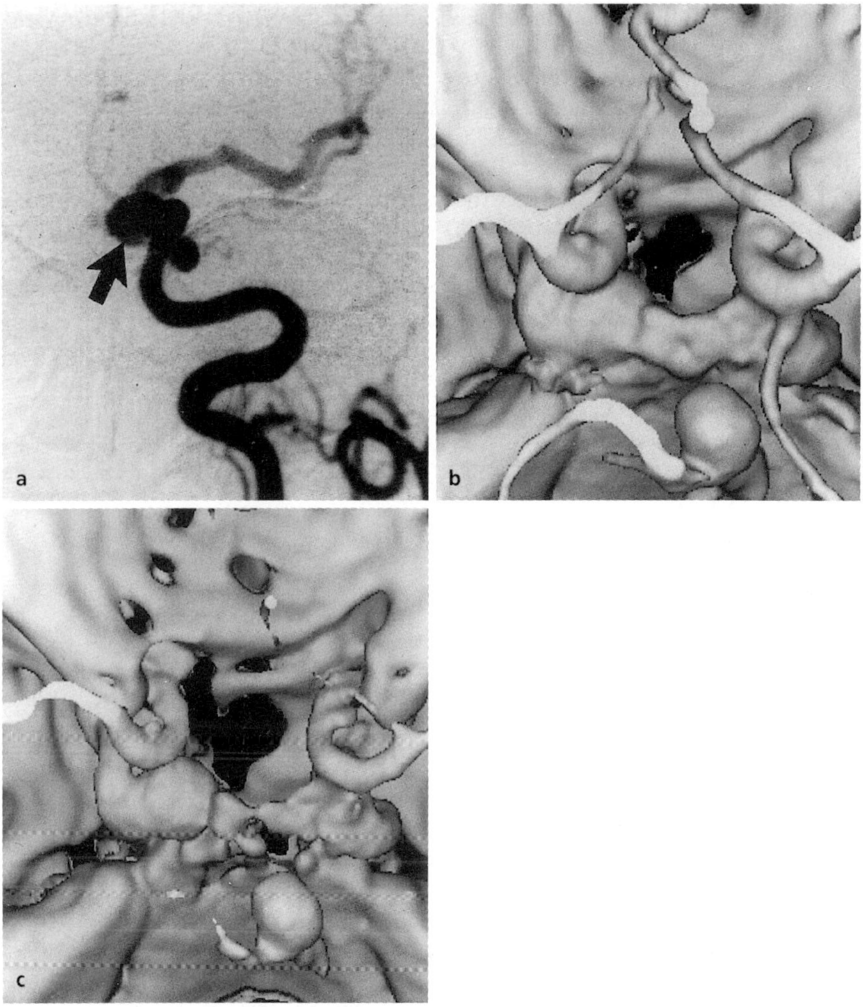

Fig. 8.5a–c. ICA cavernous aneurysm (15 mm in diameter).
a DSA; **b** CTA (SSR image at threshold level of 150 HU); **c** CTA (SSR image at threshold level of 250 HU)

fails to give information about the blood flow characteristics. The final and major disadvantages are the necessity for intravenous iodinated contrast medium and the possible side effects of irradiation.

8.4 Role of CTA in Surgical Planning: Is DSA Necessary?

Based on previous experiences and the definite advantages of CTA, we aimed to investigate the possibility of aneurysmal clipping after only referring to images obtained by CTA. Between January 1995 and August 1997, 42 cerebral aneurysms in 29 patients were diagnosed with CTA, including five patients (eight aneurysms) with SAH. Among these cases, 17 patients with 22 cerebral aneurysms underwent surgery; five of these aneurysms were located on the anterior communicating artery, 12 on the MCA, and five on the ICA. The majority of aneurysms were less than 11 mm in size. All aneurysms detected with CTA were proved under direct observation during surgery. In comparison with intraoperative findings, the exact size of the aneurysm, its shape, and the relationship of the parent artery and its branches to the aneurysmal sac were highly consistent with three-dimensional reconstruction CTA images.

For surgical planning, SSR images provide a good three-dimensional presentation of the aneurysmal lesion. In patients with aneurysms of the anterior communicating artery, information about the direction of the aneurysm, the distance from the planum sphenoidale, and its relationship with both A2 segments of the ACA and fenestrations of the anterior communicating artery were indispensable for direct clipping (Fig. 8.6). Anatomical relationships with M1 and M2 segments

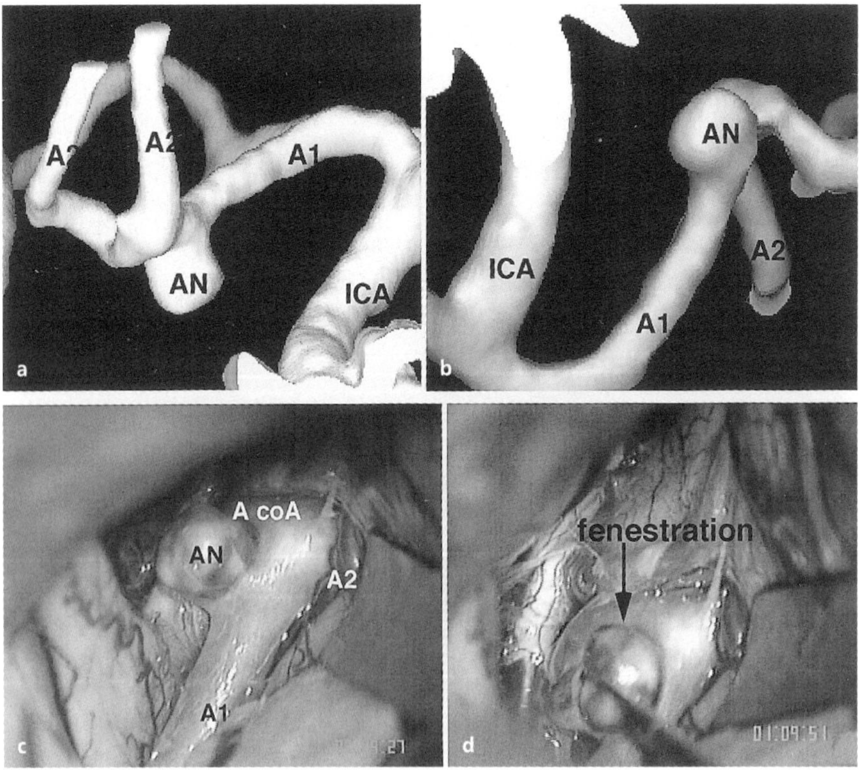

Fig. 8.6a–d. Anterior communicating artery aneurysm (5 mm in diameter). **a** CTA (anteroposterior view); **b** CTA (surgical simulation image); **c, d** operative findings

and the sylvian veins were easily understood for clipping of MCA aneurysms (Fig. 8.7). As mentioned before, SSR images facilitated anatomical understanding of surrounding bony structures near the ICA aneurysms.

During the same period, DSA was performed on 15 patients with 24 unruptured cerebral aneurysms for various reasons. Fifteen aneurysms were located on the ICA, one on the MCA, seven on the BA. and one on the VA. Nine of the 15 aneurysms were over 14 mm in diameter. One of the reasons why DSA was carried out was that the assessment of hemodynamics during the proximal occlusion was essential for direct clipping in ten cases (Fig. 8.8). Other reasons were routine inspection in three cases, coexistence with a petroclival meningioma in one case, and an inquiry into the presence of perforating arteries around the BA top aneurysm in one case.

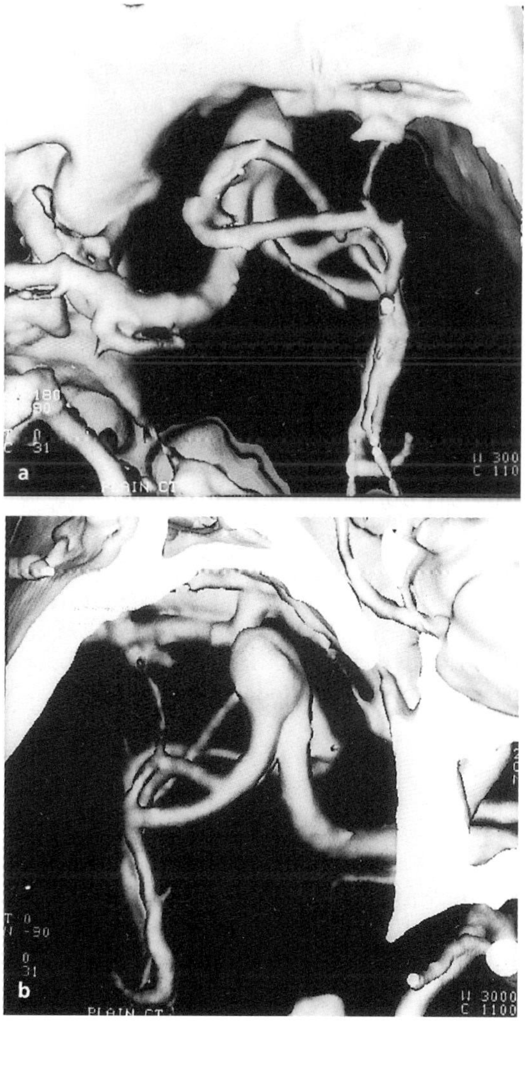

Fig. 8.7a, b. Middle cerebral artery aneurysm (8 mm in diameter). **a** CTA (superoinferior view); **b** CTA (inferosuperior view)

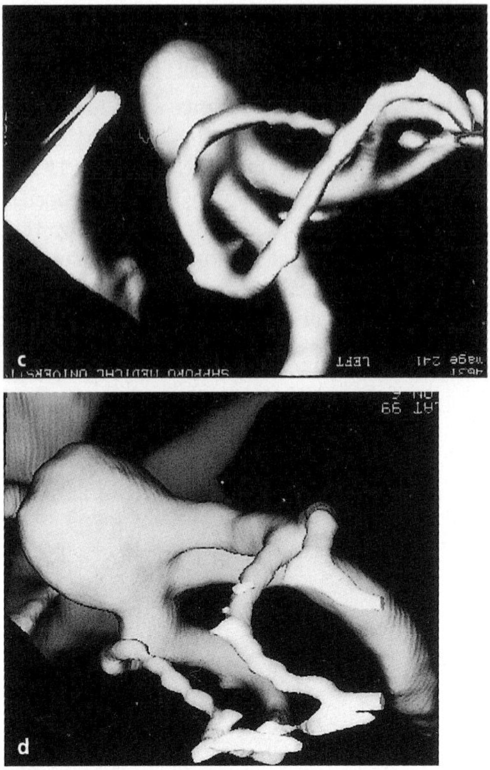

Fig. 8.7c, d. Middle cerebral artery aneurysm (8 mm in diameter). **c** target CTA (superoinferior view); **d** target CTA (inferosuperior view)

From these results, it seems clear that CTA will eventually be able to replace DSA in the assessment of selected patients with small and medium-sized aneurysms located on the anterior part of the circle of Willis. For the time being, however, in patients with large aneurysms more than 14 mm in size, DSA is indicated for hemodynamic evaluation, since intraoperative temporary occlusion of the parent artery is expected.

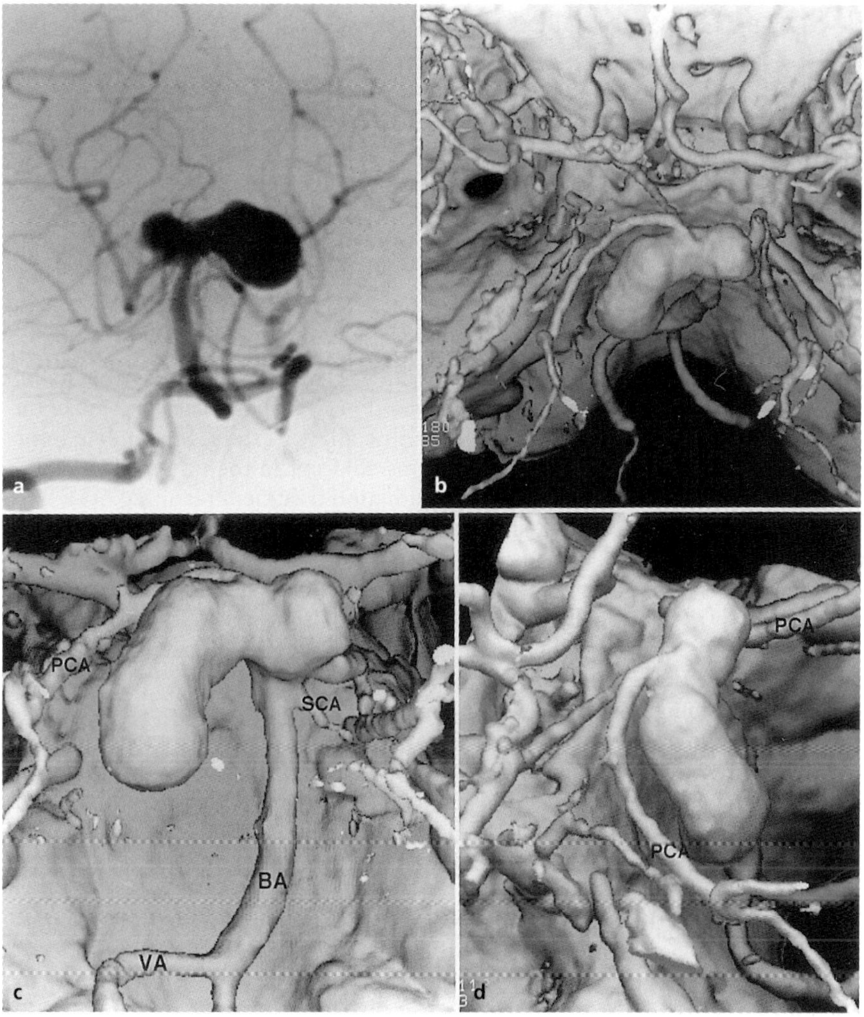

Fig. 8.8a–d. Giant thrombosed basilar artery aneurysms [BA-SCA (32 mm in diameter), BA top (11 mm in diameter)]. **a** DSA; **b** CTA (superoinferior view); **c** target CTA (posteroanterior view); **d** target CTA (superoinferior view)

9 Spiral CT vs. Subsecond Conventional CT in Head and Neck Malignancies

R. MAROLDI, G. BATTAGLIA, P. MACULOTTI, D. FARINA, F. CODAZZI, A. CHIESA

9.1 Introduction

Motion, respiration artifacts, and swallowing very often affect the image quality of conventional CT (CCT) studies of head and neck malignancies and make impossible to obtain a detailed assessment of neoplastic extent. Incomplete information about the involvement of structures adjacent to the tumor may lead to both inadequate resection and defective radiation treatment planning.

To avoid these artifacts the shortest possible scanning time is required. Because spiral CT (SCT) allows fast volumetric data acquisition, it should permit the imaging of even large areas with minimal artifacts due to reduced patient cooperation [1]. Additionally, 2D and 3D reconstructions can be calculated out of the data set, providing high-quality images [2, 3]. Moreover, reduced contrast material (CM) doses are required to obtain adequate or better vascular and tissue enhancement compared to CCT [4].

Previous studies demonstrated that CM can be used more efficiently on SCT of the lung and the abdomen. Because of its relative short scan duration the entire liver can be imaged during both the arterial and portal phases without scanning during the equilibrium phase of enhancement. As a result, improved depiction of hepatic lesions has been demonstrated when such biphasic SCT technique is used [5].

The purpose of this study was to prospectively compare SCT with CCT for assessing the local neoplastic extent of head and neck malignancies using a fast CT equipment (0.7-s scan time) and performing a dual-phase CT technique. This combined a very short delay between CM injection and SCT scanning with a CCT obtained immediately after SCT and a second CM injection.

9.2 Patients and Methods

Sixty-one patients suspected of laryngeal-hypopharyngeal ($n=38$), oro-nasopharyngeal ($n=15$), and neck ($n=8$) abnormalities underwent CT studies, using spiral and conventional techniques. There were 41 men and 20 women; ages ranged from 29 to 78 years (mean 51.1). The distribution of lesions is given in Table 9.1. All examinations were performed on a Somatom Plus 4 (Siemens, Erlangen, Germany). Each patient had two SCT studies, plain and contrast enhanced examinations. A CM volume of 80 ml (Optiray 320, Mallinckrodt Medical) was administered by a power injector at a flow rate of 3 ml/s. Time delay

Table 9.1. Distribution of lesions ($n=61$)

	Primary tumor	Recurrent tumor
Glottis	9	1
Supraglottis	20	2
Hypopharynx	6	0
Oropharynx	8	0
Nasopharynx	7	0
Lymph nodes	6	2

between starting of injection and start of spiral acquisition was 30 s. A CCT (scanning time 0.7 s, interscan duration 8 s) was obtained immediately after the enhanced SCT along with a second CM injection (40 ml, 1 ml/s). Both CCT and SCT studies were obtained using 3-mm section collimation and 2/3-mm increments (CCT). The SCT images were also reconstructed at the same increments.

The SCT and CCT images were compared by two observers who evaluated breath and motion artifacts and enhancement of vessels and of neoplastic tissue; agreement between the observers was obtained. Artifacts were rated assessing scores of 1–3, where 1 represented more than 3 degraded images, 2 less than 3 degraded images, and 3 no artifact at all on any image. Increase in density of vessels, neoplastic tissue, and neck muscles from plain to both enhanced SCT (DHU SCT) and CCT (DHU CCT) was measured.

Differences were assessed using standard parametric statistical techniques (average scores for each parameter in both techniques and densities were compared using a two-tailed *t* test, difference was considered significant when $p<0.05$).

9.3 Results

A summary of results comparing SCT and CCT studies is presented in Table 9.2. Both techniques allowed good to excellent visualization of the anatomy in the different areas of the neck. At any level of the neck SCT had less breath and motion artifacts than CCT, this difference being greater for the glottis (2.60 vs. 2.30), the supraglottis (2.59 vs. 2.36), and the oropharynx (2.62 vs. 2.37). However, although SCT was superior to CCT, in no anatomical area of the neck was the difference between the two average scores statistically significant.

Table 9.2. Breath and motion artifacts: SCT versus CCT ($n=61$)

	SCT	CCT
Glottis ($n=10$)	2.60 ± 0.69	2.30 ± 0.67
Supraglottis ($n=22$)	2.59 ± 0.59	2.36 ± 0.65
Hypopharynx ($n=6$)	2.83 ± 0.40	2.66 ± 0.51
Oropharynx ($n=8$)	2.62 ± 0.51	2.37 ± 0.74
Nasopharynx ($n=7$)	2.85 ± 0.37	2.71 ± 0.48
Lymph nodes ($n=8$)	2.75 ± 0.46	2.62 ± 0.51

Mean enhancement (absolute HU values) of neck vessels was 209.64 ± 13.68 at SCT and 119.37 ± 10.27 at CCT for common carotid/internal carotid arteries ($p < 0.001$), 196.57 ± 12.46 (SCT) and 111.77 ± 8.87 (CCT) for the internal jugular vein ($p < 0.001$).

The enhancement of neoplastic tissue differed significantly between SCT and CCT only for hypopharyngeal neoplasms (47.83 ± 11.26 vs. 20.5 ± 7.39, $p = 0.013$; Table 9.3). In all six piriform sinus lesions, intense and rather homogeneous enhancement was detected on SCT. On subsequent CCT the density of neoplastic tissue resulted remarkably lower. A thin hyperdense rim between tumor and adjacent normal tissue was present on CCT only (Fig. 9.1). In the subset of glottic and supraglottic laryngeal neoplasms the trend was the opposite, with enhancement being superior on CCT than on SCT in most cases (Fig. 9.2). The lowest

Table 9.3. Enhancement of tumor on SCT and CCT, compared to plain SCT, DHU SCT, and DHU CCT, increased density between plain SCT and enhanced SCT or CCT

	DHU SCT	DHU CCT	p
Glottis ($n = 10$)	21.4 ± 11.87	31.6 ± 13.38	NS
Supraglottis ($n = 22$)	30.18 ± 14.29	36.9 ± 15.45	NS
Hypopharynx ($n = 6$)	47.83 ± 11.26	20.5 ± 7.39	0.013
Oropharynx ($n = 8$)	28.62 ± 12.75	17.75 ± 7.04	N
Nasopharynx ($n = 7$)	11.57 ± 4.57	19 ± 6.68	NS
Lymph nodes ($n = 8$)	16.5 ± 10.98	19.62 ± 5.80	NS

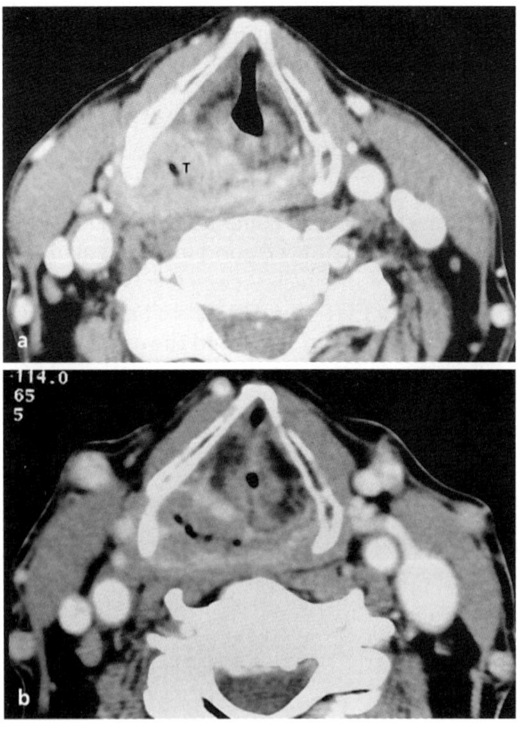

Fig. 9.1a, b. Carcinoma of the right piriform sinus, invading the thyroid cartilage. **a** SCT allows an excellent and prompt enhancement of the neoplasm (*T*). **b** On CCT the same lesion becomes hypodense. An hyperdense rim delineates the borders of the tumor

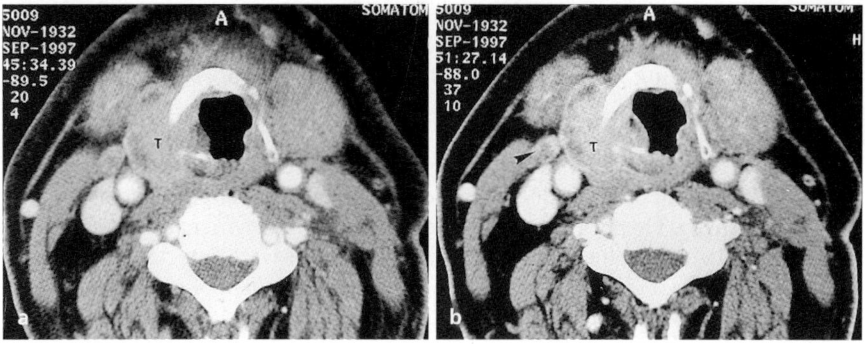

Fig. 9.2a, b. Recurrent supraglottic carcinoma after conservative surgery. **a** The submucosal lesion (*T*) shows mild enhancement on SCT. **b** It appears more hyperdense on CCT. The small lymph node (detected at level III, on the right side) demonstrates late peripheral rim enhancement (*arrowhead*)

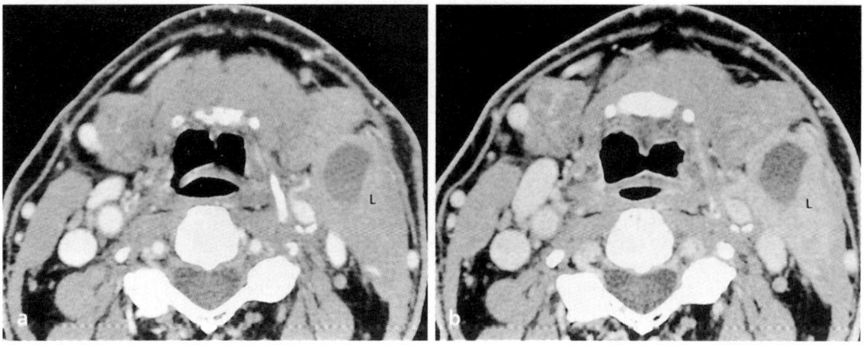

Fig. 9.3a, b. Partially necrotic laterocervical lymphadenopathy (level II–III). **a** On SCT the node (*L*), poorly enhanced, is not easily discriminated from the adjacent sterno cleidomastoid muscle. **b** CCT allows a more precise assessment of the lesion extent due to its late enhancement. Although the enhancement of neck vessels appears remarkably higher on SCT, the opacification of vessels on CCT results adequate

variations in tumor densities were observed among nasopharyngeal lesions (11.57±4.57 on SCT, 19±6.68 on CCT) and neck lymph nodes (16.5±10.98 on SCT, 19.62±5.8; Fig. 9.3). Mean enhancement of muscles was lower on SCT (5.75±2.65) than on CCT (9.12±4.08), the difference being statistically significant ($p=0.0281$).

9.4 Discussion

The results of this prospective study demonstrate an overall better image quality with SCT than with CCT. However, no abnormality was missed using CCT. These data are similar to those of Mukherji et al. [6] and Robert et al. [7] who demonstrated that anatomical information provided by SCT studies is at least equal to if not better than that from CCT. In selected lesions quiet respiration scans allowed the adequate imaging of true vocal cords and anterior and posterior commissure on CCT.

An accurate assessment of the extent of tumor is required to plan the proper treatment in head and neck malignancies. In most cases the neoplasm can be distinguished by mean of both morphological changes (mass effect, distortion) and abnormal density. Therefore notable differences of enhancement between lesions and normal tissue are effective. In this study all lesions were detected by SCT and CCT. Additionally, no significant difference in the assessment of neoplastic extent was observed between the two techniques.

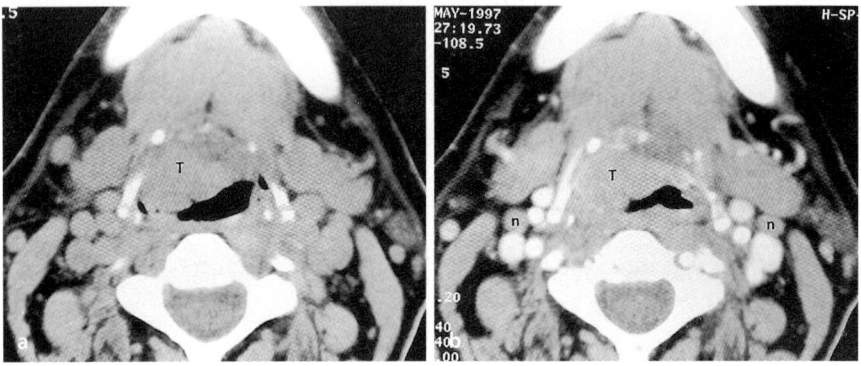

Fig. 9.4a, b. Carcinoma of the base of the tongue. **a** On plain study the lesion (*T*) results isodense to adjacent muscles. **b** After CM injection a moderate homogeneous enhancement is obtained on SCT. Small level II nodes (*n*) are easily discriminated from hyperdense surrounding neck vessels

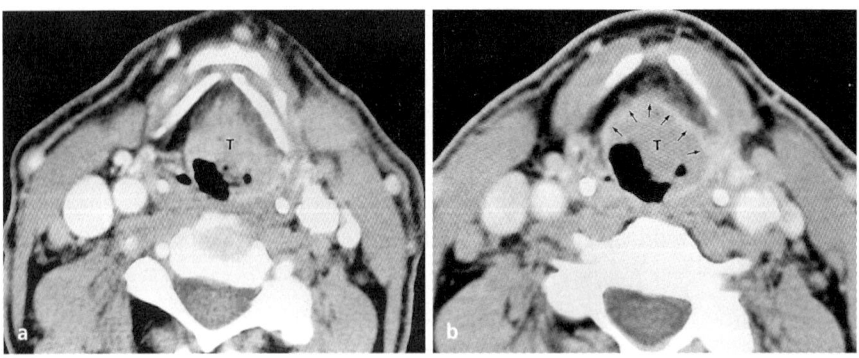

Fig. 9.5a, b. Supraglottic carcinoma arising from the infrahyoid epiglottis. **a** The neoplasm (*T*) shows a moderate and homogeneous enhancement on SCT. **b** On CCT the same lesion appears relatively hypodense, with a peripheral hyperdense rim (*arrows*). Excellent to adequate opacification of common carotid arteries and internal jugular vein can be appreciated on both SCT and CCT

The results of the investigation show that all the hypopharyngeal tumors examined (6/6), some of the oropharyngeal (2/8; Fig. 9.4), supraglottic (4/22; Fig. 9.5), and one glottic neoplasm present a prompt and fast disappearing enhancement, ranging from 37 to 69 HU (average 47.83) during SCT. On subsequent CCT the density of these tumors quickly declined. All the remaining neoplasms presented an opposite pattern, with densities being higher on CCT studies. These data suggest that squamous cell carcinomas arising from a very restricted area made up of pharynx and adjacent mucosa of the supraglottic larynx can exhibit a very similar pattern of tissue enhancement.

Previous studies compared SCT and CCT examinations of the neck. Patterns of the enhancement of normal cervical structures (vessels, muscles) have been reported using a dual phase technique with two boluses of 50 ml CM, flow rates not exceeding 2 ml/s and a long delay (more than 3 min) [4, 8]. The results of the current study show that a lower dose (80 ml) of CM, delivered at 3 ml/s, and a shorter delay (30 s) provide an excellent opacification of neck vessels in all cases. The absolute HU values measured for carotid arteries and jugular vein are superior to those obtained by other investigators [4]. Nevertheless, SCT did not provide a superior enhancement of neoplastic tissues or muscles in comparison to CCT, except for hypopharyngeal tumors.

In conclusion, both SCT and CCT can be used to perform high-quality image examinations of head and neck malignancies. In the current study CCT images provided by a very fast subsecond equipment (0.7 s) resulted more adequate than a short delayed SCT in achieving tumor enhancement.

References

1. Suojanen JN, Mukherji SK, Wippold FJ (1994) Spiral CT of the larynx. AJNR Am J Neurorad 15 (8): 1579–82
2. Silvermann PM, Zeiberg AS, Sessions RB, Troost TR, Zeman RK (1995) Three-dimensional imaging of the hypopharynx and larynx by means of helical (spiral) computed tomography. Comparison of radiological and otolaryngological evaluation. Ann Otol Rhinol Laryngol 104 (6): 425–431
3. Hermans R, Marchal G, Baert AL (1995) Toepassingen van spiraal-CT in het hoofd- en halsgebied. J Belge Radiol 78 (2): 79–82
4. Spreer J, Krahe T, Jung G, Lackner K (1995) Spiral versus conventional CT in routine examinations of the neck. J Comput Assist Tomogr 19 (6): 905–910
5. Heiken JP, Bae AT (1997) Liver: CT contrast-enhancement techniques. RSNA categorical course in diagnostic radiology. Gastrointestinol 9163–170
6. Mukherji SK, Castillo M, Huda W, Suojanen J, Kubilis P, Tart RP, Dhillon G (1995) Comparison of dynamic and spiral CT for imaging the glottic larynx. J Comput Assist Tomogr 19 (6): 899–904
7. Robert Y, Rocourt N, Chevalier D, Duhamel A, Carcasset S, Lemaitre L (1996) Helical CT of the larynx: a comparative study with conventional scan. Clin Radiol 51: 882–885
8. Ehritt-Braun C, Ferstl F, Brehm A, Krause W, Langer M (1994) Optimierung der intravenosen Kontrastmittelbolusinjektion in der zervikalen CT diagnostik. Aktuelle Radiol 4 (5): 222–224

10 Spiral CT in Maxillofacial Trauma

C. H. BUITRAGO-TÉLLEZ, M. BOHNERT, M. KIMMIG, K. H. ALLMANN,
N.-C. GELLRICH, M. LANGER

10.1
Introduction

The development of spiral computed tomography (CT) has been a major advance in the radiological evaluation of patients suffering maxillofacial injuries in the acute setting. Because of the high-speed data acquisition of current CT scanners, detailed information about most facial bone areas may be obtained in a very short period of time, i.e., about 40–60 s.

From a clinical standpoint this is extremely important. With this reduction in examination time, polytraumatized patients with clinical signs of maxillofacial injuries may be scanned immediately after the standard CT head examination, thus defining the severity of the lesions and the timing of a necessary surgical approach. This is especially important in cases of orbital fractures, when a surgical decompression may be indicated to prevent irreversible optic nerve damage.

We present here a succint review of practical technical and clinical aspects concerning spiral CT in the evaluation of the patient with a maxillofacial trauma.

10.2
Technical and Clinical Correlation

Spiral CT differs from conventional CT in that the examined anatomical region of interest, as in this case the maxillofacial complex, can be imaged via rapid continuous scanning and patient transport. Initially some concern about image quality was discussed, taking into account the widening of section sensitivity profiles due to transport during scanning [11]. However, experimental [14] and clinical [17] studies confirmed similar diagnostic image quality using appropriate parameters. In this context, the use of narrow-width slice thickness with a collimation of 2–3 mm, a minimal table incrementation of 3 mm/s or less and a high-order interpolation algorithm seems to be essential to evaluate the partly very thin osseous structures of the maxillofacial region [14]. Concerning specific scanning parameters there are still some controversy in literature.

Some authors [14, 17] still consider spiral CT scans with 2-mm slice thickness, 3-mm table feed, and 1-mm increment as adequate for the evaluation of the craniofacial region. This approach is certainly useful in the evaluation of patients with associated facial and mandibular fractures. However, if there are no clinical signs of mandibular trauma and an adequate evaluation of visual impairment is not possible, as in unconcious patients, a transaxial approach using 1-mm slice thickness, 2-mm table feed, and 1-mm increment should be preferred (see Ta-

Table 10.1. Examination protocol in the evaluation of midfacial fractures in the acute setting

Examination technique	Primary axial scanning (compare region of interest as shown in the figure)
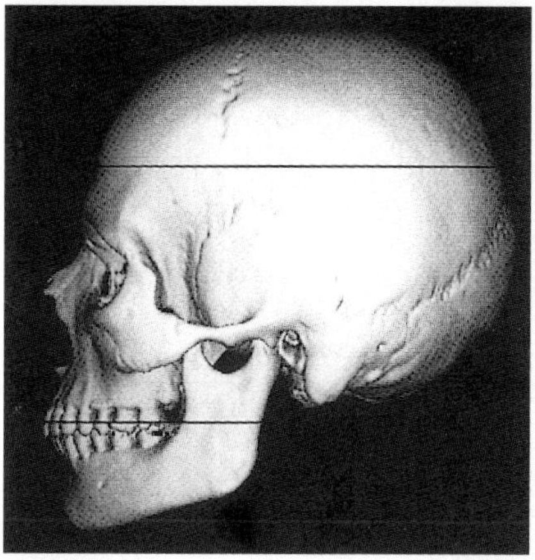	Spiral CT: Imaging parameters Slice thickness 1 (2) mm Table feed 2 (3) mm Increment 1 mm Standard: Coronal 2D-reconstructions Optional: 3D-CT reconstructions: panfacial fractures

ble 10.1). As Luka et al. [12] underlined in a clinical study including 314 patients, all dislocated fractures of the orbital floor or herniations of extraocular muscles are reliably identified using this narrow-width approach. Coronal reconstructions are mandatory in this setting beginning at the level of the clivus up to the nasal region. The increment of 1 mm is necessary to enhance longitudinal resolution. This approach also facilitates the diagnosis of orbital apex fractures with accurate delineation of fracture lines involving the optic nerve canal and surrounding regions (Fig. 10.1). Furthermore, current scanners, as the Somatom Plus 4 (Siemens, Erlangen, Germany) used in our institution, allow the examination of the entire midface including the skull base in a single spiral CT image acquisition (up to 60–70 s) depending on rotation time and mAs value.

Perhaps the most relevant clinical improvement in spiral CT data acquisition is its capability to generate high quality two-dimensional (2D) multiplanar reformatted reconstructions (MPR) as well as three-dimensional (3D) images.

3D reconstructions of the spiral CT data set may be obtained using two basic different techniques: the surface rendering and the volumen rendering technique. The surface rendering technique relies on the definition of a threshold value to eliminate voxels above or below the threshold [10]. A typical treshold value to evaluate the facial skeleton lies between 140 and 200 HU (Figs. 10.1b, Fig. 10.2). A standard reconstruction algorithm of the primary axial CT data should be preferred (Kernel AH 10–50). Illumination by virtual light sources as well as cutting overlying structures are useful processing tools.

The basic characteristic of the surface rendering technique is the need to isolate/segmentate the structure to be imaged from the data volume. On the other hand, a volumen-rendering technique does not require segmentation because it is based on projecting a data volume onto an image plane while assigning different optical transparencies or colors to different tissues [9]. Moreover, a volumen-rendering technique allows a real-time 3D visualization of the whole data volume, thus enabling a virtual endoscopy of such structures as the optic canal or the orbital region (Fig. 10.1c–e).

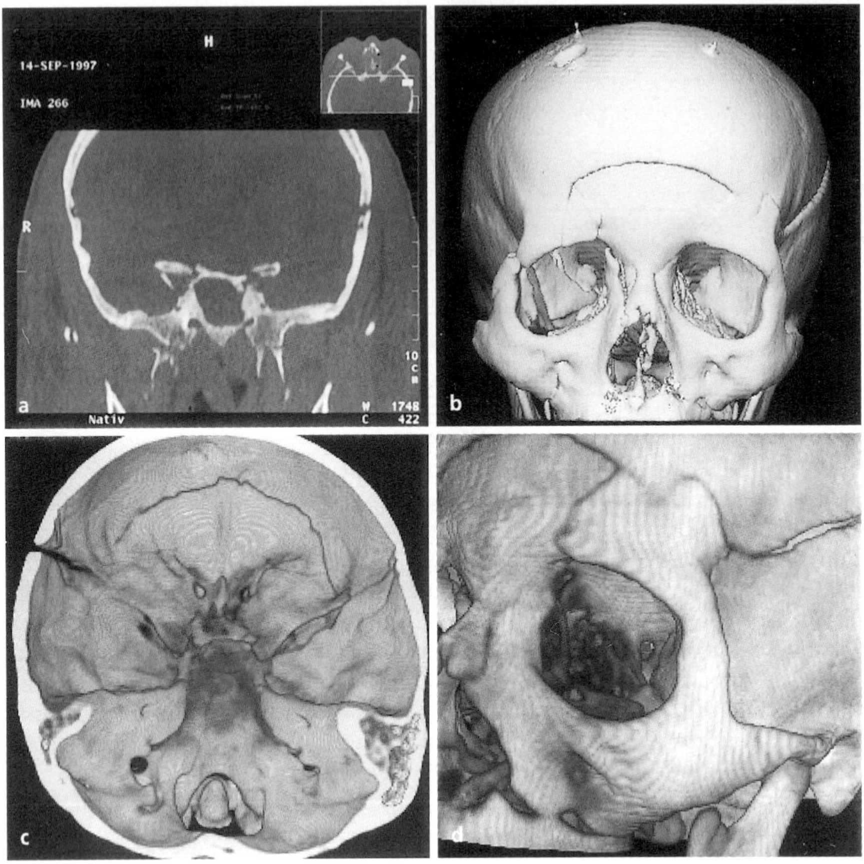

Fig. 10.1a–f. Severe craniofacial trauma. **a** Secondary 2D coronal reconstruction based on a spiral CT data set (1 × 2 × 1 mm). Note the transfacial fracture with bilateral fracture of both pterygoid processes. Note also the angulation of the fractured roof of the sphenoidal sinus. **b** Frontal 3D CT view with a surface rendering technique (threshold: 150 HU). Note complex panfacial fracture including a displaced tripod fracture as well as a heminasoethmoidal fracture on the right, an impression fracture of the frontal skull, a low maxillary fracture at the Lefort level I on the left as well as a frontoparietal calotte fracture. **c** Cranial 3D CT view using a volumen-rendering technique. Note multiple fracture lines through the frontobasis. **d** Virtual endoscopy of the orbital region based on the volumen rendering technique. Initial localization of the optic canal. **e** Fly through the optic canal shows a bone fragment partially occluding the endocranial margins of the canal. **f** Authopsy findings. One week later the patient died because of severe intracranial bleeding. Autopsy confirmed the avulsion of a fragment of the roof of the sphenoidal sinus with direct lesion of the optic nerve on the left

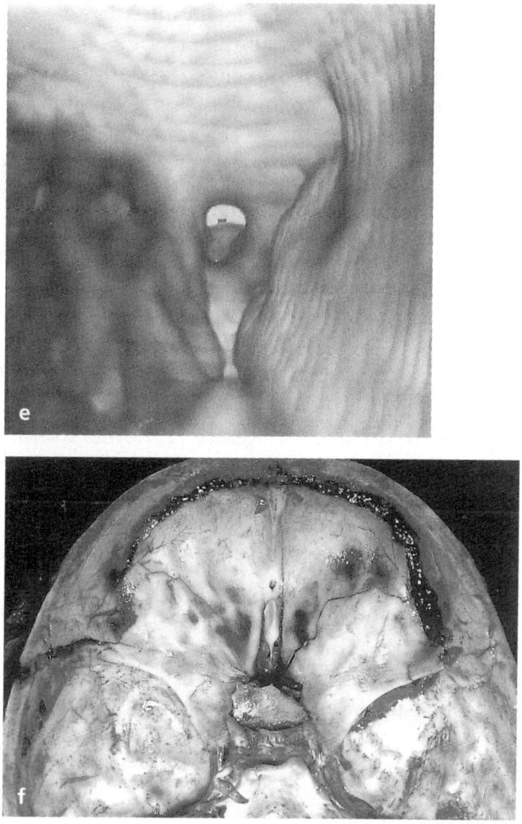

10.3 Clinical Relevance

Complex maxillofacial trauma repair requires precise surgical technique with little margin for error. The general objectives of imaging studies are therefore to define precisely the therapeutically relevant anatomical regions involved, to describe the degree of comminution or displacement of fragments, to detect osseous defects requiring bone grafts, and to allow an analysis of facial asymmetry. As Manson et al. [13] have emphasized, CT is especially accurate in defining the pattern of comminution of maxillofacial fractures [13]. Moreover, Hemmy [8] commented on the report of Manson that the appreciation of facial fractures and the devising of a correct surgical solution require a 3D comprehension.

The refinement in the technique of radiological assessment of maxillofacial fractures is achieved by spiral CT. Spiral CT allows the examination of a polytraumatized patient with associated maxillofacial injuries in a very short period of time and with the capabilities of high-quality 2D and 3D image reconstructions.

Concerning the clinical relevance of 2D MPR, there is consensus about its value in the diagnosis of orbital fractures, especially involving the orbital floor and roof. Coronal, as well as oblique reconstructions along the optic nerve are mandatory [1, 12]. Condylar fractures, luxations, and subluxations are also well detected by coronal and sagittal 2D reconstructions. Isolated evaluation of 2D MPR reconstructions are less effective than axial CT images obtained from a spiral CT data set to evaluate complex maxillofacial fractures, as demonstrated by Fox et al. [7].

Although no randomized studies have compared direct coronal CT studies with secondary 2D coronal reconstruction for the evaluation of orbital floor fractures, there is clinical evidence [12] of its usefulness using the narrow-width approach ($1\times2\times1$ mm). Moreover, metal artifacts resulting from crowns, bridges, and metal fillings do not compromise diagnostic image quality of the orbital floor, as often occurs in direct coronal CT. Another practical point is the inability of polytraumatized patients to be examined in prone position.

Concerning the clinical relevance of high-quality 3D reconstructions there is still some controversy [1–5, 7, 12, 15]. After the publication of the first 3D reconstructions based on spiral CT data [6] several research groups addressed this question. Disadvantages of 3D CT reconstructions using the surface rendering technique include their inability to display nondisplaced fractures and the presence of pseudoforamina in the thin lamellar bones of the medial orbital wall, floor, and roof as well as in the walls of the maxillary sinuses [1]. However, 3D CT allows an accurate evaluation of rotated fractured fragments [1], complex fractures involving multiple planes [7], asymmetries of the whole face and skull, large defects of the midface, skull vault and fractures with major dislocation [5], and condylar fractures/luxations [2].

Moreover, a standardization of 3D CT projections for mandibular and temporomandibular disorders, including trauma [2], and in the setting of maxillofacial trauma [3] has been proposed to enhance the reproducibility of 3D CT examinations for inter- and intraindividual comparison.

3D CT reconstructions are also recommended in the preoperative assessment of panfacial fractures to help the maxillofacial surgeon conceptualize the overall injury [15] and the involvement of facial buttresses (Fig. 10.2).

Finally, both 3D CT reconstructions and spiral CT datasets are the basis for producing life-size 3D stereolithographic models for preoperative planning, especially in the setting of posttraumatic deformities or osseous defects [4, 16].

3D laser stereolithography is an additive process building objects through layer-by-layer polymerization of a photosensitive resin. Combining an imaging technology such as CT with rapid prototyping technology such as laser stereolithography allows the generation of 3D hard copies of the cranium for preoperative planning. In addition, virtual-reality prosthesis design enables an exact implant design in cases of severe osseous loss. There is also the possibility of using computer-aided manufacturing to prepare artificial bone – hydroxyapatite – or

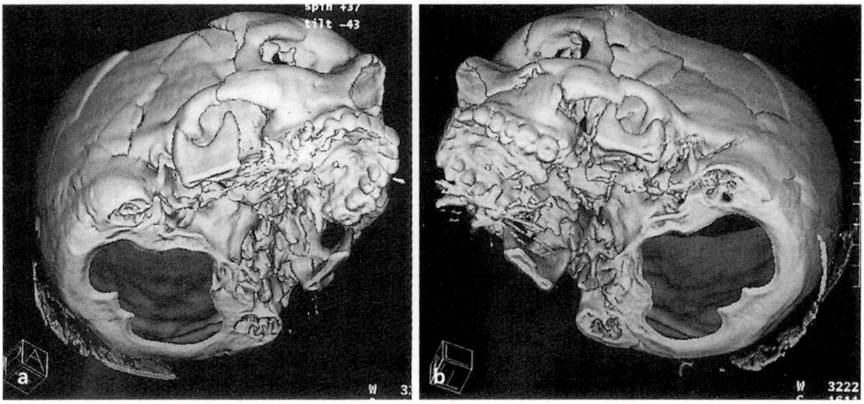

Fig. 10.2a, b. Complex craniofacial fracture after an accident in the forest. **a** Oblique 3D CT view (surface rendering technique) from the right demonstrating an isolated displacement of the zygomatico-temporal component of the zygomatic buttress. Note multiple calotte fractures. **b** Oblique 3D CT view from the left. Note displaced fractures involving the zygomatico-temporal, zygomatico-maxillary, and zygomatico-frontal components of the zygomatic buttress. Note also the fractures of the paranasal and pterygo-maxillary buttresses

titan prostheses. The advantages of those prostheses are a reduction in operation time and a decreased risk of infection secondary to reduction of dead space in the interface prostheses-bone [4].

10.4 Conclusions and Perspectives

Spiral CT represents a major advantage in examining the polytraumatized patient with associated maxillofacial injury due to its reduction of examination time and capabilities of narrow-width transaxial imaging. High-quality 2D multiplanar reconstructions, especially in the coronal plane, allow a diagnostic evaluation of orbital structures using an examination technique with thin slices.

3D CT reconstructions based on a spiral-CT data set are further indicated in the presence of panfacial fractures, rotated fractured fragments, large asymmetries or osseous defects of the midface, complex condylar injuries and posttraumatic deformities. Spiral CT scan data represent an optimal basis for 3D stereolithographic models in cases of posttraumatic deformities or osseous defects.

The 3D volumen-rendering technique based on axial spiral CT data with narrow-width approach allows a real-time evaluation of complex maxillofacial fractures with the capabilities of a virtual endoscopy of the orbital region, especially evaluating the osseous margins of the optic canal. This may play a role in the preoperative planning of endoscopic orbital decompression procedures.

Spiral CT data obtained with special designed reference markers allow the clinical use of navigation systems in surgical procedures involving the maxillofacial complex.

References

1. Buitrago-Téllez CH, Wächter R, Ferstl F, Stoll P, Düker J, Langer M (1994) 3D-CT zur Befunddemonstration bei komplexen Gesichtsschädelverletzungen. Fortschr Rontgenstr 160: 106–112
2. Buitrago-Téllez CH, Wächter R, Ferstl F, Stoll P, Langer M (1994) Mandibular and temporomandibular joint pathology: standard approach with the Somatom Plus 3-D CT software programm. In: Pokieser H, Lechner G (eds) Advances in CT III. Springer, Berlin Heidelberg New York, pp 183–192
3. Buitrago-Téllez CH, Wächter R, Gufler H, Beschnidt M, Stoll P, Langer M (1996) Reproducible 3D-CT of the maxillofacial complex for preoperative planning. In: Lemke HU et al (eds) Computer assisted radiology CAR '96. Elsevier Science, Amsterdam, pp 975–980
4. Buitrago-Téllez CH, Zollikofer CPE, Cantini J. L, Gufler H, Kimmig M, Stoll P, Langer M, Matter P (1997) Preoperative planning of complex craniofacial fractures. AO-Dialogue 10:18–19
5. Carls FR, Schuknecht B, Sailer HF (1994) Value of three-dimensional computed tomography in craniomaxillofacial surgery. J Craniofac Surg 4:282–288
6. Fox LA (1993) Three-dimensional CT diagnosis of maxillofacial trauma. N Engl J Med 329: 102
7. Fox LA, Vannier MW, West OC, Wilson AJ, Baran GA, Pilgram TK (1995) Diagnostic performance of CT, MPR and 3DCT imaging in maxillofacial trauma. Comput Med Imag Graphics 19:385–395
8. Hemmy DC (1990) Discussion of "Toward CT-based facial fracture treatment" by P. Manson et al. Plast Reconstr Surg 85:213–214
9. Hemmy DC, Zonneveld, Lobregt S, Fukuta K (1994) A decade of clinical three-dimensional imaging: a review. I. Historical development. Invest Radiol 29:489–496
10. Herman GT (1988) Three-dimensional imaging on a CT or MR scanner. JCAT 12:450–458
11. Kalender WA, Seissler W, Klotz E, Vock P (1990) Spiral volumetric CT with single-breathhold technique, continuous transport, and continuous scanner rotation. Radiology 176: 181–183
12. Luka B, Brechtelsbauer D, Gellrich N, König M (1995) 2D and 3D CT reconstructions of the facial skeleton: an unnecessary option or a diagnostic pearl? Int J Oral Maxillofac Surg 24: 76–83
13. Manson P, Markowitz P, Mirvis S, Dunham M, Yaremchuk M (1990) Toward CT-based facial fracture treatment. Plast Reconstr Surg 85:202–212
14. McEnery KW, Wilson AJ, Murphy WA Jr (1994) Comparison of spiral computed tomography versus conventional computed tomography multiplanar reconstructions of a fracture displacement phantom. Invest Radiol 29:665–670
15. Moritz M, Niederdellmann H, Held P, Feuerbach S (1994) Indications et pertinence de la tomodensitometrie 3D lors de fractures panfaciales. Acta Stomatol Belgica 91:163–168
16. Ono I, Gunji H, Suda K, Kaneko F (1994) Method for preparing an exact-size model using helical volumen scan computed tomography. Plast Reconstr Surg 93:1363–1371
17. Tello R, Suojanen J, Costello P, McGinnes A (1994) Comparison of spiral CT and conventional CT in 3D visualisation of facial trauma: work in progress. Comput Med Imag & Graphics 18:423–427

Part III
Chest

Moderators: E. K. Fishman, M. Reiser

11 Optimizing CT Angiography of the Chest

C. M. SCHAEFER-PROKOP, M. PROKOP, C. ENGELKE, M. GALANSKI

11.1 Introduction

Computed tomography angiography (CTA) is a well-established minimally invasive tool for imaging of the aorta and the supra-aortic side branches as well as the pulmonary vasculature. Thoracic applications of CTA were suggested very early on [5, 9, 13]. Several publications document that CTA can yield excellent results, both for aortic disease and the diagnosis of pulmonary embolism [8, 15]. Since the various types of pathology place varying demands on spatial and contrast resolution, the examination technique has to be adapted accordingly.

We will discuss the most important factors that influence image quality and give suggestions for examination techniques with the Somatom Plus 4A. We will suggest how classical problems such as streak artifacts in the brachiocephalic veins or pulsation effects in the ascending aorta can be reduced, and how the faster tube rotation can be used to improve spatial resolution, to improve vascular contrast, or reduce the total amount of contrast agent.

11.2 Imaging Technique

With respect to imaging techniques, we distinguish three major groups of examinations:

1. Examinations that place few demands on technique, such as the evaluation of aneurysms of the ascending aorta.
2. Scans that place moderate demands on spatial resolution but high demands on intravascular contrast, since various types of three-dimensional displays may be required. This group includes more complex types of aortic disease, especially disease that might involve the aortic arch.
3. Evaluation of the central pulmonary arteries, mainly for acute and chronic pulmonary thrombembolism.

Since there is a multitude of variable parameters that determine the spiral scan and reconstruction and the mode of contrast application, it is important to provide a simple and intuitive way to describe them. In clinical routine practice, we have found the abbreviations given in Table 11.1 most helpful for defining examination protocols. Since these abbreviations contain the most relevant parameters that influence image quality in a spiral scan, this mode of description allows for a fast and individualized prescription of examination protocols. Table 11.1

Table 11.1. Scan parameters

Spiral scan	SC/TF/RI	Contrast injection	V/F/DX
Precontrast scan (r/o bleeding)	7/12/6	↑	–
Protocol A: low technical requirements			
Aorta (e.g., ascending aortic aneurysm)	7/12/6	↑	50 + 50/2/10P
Protocol B: three dimensional visualization			
Aorta (e.g. aneurysm of aortic arch)	3/5/2	↑	120 + 60/4/5A
Aorta (complex pathology, femoral injection)	3/5/2	↓	120 + 60/4/5A
Aortic arch and supra-aortic arteries (40–60 s)	2/4/2	↑	150 + 40/4/5RV
Protocol C: pulmonary vasculature			
Pulmonary embolism	2/4/2	↑	120 + 60/4/5RV

Contrast concentration, 300 mg iodine/ml.
SC, slice collimation (mm); TF, table feed (mm per tube rotation); RI, reconstruction increment (mm); ↑↓, scan direction (caudocranial/craniocaudal), 30-s breathhold phase; V, contrast volume (ml); F, flow rate (ml/s); D, start delay (s); X, region of interest (ROI) for bolus triggering; P, pulmonary artery; A, ascending aorta; RV, right ventricle).

summarizes the scan parameters that we suggest for the three imaging tasks defined above.

11.2.1 Slice Collimation and Pitch Factor

Depending on the imaging task, the scan protocol has to be adapted to the required spatial resolution along the *z*-axis. For simple aneurysms of the ascending aorta, the *z*-axis resolution is not a critical factor, since the structures of interest are large and can be adequately displayed independent of slice thickness and vascular contrast. The spatial resolution along the *z*-axis should be higher for patients with aortic dissection or complex aortic anatomy, especially in the region of the aortic arch and the supra-aortic vessels. The highest *z*-axis resolution is necessary for the display of peripheral pulmonary vessels whenever pulmonary embolism needs to be be ruled out. The higher the *z*-axis resolution, the more subsegmental vessels can be evaluated even if they run parallel or oblique relative to the scan plane [11].

For maximum spatial resolution, small collimation and large pitch factors are best suited. In general, pitch factors greater than 1.5 should be used [12].

11.2.2 Raw Data Interpolation

The "slim2" raw data interpolation is preferable to the "slim" interpolation, since spatial resolution along the *z*-axis is similar and noise is reduced by 23% (see Chap. 3, this volume). "Wide" may be helpful to decrease pulsation in the ascending aorta [2].

11.2.3 Reconstruction Increment

For simple imaging tasks, reconstruction increment (RI) is not a limiting factor. However, whenever three-dimensional image displays are considered, highly overlapping reconstruction is advisable. RI of 1–3 mm will optimize spatial resolution along the *z*-axis [3].

11.2.4 Scan Length and Scan Time

Total scan time (TI) is generally limited by the breathhold period. Given proper instruction prior to the spiral scan, most patients will tolerate a 30-s breathhold. In those patients who are not able to hold their breath for more than 15 s, quiet respiration should be preferred to attempting a breathhold examination, as sudden inspiratory movements cause major artifacts if the patients starts to breathe too early.

TI and scan length (L) are directly related to the maximum possible spatial resolution along the *z*-axis: The table speed (TS, table feed per s) is determined by the following equation:

$$TS = L/TI \tag{1}$$

The table feed (TF, per rotation) can be calculated from Eq. 1 using the rotation time (RT) per tube revolution according to the following equation:

$$TF = TS/RT = L/(TI \times RT) \tag{2}$$

Since table feed and spatial resolution along the *z*-axis are closely linked, it is obvious that a shorter scan length will allow for a higher resolution along the *z*-axis.

Whenever a high spatial resolution along the *z*-axis is necessary, the scan length should be kept as small as possible. For three-dimensional imaging of the thoracic aorta, it is therefore advisable to perform a low-resolution precontrast scan (see Table 11.1) in order to determine the scan length. Usually, the portion of the descending aorta that lies immediately above the diaphragmatic hiatus may be excluded from the scan volume: rapid changes of the aortic width are a rarity, and dissecting membranes continuously pass through this region without demonstrating sudden changes in pathology. For most examinations of the thoracic aorta, it will be therefore sufficient to start the scan just below the aortic root and end well above the aortic arch.

For examinations of the pulmonary vasculature, the scan may start just above the diaphragm and end immediately above the aortic arch [9]. This is reasonable, since visualization of small pulmonary arteries is limited by partial volume effects that are most prominent for the periphery of the lungs.

11.2.5 Subsecond Scanning

With the Somatom Plus A, one should take advantage of the 0.75-subsecond rotation of the tube detector system (see Eq. 2). This allows for 40 rotations within the usual breath hold period of 30 s.

As compared to scanners with a tube rotation time of 1 s, the scan duration may be reduced by 25% (instead of 30 s breathhold time only 23 s) to cover a certain scan volume or to increase the scan length by 25% within the same breathhold time (e.g., 20 cm instead of 15 cm). The latter effect can be used to routinely include the whole chest in a CTA scan protocol with 3-mm slice collimation and 5–6 mm table feed.

Faster data acquisition has the additional advantage of reducing the acquisition time for a single image. As a result, diastolic images suffer less from pulsation than with a rotation time of 1 s, even at higher heart rates (Fig. 11.1).

11.2.6 Scan Direction

Scan direction may have a major impact on the quality of CTA of the chest. Since problems with breathholding occur most frequently at the end of a scan, diaphragmatic movements produce major motion artifacts if a craniocaudal scan

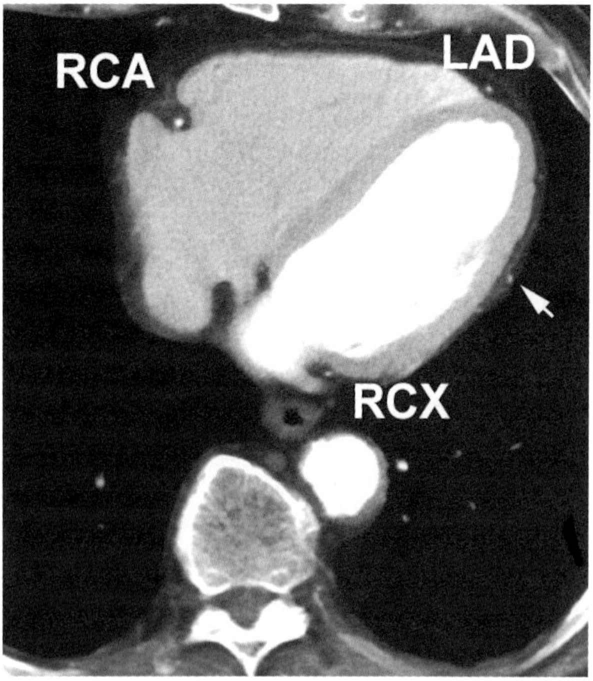

Fig. 11.1. Subsecond scanning reduces the amount of pulsation artifacts in the diastolic phase. In this patient, the various coronary branches can be distinguished: right coronary artery (*RCA*), left anterior descending (*LAD*), and circumflex branch (*RCX*) as well as diagonal branch (*arrow*) of the left coronary artery

direction is employed. In order to ensure the least amount of motion artifacts, scans should generally be performed in a caudocranial direction. This approach also reduces the amount of streak artifacts due to inflow of high concentrations of contrast medium in the brachiocephalic veins or the superior vena cava (Fig. 11.2). Due to washout effects, the contrast concentration in these veins is reduced close to the end of the scan.

Only with femoral injection of contrast medium is a craniocaudal scan direction advantageous. The rapid opacification of the jugular veins leads to superimposition of arterial and venous structures in the supra-aortic region if a caudocranial scan direction is chosen. This can virtually be eliminated if the scan direction is inversed.

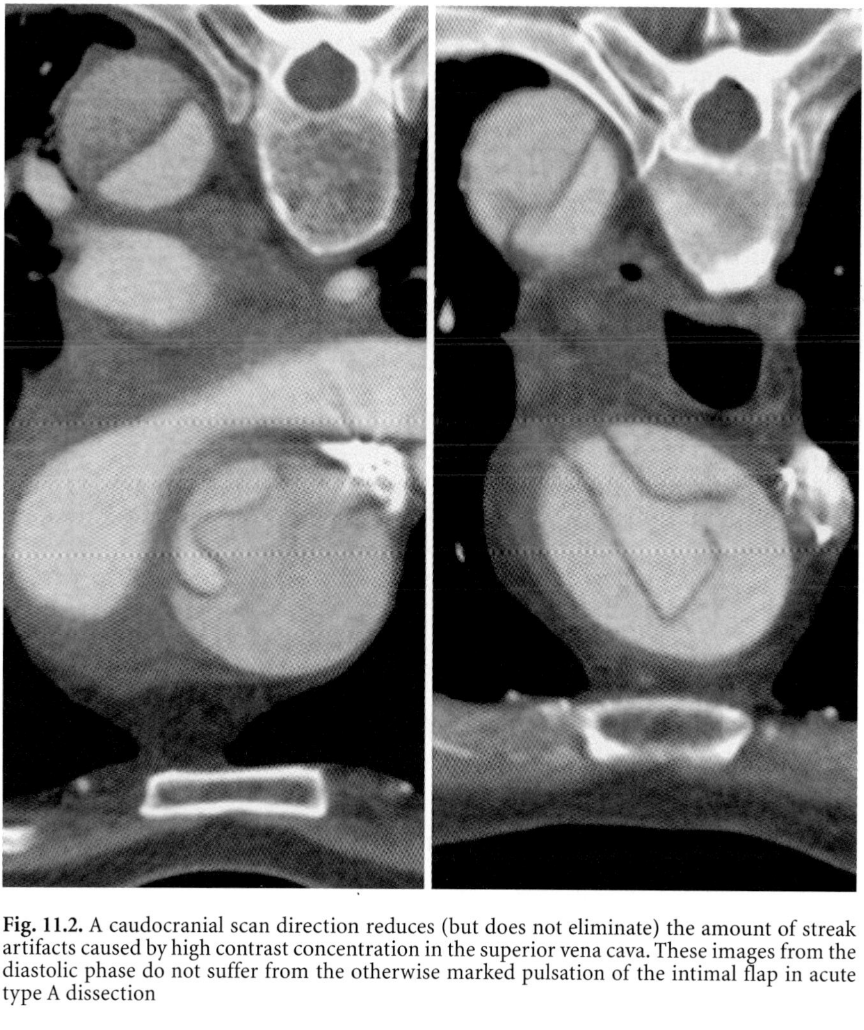

Fig. 11.2. A caudocranial scan direction reduces (but does not eliminate) the amount of streak artifacts caused by high contrast concentration in the superior vena cava. These images from the diastolic phase do not suffer from the otherwise marked pulsation of the intimal flap in acute type A dissection

11.3 Contrast Administration

Like the choice of scan parameters, the administration of intravenous contrast medium depends on the imaging task. While simple imaging tasks do not require a large amount of contrast agent (a resulting intravascular contrast of 50 HE is generally sufficient to demonstrate mural thrombus and the presence of a dissecting membrane), most applications require at least 100 ml intravenous contrast medium in order to obtain an intravascular contrast of at least 150 HE.

11.3.1 Flow Rate

The flow rate of the contrast injection determines the maximum opacification of the aorta or the pulmonary vessels. With current scanners, a flow rate of 4 ml/s ensures constant and high contrast in the aorta and pulmonary arteries. Higher flow rates further increase the vascular contrast but require very precise timing of the contrast bolus in order to avoid nondiagnostic contrast at the beginning or the end of the spiral scan. Lower flow rates are possible whenever the imaging task is not too complex (e.g., aortic aneurysms) and the quality of three-dimensional images is not critical. The display of complex aortic anatomy or complex aortic dissections requires high contrast. In particular, the display of the supra-aortic branches in aortic dissection is heavily dependent on optimum contrast in these vessels.

11.3.2 Saline Chaser Bolus

In analogy to the injection protocols for intravenous digital subtraction angiography (DSA), we suggest the use of a 40- to 60-ml saline chaser bolus to push the contrast forward and flush the brachiocephalic veins [7]. With this protocol and a caudocranial scan direction, the brachiocephalic veins are scanned when most of the contrast medium has been flushed out. As a result, the number of streak artifacts is considerably reduced.

For the abdomen, it was shown that a 10-ml saline chaser bolus increases the length of the contrast plateau by 8 s [7]. This can be expected to also be true for the chest. The effect can be used to improve the vascular contrast close to the end of the scan or to reduce the amount of contrast medium.

In practice, a saline chaser bolus can be produced by first loading normal saline into the injection syringe followed by the chosen amount of contrast material. During the injection, the contrast material will be injected first, immediately followed by the saline.

11.3.3 Bolus Triggering (C.A.R.E. Bolus)

Precise timing of the contrast bolus saves contrast medium and ensures a consistent opacification of the vasculature within the whole target volume. For this reason, bolus triggering should be performed.

In our institution, we set the threshold level for the C.A.R.E. bolus program to 50 HU. For imaging of the aorta, the smallest possible trigger delay should be chosen and the region of interest (ROI) should be placed in the ascending aorta. In young patients with a high cardiac output, the trigger ROI may be placed in the

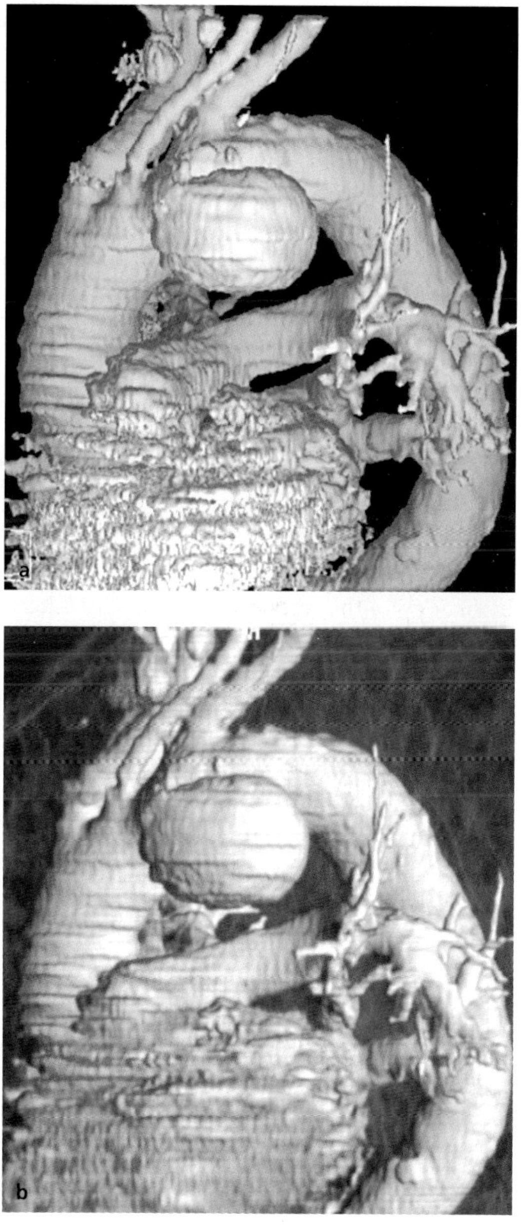

Fig. 11.3a, b. In this patient, preoperative three-dimensional surface displays in an LAO view were performed using **a** shaded surface display (SSD) and **b** volume ray tracing (VRT). A femoral contrast injection with a craniocaudal scan direction was chosen to avoid superimposition of the brachiocephalic vein. Pulsation of the heart is less prominent with VRT. However, neither technique is able to directly display the extensive thrombus in this aneurysm of the aortic arch (indirect sign: displacement of the pulmonary artery)

left ventricle. For the pulmonary arteries, the ROI can be placed either in the pulmonary outflow tract (older patients) or the right ventricle (younger patients). The trigger delay should be set to the minimum (currently 5 s).

11.3.4 Injection Sites

For most routine applications of CTA of the thoracic aorta, a cubital venous approach via a 18-gauge needle is sufficient.

The display of complex aortic anatomy or complex aortic dissections benefits from a femoral venous approach. This approach has the advantage of virtually no artifacts from brachiocephalic veins or the superior vena cava. Together with a craniocaudal scan direction, it guarantees improved three-dimensional displays of the supra-aortic vessels without superimposition of venous structures (Fig. 11.3). Excellent contrast in all thoracic vessels is found, and streak artifacts are almost completely absent in critical regions [6]. In general, however, a femoral venous access is much more cumbersome than a cubital injection site and requires the placement of a venous access catheter.

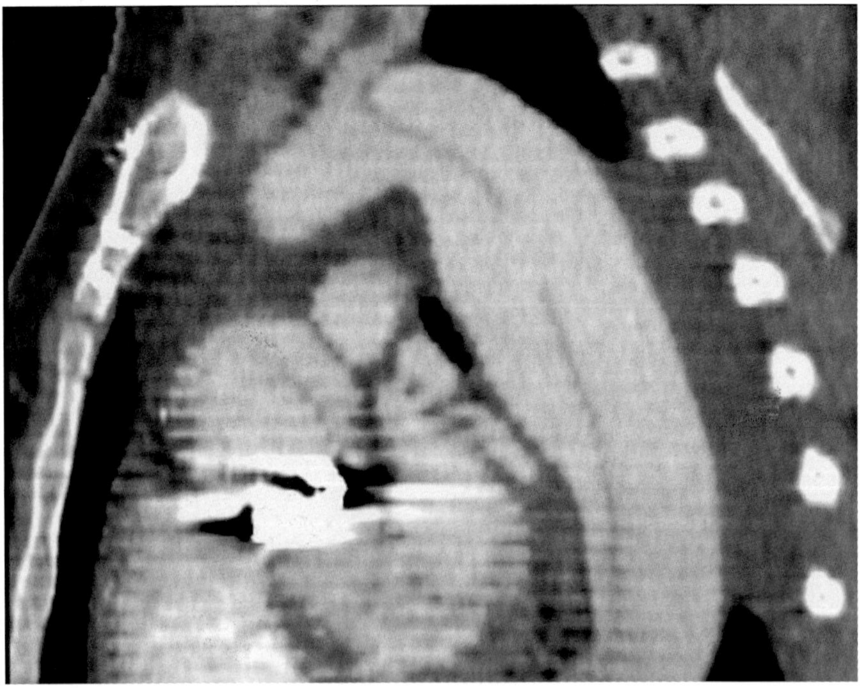

Fig. 11.4. This multiplanar reformat of a type B aortic dissection demonstrates the entry to the false channel more clearly than axial images alone. Pulsation artifacts lead to serrated contours of the heart and the ascending aorta

11.4 Image Processing

11.4.1 Multiplanar Reformats

Multiplanar reformats (MPR) may be helpful for displaying the aortic arch and the supra-aortic branches. Especially in aortic dissections, MPR of these regions are clinically relevant to display the course of the membranes [16].

For the evaluation of pulmonary embolism, MPR are important in those cases in which there are problems in differentiating between hilar lymph nodes and mural thrombi [10].

MPR of the ascending aorta, the proximal portion of the aortic arch, and the central pulmonary arteries suffer from marked pulsation that results in serration in the affected regions (Fig. 11.4).

11.4.2 Maximum-Intensity Projection

In simple cases, maximum-intensity-projections (MIP) are well suited to display the anatomy of the aortic arch. In cases with superimposition of vessels (e.g., superposition of the aorta by the pulmonary vasculature) or complex situations, MIP is not the method of choice. Thin-slab MIP [4] reduce the amount of overlying structures and may be helpful in these critical situations.

11.4.3 Shaded Three-Dimensional Surface Displays

For clinical routine, three-dimensional surface displays of the aorta are more important than other display techniques. For the pulmonary vasculature, SSD does not play a major role, since many emboli are not displayed.

The technique can be performed in a "quick" version, in which no major editing procedures are used with the exception of partial removal of some skeletal structures by cutting procedures. In most cases, a threshold of 150 HU will suffice. In our experience, the 45° LAO projection is sufficient in many cases to give the surgeon an overview of the anatomy (Fig. 11.3a).

In more complex cases in which optimum display techniques are required, three-dimensional editing has to be used to remove skeletal structures or even overlying veins. Even with the slab editor and three-dimensional region-growing algorithms, this procedure is still cumbersome and time-consuming. One of the problems is to separate the first rib and the clavicles from the adjacent vessels. Clipping artifacts are often unavoidable.

11.4.4 Volume Rendering Technique

Volume rendering technique (VRT) is a way of displaying the aorta and pulmonary vasculature in a semitransparent fashion. It can be used instead of SSD. For the aorta, good results are obtained for LAO and RAO views (Fig. 11.3b). For other views, cutting or relatively extensive preediting may be necessary.

For the pulmonary vasculature, the results of VRT are superior to SSD or MIP but require the display of rather thin subvolumes to reduce the distraction by too many superimposing vascular structures.

The major drawback of the procedure is that it requires online control of parameter settings or cutting procedures in order to achieve acceptable images within a reasonable amount of time. For this reason, it is currently not practicable on a Magic View workstation, but it may be employed on the new Silicon Graphics O_2-based platforms.

11.5 **Artifacts**

11.5.1 Pulsation

One major source of artifacts in the chest is the pulsation of the heart and ascending aorta. This is much more prominent in young patients with elastic arterial walls than in older patients with artherosclerotic wall disease.

On axial sections, pulsation may simulate dissecting membranes (Fig. 11.5a) and may distort vascular contours. On MPR, SSD, or MIP, pulsation causes irregular contours of the heart, ascending aorta, and aortic arch. VRT images are less affected given proper display parameters (Fig. 11.3).

The effect of pulsation can be reduced using the 360° reconstruction algorithm instead of the 180° algorithm. With this interpolation, pulsation artifacts are less prominent due to the stronger data interpolation over a longer time interval. At the same time, however, the spatial resolution along the *z*-axis is reduced.

Electrocardiogram (ECG)-triggered interpolation promises even better results [3]. Since ECG-triggered interpolation is not yet generally available, highly overlapping image reconstruction and selection of only those images in which pulsation is least obvious (diastolic phase) may improve the results of three-dimensional displays. This is possible since subsecond scanning reduces the acquisition time per single image and thus almost eliminates pulsation effects in those frames that are acquired during the diastolic phase (Figs. 11.1, 11.2). This procedure, however, is very time-consuming and can only be recommended in selective cases.

11.5.2 Streak Artifacts

Streak artifacts occur whenever there is highly concentrated contrast medium within the scan plane. Thus scanning the chest in a craniocaudal direction while injecting iodinated contrast agents will always lead to streak artifacts from high concentrations of contrast medium in the brachiocephalic veins or the superior vena cava.

Streak artifacts may reduce the quality of three-dimensional displays and may simulate dissecting membranes (Fig. 11.5b).

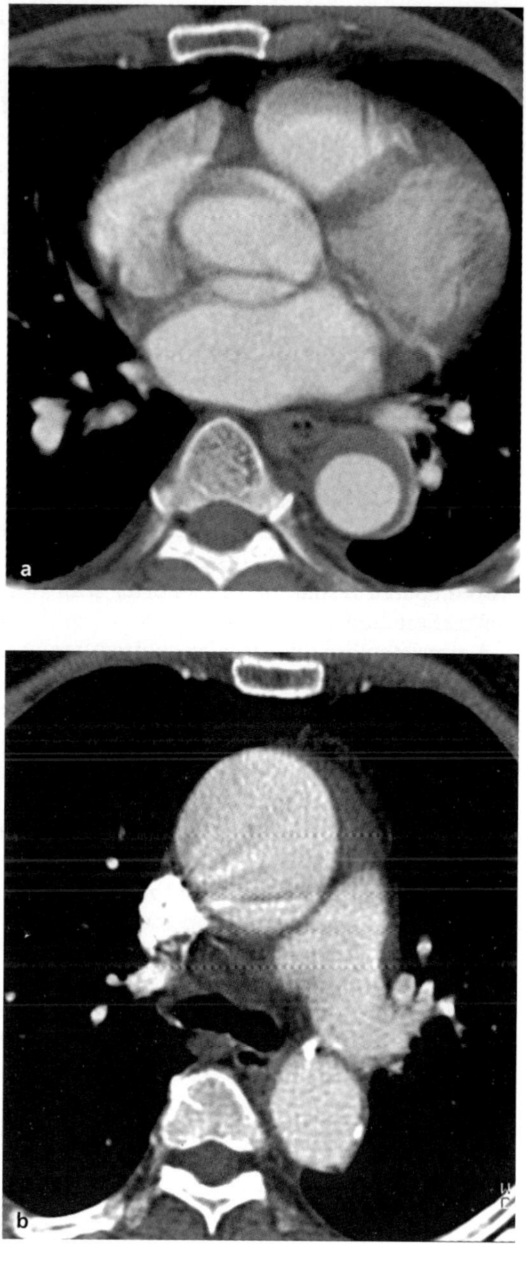

Fig. 11.5a, b. Artifacts simulating aortic dissection may be due to **a** pulsation or **b** high concentration of contrast medium in the superior vena cava. They can be distinguished from real disease by comparing the findings in adjacent sections

As has been pointed out, streak artifacts are almost completely eliminated if a femoral injection site is chosen. They can be reduced substantially if a saline chaser bolus is employed and a caudocranial scan direction is chosen.

11.6 Discussion

Since 1991 we have used CTA for all diagnostic CT examinations of the aorta. The number of diagnostic DSA examinationssy almost instantaneously dropped to less than ten a year. At present, we perform intra-arterial DSA only in those cases in which we suspect a lesion that can be immediately treated angiographically.

CTA has a high acceptance among surgical colleagues, since it is a procedure that is fast and easy to perform and allows for immediate access to a critically ill patient. Three-dimensional displays are preferred to convey the findings to the surgeon.

In order to be able to provide consistent image quality, optimization of scan parameters is necessary for most of these imaging tasks. Only simple tasks such as the evaluation of ascending aortic aneurysms are not critically influenced by the chosen scan parameters and the parameters for contrast injection. In all other cases, both spatial resolution and intravascular contrast have to be optimized.

A high spatial resolution along the z-axis can be achieved by limiting the scan volume and choosing a small slice collimation, a large pitch factor, and a small reconstruction increment. Taking advantage of subsecond scanning leads to improved spatial resolution or a shorter scan time (and thus potential savings in contrast medium).

A consistently high vascular contrast requires sufficient amounts of contrast medium (>100 ml), high flow rates (4 ml/s), and individualized start delays that should be determined by bolus triggering (C.A.R.E. Bolus). A saline chaser bolus improves vascular contrast for small volumes of contrast medium but, most importantly, also prolongs the length of the plateau phase and reduces streak artifacts in the brachiocephalic veins.

MPR are useful for the aortic arch and the supra-aortic vessels as well as for the central pulmonary arteries. MIP play a minor role for aortic disease, while thin-slab MIP may be useful for the evaluation of pulmonary embolism. For the aorta, SSD can at present be considered the display technique of choice. In the future, this will probably change in favor of VRT. This technique, however, is still limited to special workstations.

Artifacts from pulsation of the heart and major vessels may be reduced by employing a 360° LI interpolation algorithm or using ECG-gated interpolation. Streak artifacts from highly concentrated contrast medium in the brachiocephalic veins or the superior vena cava can be avoided by choosing a femoral vein for contrast injection or by using a saline chaser bolus together with a caudocranial scan direction.

Given optimized scanning protocols, CTA of the chest is a reliable technique that provides consistent results for imaging of the aorta and the pulmonary vasculature.

References

1. Costello P, Ecker CP, Tello R et al (1992) Assessment of the thoracic aorta by spiral CT. AJR 158:1127–1130
2. Galanski M, Prokop M (1998) Ganzkörper-Computertomographie. Thieme, Stuttgart
3. Kalender WA (1995) Principles and performance of spiral CT. In: Goldman LW, Fowlkes JB (eds) Medical CT and ultrasound: current technology and applications. American Associaton of Physicist in Medicine, pp 379–410
4. Napel S, Rubin GD, Jeffrey RB (1993) STS-MIP: a new reconstruction technique for CT of the chest: J Comput Assist Tomogr 17:832–838
5. Prokop M, Schaefer C, Doehring W, Laas J, Nischelsky J, Galanski M (1991) Spiral CT for three dimensional imaging of complex vascular structures. Radiology 181(P):293
6. Prokop M, Schaefer C, Leppert AGA, Galanski M (1993) Spiral CT angiography of thoracic aorta: femoral or antecubital injection site for intravenous administration of contrast material? Radiology 189(P):111
7. Prokop M, Engelke C, Schaefer-Prokop C, Jörgensen M (1995) Optimierung der Gefäßkontrastierung bei der Spiral CT Angiographie durch NaCl-Bolus. Radiologe 35(4): S167
8. Rémy Jardin M, Rémy J, Deschildre F et al (1996) Diagnosis of pulmonary embolism with spiral CT. Comparison with pulmonary angiography and scintigraphy. Radiology 200: 699–706
9. Rémy Jardin M, Rémy J, Wattine L, Giraud F (1992) Central pulmonary thrombembolism: diagnosis with spiral volumetric CT with the single breathhold technique: comparison with pulmonary angiography. Radiology 185:381–387
10. Rémy Jardin M, Rémy J, Cauvain O, Petyt L, Wannebrouq J, Beregi JP (1995) Diagnosis of central pulmonary embolism with helical CT: role of two-dimensional multiplanar reformations. AJR 165:1131–1138
11. Rémy-Jardin M, Rémy J, Artaud D et al (1997) Peripheral pulmonary arteries: optimization of the spiral CT acquisition protocol. Radiology 204:157–163
12. Rubin GD, Napel S (1995) Increased scan pitch for vascular and thoracic spiral CT. Radiology 197:316–317
13. Schaefer C, Prokop M, Nischelsky J, Reimer P, Bonk K, Galanski M (1992) Vascular imaging with spiral CT. In: Felix R, Langer M (eds) Advances in CT II. 2nd European Scientific User Conference SOMATOM PLUS, Berlin. Springer, Berlin Heidelberg New York, pp 109–115
14. Schnyder P, Meuli R, Wicky S, Mayor B (1995) Injection techniques. In: Rémy-Jordin M, Remi J (eds) Spiral CT of the chest. Springer, Berlin, Heidelberg, pp 57–99
15. Sommer T, Fehske W, Holzknecht N et al (1996) Aortic dissections: a comparative study of diagnosis with spiral CT, multiplanar transesophageal echocardiography, and MR imaging. Radiology 199:347–352
16. Zeman RK, Berman PM, Silverman PM et al (1995) Diagnosis of aortic dissections: value of helical CT with multiplanar reformations and three-dimensional rendering. AJR 164: 1375–1380

12 The Diagnostic Impact of Spiral CT for Pulmonary Embolism

A. K. Dixon, J. J. Cross, C. D. R. Flower

12.1 Introduction

Many departments around the world are performing more and more spiral CT investigations for suspected pulmonary embolism. Direct visualisation of the embolus [1], with no more invasion than an intravenous injection of contrast medium, carries obvious and immediate appeal. What is not yet clear is whether spiral CT is being performed in place of ventilation perfusion lung scintigraphy, in place of pulmonary angiography or as an additional investigation [2]. There is considerable controversy as to the optimal investigative sequence and guidelines are not definitive in this setting [3, 4]. However, such controversy is common enough during the introduction of new diagnostic investigations. Very few have been subjected to rigorous randomised clinical trials. Most are introduced before formal cost-effectiveness studies have been performed. The diagnostic investigations which they replace tend to atrophy slowly rather than being stopped forthwith.

There is a certain inevitability about the sequence of events described above. The technical performance of spiral CT was quickly established [5, 6]. Several workers cleverly appreciated the diagnostic potential for pulmonary embolism, first in the chronic [7, 8] and then in the more acute setting [9–11]. The diagnostic performance was established in these settings, usually in teaching hospitals with a somewhat atypical prevalence of positive findings, excellent CT equipment and dedicated radiologists with great expertise in thoracic CT. As the initial trials are now being completed, many clinicians have become accustomed to having the diagnosis established by spiral CT. They no longer trust some of their therapeutic decisions based on VQ scintigraphy alone. They know that there is a less invasive alternative to pulmonary angiography. It becomes difficult to stop the demand for the new technique – so much so that it is ethically difficult to withhold the investigation in the appropriate clinical setting, even if CT units are already running at full capacity and health purchasers are reluctant to spend more money on the diagnosis of pulmonary embolus. Certainly ethical committees would now have difficulty in granting approval to a randomised study in which one arm is denied access to spiral CT in an institution where appropriate facilities are available on site.

But there are established methods for assessing the effectiveness of new diagnostic techniques, based on a hierarchical evaluation of technical performance, diagnostic performance, diagnostic impact, therapeutic impact and impact on health status [12–14]. And many of these aspects have been and are being pursued for the use of spiral CT in the diagnosis of pulmonary embolus. When these studies are finally complete, there should be a strong body of evidence pointing out the cost-effectiveness and societal benefit of this exciting diagnostic technique. This chapter addresses some of these issues with particular emphasis on the way in which spiral CT influences the diagnostic thinking of the referring clinician (diagnostic impact).

12.2 Technical Performance

All modern spiral CT systems have a 1-s (or shorter) data acquisition time per revolution and a tube capacity capable of examining the whole chest during a single breathhold. All CT units with a fast spiral CT system should possess a pump injector to facilitate continuous injection of contrast medium at a constant flow rate. Suitable flow rates and CT protocols have been developed. Numerous technical problems and anatomical pitfalls have been encountered [15] and ironed out so that now most CT units use a fairly standard technique [16]. That employed in our own Unit [17] is the Siemens Somatom Plus 4 System:

- 100 ml 300 mg/ml iopamidol (Niopam, Merck) mixed with 20 ml normal saline injected via
- Intravenous cannula, ideally in an antecubital vein
- Flow rate of 3.5 ml/s with a Medtron (Mallinckrodt Medical) pump
- Data acquisition started after a delay of 15 s (20 s for wrist injection)
- Slice thickness 3 mm with table feed of 4.5 mm/s with 3 mm contiguous image reconstruction
- Data acquisition from 2 cm cranial to the more inferior hemi-diaphragm up to the aortic arch
- Total data acquisition time depending on body habitus, but up to 30 s
- Patient suspending breathing in comfortable inspiration

12.3 Diagnostic Performance

It is in this area (sensitivity, specificity, accuracy) that most evidence is available, often with angiographic correlation. However, some studies accept CT or scintigraphic evidence of pulmonary embolus as a final diagnosis. Even at angiography there is significant intra- and inter-observer variation for the diagnosis of peripheral emboli. However, such difficulty with regard to final diagnosis is not unique to the radiological diagnosis of pulmonary embolus; it is inevitable for any disease process where surgery is rarely performed and correlative post-mortem evidence is scanty.

Given these caveats, spiral CT has particularly good diagnostic performance in chronic pulmonary embolism where the pulmonary arteries may be large, the flow through the great vessels is relatively slow, and the emboli are often static and adherent to the pulmonary arterial walls. Such patients were the subject of initial attention, and the accuracy seems very high [8] unless the embolus has become calcified.

The determination of accuracy in the acute situation raises various problems. The acutely distressed patient may find it difficult to keep still. The fitter, younger patient, especially one with no pulmonary disease, exhibits rapid transit of contrast medium and considerable vascular motion artefact, all hindering interpretation; the use of test injections or bolus tracking may help ensure optimal timing here. Angiographic proof is not available in every patient as some clinicians base their management decisions on VQ scintigraphy or CT results. Despite these problems numerous excellent studies have now been published, all pointing to a very acceptable accuracy. In the classical paper by Remy-Jardin et al. [10], the prospective sensitivity of CT was 91% overall, with a sensitivity of 78%; in their series the predictive value of a positive CT was 100% and of a negative CT 89%. When only zones which were adequately depicted by both CT and angiography were compared, the sensitivity rose to 98% and the specificity to 99%. They concluded that 'spiral CT can reliably depict central pulmonary emboli and may be introduced into diagnostic algorithms'. Van Rossum's group is more forthcoming [11] and quote an overall sensitivity for spiral CT of 95% and specificity of 97%; in their series the predictive values for positive and negative tests were both 97%. They conclude that 'CT is a relatively non-invasive test for pulmonary embolism ... which may serve as an alternative to ventilation scintigraphy and possibly to pulmonary angiography'.

There are, of course, continuing questions about isolated subsegmental emboli which may be missed at cross-sectional imaging [18], and this debate will continue for some time, largely because the diagnosis of such emboli is open to intra- and inter-observer variation. However such discrepancy in observation is a problem for all imaging techniques and may be lower for spiral CT than VQ scintigraphy or angiography. Whether the problem of the isolated subsegmental embolus will be extensively pursued in the future may depend on clinicians' attitude to the correct therapeutic approach.

12.4 Diagnostic Impact

This is a measure of the extent to which the result of the radiological investigation alters the referring clinician's working diagnosis. Ideally this necessitates the working diagnosis (and confidence thereof) being stated before and after the result of the radiological investigation. Such a prospective study requires considerable physician cooperation and, in practice, is rarely fully achieved. But the nuclear medicine community has been in the forefront here and has long advocated that VQ scintigram results should be interpreted in the light of the pre-test clinical probability (low, intermediate or high). Thus these data are usually available at the time the investigations are performed (VQ scintigraphy, spiral CT, etc.). However, it is much more difficult to establish what the post-test working diagnosis is. Just because the patient is treated with anticoagulants, it does not follow that the physician is 100% certain that the patient has had a pulmonary embolus. This is apparent from scrutiny of the recent report by Kember et al. which followed up 111 patients with intermediate VQ scintigraphic findings [19].

What is needed is a study measuring the clinician's confidence in the diagnosis immediately before and after imaging.

A point which is not always fully recognised is that patients do not present with a label pulmonary embolus. Their symptoms are often non-specific and range from unexplained chest pain to dyspnoea and haemoptysis. Note the number of patients in whom pulmonary embolism is discovered by serendipity [20] (Fig. 12.1). In many cases the physician has treated the patient for pneumonia or pleurisy for a while. At some later stage the clinical progress is questioned. Then the differential diagnosis may be extended. Finally, more investigations are performed which may reveal pulmonary embolism or identify another cause which could explain the patient's symptoms.

To put the difficulty of the clinical diagnosis in perspective, it is worth considering the findings in a recent study from our own institution [21]. Amongst 77 patients referred for imaging with possible pulmonary embolism (clinical likelihood high in 22, intermediate in 31, low in 24), pulmonary embolism was confirmed as the final diagnosis in only 13 (overall prevalence of 17%). Even in those patients with a high pre-test clinical probability the prevalence was only 36% (8/22). Although the pre-test clinical likelihood was correlated with the presence of embolism at imaging, the correlation is not really strong enough to be all that useful for an individual patient. This is in keeping with the findings in the PIOPED study [22]. The prevalence of pulmonary embolism was lower in our study than in the PIOPED study, which may have been weighted towards more severe clinical situations because of the inclusion of pulmonary angiography in all patients. It is likely that our relatively low prevalence is more in line with typical referrals in many hospitals worldwide.

What of the patients referred with a possible pulmonary embolism who do not have an embolism? This is where spiral CT really comes into its own. In our pros-

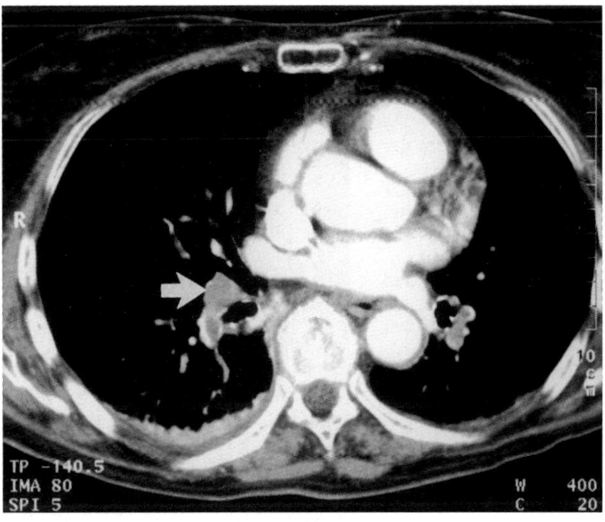

Fig. 12.1. A patient referred with severe chest pain and suspected aortic dissection. Multiple pulmonary emboli were demonstrated. A large filling defect occupies much of the artery in the right lower lobe (*arrow*). Smaller emboli in the left lower lobe also

pective study [21], where patients were randomly assigned to VQ scintigraphy or spiral CT as the initial investigation, spiral CT was able to offer the clinician an alternative explanation for the symptoms in 23 of 51 such patients (45%). These diagnoses included consolidation, effusion, emphysema and in one patient an unsuspected pulmonary mass. This clearly demonstrates the advantage of an investigation (CT) which can directly demonstrate several alternative diagnoses. Indeed the patient shown in Fig. 12.1 illustrates just this point: a patient is referred for possible aortic dissection because of rather non-descript chest pain; spiral CT elegantly demonstrates a pulmonary embolus. This inherent advantage of cross-sectional imaging is now well recognised elsewhere in the body. Who would still use an organ-specific investigation such as a barium enema as the first investigation for an abdominal mass?! It is perhaps the facility to provide a range of alternative diagnoses, rather than merely confirmation or rebuttal of a suspected diagnosis, which represents the greatest diagnostic impact of spiral CT (Fig. 12.2).

Another rather indirect measure of the diagnostic impact of a new radiological investigation is the extent to which it displaces other diagnostic investigations. At present there is a risk that spiral CT may be used as an 'add on' to the investigative sequence [2]. The most radical approach has been proposed by Goodman and Lipchik who suggest that VQ scintigraphy should be abandoned for patients with suspected pulmonary embolism [23]. In the United Kingdom few hospitals have sufficient CT capacity to take on this additional work in anything other than over a gradual transition. Our randomised study [21] suggested a less radical approach, namely that patients with no underlying cardio-respiratory disease should continue to be investigated by VQ scintigraphy. Patients with known cardio-respiratory disorders (e.g. abnormal CXR), in whom VQ scintigraphy is likely to give an indeterminate report, should have spiral CT as the initial investigation. Certainly spiral CT will be increasingly used in place of pulmonary angiography.

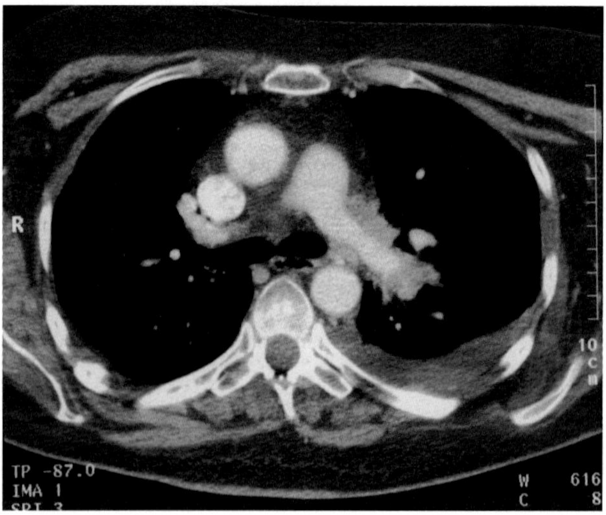

Fig. 12.2. A patient with known breast carcinoma and increasing breathlessness. VQ scintigraphy had shown considerable mis-match on the left, suggesting embolism. CT shows that the left main pulmonary artery is encased by tumour and demonstrates a left sided pleural effusion. This neatly demonstrates the advantages of cross-sectional imaging

12.5 Therapeutic Impact

Assessment of therapeutic impact, again, requires close physician cooperation. They must theoretically define the therapeutic approach before and after imaging. However, in the United Kingdom most patients have for many years been managed on the basis of VQ scintigraphy alone. If a study were carried out with the main aim of assessing the therapeutic impact of spiral CT when used as the first investigation for possible pulmonary embolism, the results should show that many patients are moved from the 'further investigation' category to 'medical treatment'. However, this would probably differ little from the results when using VQ scintigraphy. What might differ is the proportion of patients receiving anticoagulation. For example, in the randomised study performed at our institution [21], several of the intermediate results in patients investigated first by scintigraphy were converted into definite pulmonary embolism or definitely normal after CT, with appropriate alteration in management. The greater confidence in the diagnosis provided by spiral CT could also be reflected in the duration of anticoagulant therapy; for example 'direct visualisation' [1] of the embolus at CT might mean that the physician continued anticoagulation therapy for longer than after an intermediate probability report at VQ scintigraphy. More work is needed to assess this aspect.

12.6 Impact on Health

Evaluation of the impact on health brought about by a new investigation, the final outcome measure [12–14], is always the most difficult area for health technology assessment. Health economists might well argue that a new investigation is not really justified unless patients obtain better as a result! In the case of pulmonary embolus, unlike in many other areas of radiology, there is at least a tangible outcome – namely death of the patient. However, once the referring physician has thought of pulmonary embolus as a possible diagnosis, the therapeutic options are under scrutiny. Many patients are put on anticoagulant therapy pending the results of investigations, and this causes only little morbidity. More sophisticated measures (IVC filters, thrombolytic therapy, etc.) all have their advocates, but it is unlikely that the diagnostic method by which the diagnosis is obtained (Dimer testing, scintigraphy, CT, MRI, angiography, etc.) would have much influence on outcome. Of course the institution of appropriate therapy in patients shown to have unsuspected pulmonary embolism (e.g. Fig. 12.1) could contribute to improved overall survival.

Because of the likely difficulties in showing that spiral CT improves survival in patients with pulmonary embolism [24], radiologists have correctly turned to demonstrating its cost-beneficial aspects [25]. Chief amongst these is the financial advantage of obtaining an accurate and confident diagnosis in a timely fashion. As far as the patient is concerned, there is little to choose between scintigraphy and CT in terms of risk, discomfort and price. However, catheter angiography is clearly more uncomfortable and carries a higher (although probably exaggerated) morbidity. Several studies have now shown some of the advantages of spiral CT, and it is pleasing to see that there is general enthusiasm for a proposed multicentre European study to pursue these aspects [26, 27] further. One feature that will have to be watched is a general increase in the number of investigations for possible pulmonary embolus. Given that there is now a highly credible, accurate and relatively cheap investigation, namely spiral CT, it is almost inevitable that there will be an increase in the number of investigations requested. History has proved this time and time again. Just look at the number of MRI studies now performed for possible lumbar spine disease compared with the number of radiculograms of old!

Acknowledgements. The randomised study quoted [21] was funded with the aid of a pump priming grant from the Royal College of Radiologists and generous support for contrast media from Merck. Barbara Housden and Helen Clarke performed most of the CT studies. Paul Kemp and Geraldine Walsh also assisted in that study.

References

1. Gurney JW (1993) No fooling around: direct visualisation of pulmonary embolism. Radiology 188:618–619
2. Hansell DM, Padley SP (1996) Continuous volume computed tomography in pulmonary embolism: the answer or just another test? Thorax 51:1–2
3. Royal College of Radiologists (1995) Making the best use of a department of clinical radiology: guidelines for doctors, 3rd edn. Royal College of Radiologists, London
4. British Thoracic Society, Standards Care Committee (1997) Suspected acute pulmonary embolism: a practical approach. Thorax 52:S1–24
5. Kalendar WA, Seissler W, Klotz E, Vock P (1990) Spiral volumetric CT with single breathold technique, continuous transport and continuous scanner rotation. Radiology 176:181–183
6. Hacking JC, Dixon AK (1992) Spiral versus conventional CT in soft tissue diagnosis. Eur J Radiol 15:224–229
7. Remy-Jardin M, Remy J, Wattinne L, Giraud F (1992) Central pulmonary thromboembolism: diagnosis with spiral volumetric CT with single breath-hold technique – comparison with pulmonary angiography. Radiology 185:381–387
8. Tardivon AA, Musset D, Maitre S et al (1993) Role of CT in chronic pulmonary embolism: comparison with pulmonary angiography. J Comput Assist Tomogr 17:345–351
9. van Rossum AB, Pattynama PM, Truerniet FE, Schepers R, Kieft GJ (1995) Spiral CT angiography for pulmonary embolism: validation in 124 patients. Radiology 197 (P):303
10. Remy-Jardin M, Remy J, Deschildre F et al (1996) Diagnosis of pulmonary embolism with spiral CT: comparison with pulmonary angiography and scintigraphy. Radiology 200: 699–706
11. van Rossum AB, Treurniet FE, Kieft GJ, Smith SJ, Schepers-Bok R (1996) Role of spiral volumetric computed tomographic scanning in the assessment of patients with clinical suspicion of pulmonary embolism and an abnormal ventilation/perfusion lung scan. Thorax 51: 23–28
12. Fineberg HV, Bauman R, Sosman M (1977) Computized cranial tomography: effect on diagnostic and therapeutic plans. JAMA 238:224–227
13. Hillman BJ (1994) Outcomes research and cost effectiveness analysis for diagnostic imaging. Radiology 193:307–310
14. Mackenzie R, Dixon AK (1995) Measuring the effects of imaging: an evaluative framework. Clin Radiol 50:513–518
15. Oser R, Zuckeman DA, Gutierrez, FR, Brink JA (1996) Anatomic distribution of pulmonary emboli at pulmonary angiography: implications for cross-sectional imaging. Radiology 199:31–35

16. Remy-Jardin M, Remy J, Artaud D, Deschildre F, Duhamel A (1997) Peripheral pulmonary arteries: optimization of the spiral CT protocol. Radiology 204:157–63
17. Cross JJL, Kemp PM, Flower CDR (1997) Diagnostic imaging in pulmonary embolic disease. Br J Hosp Med 58:93–96
18. Mayo JR, Remy-Jardin M, Muller N et al (1997) Pulmonary embolism: prospective comparison of spiral CT with ventilation-perfusion scintigraphy. Radiology 205:447–452
19. Kember PG, Euinton HA, Morcos SK (1997) Clinicians' interpretation of the indeterminate ventilation-perfusion scan report. Br J Radiol 70:1109–1111
20. Verschakelen JA, Vanwijck E, Bogaert J, Baert AL (1993) Detection of unsuspected central pulmonary embolism with conventional CT. Radiology 188:847–850
21. Cross JJL, Kemp PM, Walsh CG, Flower CDR, Dixon AK (1998) A randomised trial of spiral CT and ventilation perfusion scintigraphy for the diagnosis of pulmonary embolus. Clin Radiol 53:177–182
23. Goodman LR, Lipchik RJ (1996) Diagnosis of acute pulmonary embolism: time for a new approach. Radiology 199:25–27
24. Ferretti GR, Bosson J-l, Buffaz P-D et al (1997) Acute pulmonary embolism: role of helical CT in 164 patients with intermediate probability at ventilation-perfusion scintigraphy and normal results at Duplex US of the legs. Radiology 205:453–458
25. van Erkel AR, van Rossum AB, Bloem JL, Kievit J, Pattynama PMT (1996) Spiral CT angiography for suspected pulmonary embolism: a cost-effectiveness analysis. Radiology 201:29–36
26. Hunink MGM (1996) Outcomes research and cost-effectiveness analysis in radiology. Eur Radiol 6:615–620
27. Dalla-Palma L, Dixon AK, Durand-Zaleski I, Reiser M, Soimakallio S (1996) An overview of cost-effective radiology. Eur Radiol 7:147–150

13 Cost-Effectiveness Analysis of Diagnostic Management of Pulmonary Embolism

M. Oudkerk, E. J. R. van Beek, A. H. H. Bongaerts

13.1 Introduction

The diagnosis of pulmonary embolism (PE) is a challenging task for any physician. Annually, two to three per 1000 inhabitants present with symptoms suggesting the presence of venous thromboembolic disease, the common denominator for deep vein thrombosis and PE [1, 2]. The range of diagnostic procedures that physicians have at their disposal varies from clinical history and physical examination – often supplemented with blood gas analysis, chest radiography and electrocardiography – to lung scintigraphy and pulmonary angiography. However, their exact role and place in a diagnostic strategy remain controversial and have been a matter of discussion in recent years [3–18].

Why this interest in the diagnostic management of PE? Firstly, because it is a potential killer: it has been estimated that up to 10% of patients with acute PE die within the first hour [19]. Furthermore, if the diagnosis is missed and patients remain untreated, up to 30% will die of subsequent recurrent pulmonary emboli, while a further 30% may sustain non-fatal recurrent embolism [19, 20]. These complications may be reduced significantly with adequate anticoagulant therapy, resulting in fatal and non-fatal PE in approximately 2% [21, 22]. Similar comparisons are available for deep vein thrombosis, with fatal PE reported in 12% of treated patients and 0.7% of untreated patients [21–23]. Non-fatal PE was encountered in 15% and 2% of untreated and treated patients with deep vein thrombosis, respectively [21–23].

Thus there is a general fear of missing the diagnosis, which predisposes physicians to institute anticoagulation therapy. However, it is important to realize that anticoagulant therapy is not without risks: 3 months of therapy are associated with a mortality rate of 0.25%, while major bleeding complications occur in 1% of patients receiving oral anticoagulants for 3 months [24–28]. This gives rise to the need for differentiating patients who have venous thromboembolic disease and require anticoagulant therapy from those in whom the risks of anticoagulants should be avoided. As shown by pulmonary angiography, the prevalence of PE in patients with clinical symptoms suggesting its presence is approximately 30% [29–32]. Therefore, the exclusion of venous thromboembolic disease is as important as proving the presence of thrombi.

13.2 Clinical Diagnosis

The presenting signs and symptoms of patients with PE vary from the classic triad of acute onset dyspnea, pleuritic chest pain and hemoptysis to non-specific complaints [33, 34]. However, the diagnosis should be considered in any patient with unexplained dyspnea.

The physical examination usually yields non-specific signs, such as tachypnea, crepitus or pleural rub, tachycardia, subfebrile temperature and rare signs of deep vein thrombosis [34]. Thus, history and physical examination are unable to differentiate patients with PE from those without the disease.

Several non-invasive diagnostic tools are available for diagnosing PE, including blood gas analysis, chest radiography and electrocardiography. These methods were shown to be of limited use for the diagnosis of PE and are more useful for assessing disorders that mimick PE (e.g. myocardial infarction, pneumonia, pneumothorax) and to evaluate possible oxygen requirements [35, 36].

13.3 Pulmonary Angiography

Although pulmonary angiography is generally regarded as the procedure of choice for diagnosing PE, it is not perfect [29, 30, 37, 38]. Several long-term follow-up studies have demonstrated that the sensitivity and specificity are 98% and 96%, respectively [29, 39–41]. With the introduction of intra-arterial digital subtraction techniques, diagnostic accuracy may have improved. More importantly, however, a normal pulmonary angiogram effectively excludes the presence of clinically significant PE, and anticoagulants may be safely withheld in these patients [39, 41]. As with any invasive technique, complications may arise. Deaths as a result of the procedure have been reported in approximately 0.2%, while non-fatal complications (defined as severe allergic reaction, cardiac perforation and rhythm disturbances requiring treatment) were reported in around 1.9%. [29, 41–43] The risks of complications have rendered this an unpopular, yet necessary, procedure for the diagnostic management of venous thromboembolism. Furthermore, refinements in catheterization techniques, contrast agents used and adequate identification of high risk patients most probably result in a much improved angiographic outcome [44, 45].

13.4 Perfusion/Ventilation Lung Scintigraphy

Lung scintigraphy is generally considered the screening test of choice for patients with clinically suspected PE. It is non-invasive, has no associated complications and can provide a basis for therapeutic decisions. Firstly, long-term follow-up studies have demonstrated that a normal perfusion lung scan effectively excludes clinically significant PE, and it is safe to withhold anticoagulants in these patients [46, 47]. The chance of obtaining a normal perfusion scan in the presence or absence of PE was reported in the PIOPED study to be 0.2% or 20%, respectively [29, 27]. Secondly, a high-probability lung scan (one or more segmental perfusion defects with normal ventilation) may be regarded as sufficient reason to institute long-term oral anticoagulant therapy [48, 49]. The chance of obtaining a high-probability lung scan was reported in the PIOPED study to be 41% if pulmonary emboli are present and 2% if they are absent [29, 48, 49].

Unfortunately, lung scintigraphy appeared to be "non-committal" in 40%–70% of patients, and the term "non-diagnostic" is being used increasingly to denote this outcome. In this category of lung scan results, PIOPED patients with pulmonary emboli had a 42.8% chance of having subsegmental perfusion defects and a 16% chance of having matched segmental perfusion/ventilation defects (together classified as non-high-probability scan) [29, 48, 49]. In the absence of pulmonary emboli, these chances are 62% and 16%, respectively [29, 48, 49]. Thus 40%–60% of patients will have lung scan results on which clinical decisions may be based.

13.5 Deep Vein Thrombosis Tests

The rationale for tests for deep vein thrombosis is derived from the fact that in a substantial proportion (ranging from 30% to 70%) of patients with proven PE, thrombi may be detected by contrast venography of the lower limbs [48, 50, 51]. Real-time B-mode compression ultrasonography (US) is regarded as the most sensitive non-invasive test for detecting deep vein thrombosis in patients with leg symptoms [52]. For PE, this situation is probably less favourable, since many thrombi are asymptomatic and one third are confined to the calf veins. Thus, by adapting available data from studies in patients with suspected deep vein thrombosis, the sensitivity and specificity of this method for all thrombi in patients with clinically suspected PE were calculated to be 79% and 99%, respectively [53].

13.6 Spiral Computed Tomography

Many studies have been performed to assess the potential use of spiral computed tomography (CT) (Fig. 13.1) for the diagnostic management of PE [54–60]. Nearly all studies were performed in selected patient populations with a relatively high prevalence of PE, and only one management study has come to light thus far. The results obtained ranged in sensitivity from 54% to 100% and in specificity from 67% to 100%. These findings are mainly related to patient selection, with lower accuracy figures in less selected series of patients. Furthermore, their sensitivity is significantly better in patients with large and central emboli, compared to those with emboli in subsegmental arteries. More recent literature indicates specificity values lower than 95% and a sensitivity range from 75% to 90%.

This modality was considered not to cause serious complications, and the costs were estimated at 200 ECU.

13.7 Cost-Effectiveness Analysis

When performing a cost-effectiveness analysis, one may either use data as obtained in a large study or use assumptions derived from the literature. We published such an analysis for the diagnostic management of PE, which was based on data from the literature and on a survey on costs in a dozen hospitals throughout the world [6]. We have now updated the analysis by introducing management strategies including spiral CT. This again resulted in a number of baseline vari-

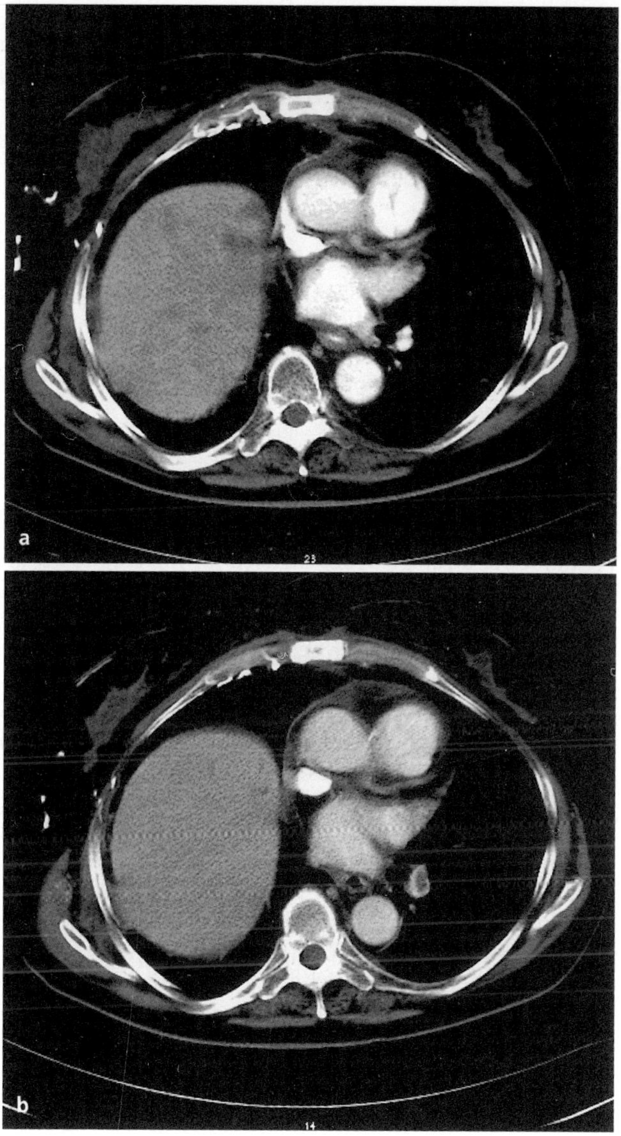

Fig. 13.1a, b. Two consecutive spiral CT axial images of the thorax at the level of the cardiac root, both obtained in context of oncologic follow-up (metastases not shown) without information of clinical suspicion of pulmonary embolism diagnosed just before the second scan was obtained some months after the first scan. The first scan top (**a**) shows homogeneous enhancement of the dividing pulmonary arteries to the mediobasal segment of the left lower lobe. The control scan bottom (**b**) shows nearly complete filling defects of these vessels (which also were visible on neighbouring consecutive scans)

Table 13.1. Diagnostic and therapeutic costs used in the analysis

Method	Costs (ECU)
Pulmonary angiography (bilateral)	500
Perfusion lung scintigraphy	100
Spiral CT	200
Ventilation lung scintigraphy	250
B-mode ultrasonography	65
Therapeutic costs	2165

ables. A summary of costs is given in Table 13.1. The costs of therapy were based on 7 days of hospitalization followed by 3 months of oral anticoagulant therapy. To assess the influence of various assumptions, a sensitivity analysis is performed that manipulates one variable at a time. If the analysis is robust, very few changes will be seen.

13.7.1 Diagnostic Strategies

A number of strategies may be used for the diagnostic and therapeutic management of PE. The simplest would be to treat every patient in whom PE is suspected. The advantage of this strategy would be the lack of diagnostic tests required, whereas a disadvantage would be that a large number of patients would be treated incorrectly, i.e. those who do not have pulmonary emboli would be at risk of developing fatal and non-fatal bleeding complications. Several other strategies may be compiled from the diagnostic tests already described. These range from the use of only non-invasive tests (lung scintigraphy with or without US of the leg veins) or spiral CT to the use of pulmonary angiography in all patients. The outcome of any diagnostic strategy in PE will influence the treatment decision and consequently will influence mortality and morbidity rates and costs associated with the chosen diagnostic/therapeutic approach. We analysed nine strategies for which we calculated effectiveness in terms of mortality, morbidity, numbers of patients with adequate or inadequate therapy and the number of patients requiring angiography. Furthermore, we determined cost-effectiveness by calculating costs per extra life saved (compared with the natural history, i.e. no anticoagulant therapy) [6]. It should be noted that all strategies that used lung scanning used ventilation scintigraphy only if at least one segmental perfusion defect was detected.

13.7.2 Results

Three groups of strategies were identified:

- A group in whom only non-invasive diagnostic tests were used (group A), i.e. spiral CT or ventilation/perfusion scintigraphy
- A group in whom a combination of tests was used that always included pulmonary angiography (group B)
- A group in which most patients were treated with anticoagulants (group C)

The results of our extended analysis show that the mortality in group A was significantly higher than groups B and C. Thus, a mortality rate of 2%–5% was sustained when perfusion/ventilation scintigraphy or spiral CT was used with or without US. In groups B and C, the mortality rates varied between 0.8% and 0.9%. A similar pattern could be discerned with regards to morbidity, i.e. non-fatal PE. Treatment decisions based on the strategies in group A resulted in both undertreatment (8%–18%) and overtreatment (2%–5%), while this was completely the opposite in group C, where 50%–70% of patients inappropriately received anticoagulant therapy. In group B, fewer than 1% of patients were missed, while less than 5% received anticoagulants inappropriately.

The costs were a direct reflection of treatment decisions. Thus, in group C, treatment for an average patient would cost 2000 ECU, which decreased to about 1300 ECU in group B, a cost reduction of 35%. Although group A costs were even less, the resulting mortality and morbidity make this approach unacceptable.

When we assessed cost-effectiveness, large differences between the groups became apparent. The ultimate choice of which strategy should be endorsed does not depend solely on costs, but should initially be dependent on overall mortality. Thus, the use of only non-invasive tests (group A) became indefensible as a result of a three- to five-fold higher mortality rate when compared to groups B and C (Table 13.2). Furthermore, since the treatment for group C was so much more expensive, we decided that a choice should be made from the strategies in group B.

For group B, the most economical strategy would be angiography alone. However, since there is a general aversion to this invasive test, we opted for a combination of non-invasive and invasive diagnostic techniques. US was highly cost-effective, but had one main drawback: Physicians had to start testing patients' legs when the presenting symptom was chest discomfort. However, the strategy that employed both lung scintigraphy and US before pulmonary angiography reduced the number of patients requiring the invasive procedure by 20%. However,

Table 13.2. Mortality per 1000 patients and costs as compared to the natural history of pulmonary embolism

Strategy	Mortality per 1000 patients	Costs (ECU, millions)
Natural history	78.1	0
P-SCT-A[a]	8.0	1.32
PV-US-A[b]	8.3	1.29
Perfusion scan, treat if abnormal	8.3	1.96
Treat everyone	8.5	2.16
Angiography, treat if abnormal	9.0	1.20
Spiral CT, treat if abnormal	22.0	0.76
PV scan, treat if high probability	46.0	0.47

[a] Perfusion scan, followed by spiral CT if perfusion scan is abnormal, followed by angiography if spiral CT does not show PE. Treatment of patients with either an abnormal spiral CT or angiogram.

[b] Perfusion/ventilation scan, followed by ultrasonography if non-high-probability scan result is obtained, followed by angiography if a normal ultrasound test is obtained. Treatment of patients with either a high-probability lung scan or an abnormal ultrasound test or an abnormal angiogram (Dutch consensus strategy).

the strategy combining perfusion scanning, spiral CT and angiography further reduced mortality and appeared almost as cost-effective as the Dutch consensus strategy [61].

A study performed by Van Erkel et al. [62] concluded that all of the best strategies included spiral CT; furthermore, in their analysis, algorithms including pulmonary angiography also yielded a lower mortality, but no superior cost-effectiveness [62].

13.8 Conclusion

Any cost-effectiveness analysis based on the literature is up to date for a limited period. Newer approaches become available, such as the introduction of clinical decision rules or new management strategies that incorporate non-invasive techniques, e.g. serial tests for deep vein thrombosis or plasma D-dimer concentration measurement. Furthermore, newer imaging techniques are under evaluation that may (partly) replace lung scintigraphy and/or pulmonary angiography, such as electron beam tomography and magnetic resonance imaging angiography. Although these techniques are promising, management studies using long-term follow-up to demonstrate their safety for the exclusion of PE have yet to be performed.

The use of an extensive strategy employing lung scintigraphy, B-mode US, pulmonary angiography or a strategy combining perfusing scanning, spiral CT and pulmonary angiography are the best strategies available for the diagnostic management of patients with suspected PE. The implementation of a spiral CT strategy without conventional pulmonary angiography should be avoided.

References

1. Gjöres JE (1988) The incidence of venous thrombosis and its sequelae in certain districts of Sweden. Acta Chir Scand 1956 [Suppl 206]:1–88
2. Anderson Jr FA, Wheeler HB, Goldberg RJ et al (1991) A population-based perspective of the hospital incidence and case-fatality rates of deep vein thrombosis and pulmonary embolism. The Worcester DVT study. Arch Intern Med 151:933–938
3. Robin ED (1977) Overdiagnosis and overtreatment of pulmonary embolism: the emperor may have no clothes. Ann Intern Med 87:775–781
4. Stein PD, Alavi A, Gottschalk A et al (1991) Usefulness of noninvasive tools for diagnosis of acute pulmonary embolism in patients with a normal chest radiograph. Am J Cardiol 67: 1117–1120
5. Hull RD, Raskob GE, Coates G et al (1991) Low-probability lung scan findings: a need for change. Ann Intern Med 114:142–143
6. Oudkerk M, van Beek EJR, van Putten WLJ, Büller HR (1993) Cost-effectiveness analysis of various strategies in the diagnostic management of pulmonary embolism. Arch Intern Med 153:947–954
7. Stein PD, Hull RD, Saltzman HA, Pineo G (1993) Strategy for diagnosis of patients with suspected acute pulmonary embolism. Chest 103:1553–1559
8. Kelley MA et al (1991) Diagnosing pulmonary embolism: new facts and strategies. Ann Intern Med 114:300–306
9. Palevsky HI et al (1991) A noninvasive strategy for the management of patients suspected of pulmonary embolism. Semin Nucl Med 21:325–331
10. Gurney JW et al (1993) No fooling around: direct visualisation of pumonary embolism. Radiology 188:618–619

11. Henschke CI et al (1994) Evaluation of competing tests for the diagnosis of pulmonary embolism in deep venous thrombosis. Clin Imaging 18:241–254
12. Hull RD et al (1994) A noninvasive strategy for the treatment of patients with suspected pulmonary embolism. Arch Intern Med 154:289–297
13. Hyers TH (1995) Diagnosis of pulmonary embolism. Thorax 50:930–932
14. Henschke CI et al (1995) Changing practice patterns in the work up of pulmonary embolism. Chest 107:940–945
15. Matsumoto AH et al (1995) Contemporary diagnostic approaches to acute pulmonary emboli. Rad Clin North Am 33:167–184
16. Rosenow EC et al (1995) Venous and pulmonary thromboembolism: an algorithmic approach to diagnosis and management. Mayo Clin Proc 70:45–49
17. Goodman LR et al (1996) Diagnosis of acute pulmonary embolism: time for a new approach. Radiology 199:25–27
18. Tapson VF et al (1997) Pulmonary embolism – new diagnostic approaches. New Engl J Med 336:1449–1451
19. Dalen JE, Alpert JS (1975) Natural history of pulmonary embolism. Progr Cardiovasc Dis 17: 259–270
20. Barritt DW, Jordan SC (1960) Anticoagulant drugs in the treatment of pulmonary embolism: a controlled study. Lancet i:1309–1312
21. Gallus A, Tillett J, Jackson J, Mills W, Wycherley A (1986) Safety and efficacy of warfarin started early after submassive venous thrombosis or pulmonary embolism. Lancet ii: 1293–1296
22. Hull R, Delmore T, Genton E et al (1970) Warfarin-sodium versus low-dose heparin in the long-term treatment of venous thrombosis. N Engl J Med 301:855–858
23. Huisman MV, Büller HR, ten Cate JW, Vreeken J (1986) Serial impedance plethysmography for suspected deep venous thrombosis in outpatients. N Engl J Med 314:823–828
24. Hull R, Hirsh J, Jay R et al (1982) Different intensities of oral anticoagulant therapy in the treatment of proximal vein thrombosis. N Engl J Med 307:1676–1681
25. Levine MN, Raskob G, Hirsh J (1989) Haemorrhagic complications of long-term anticoagulant therapy. Chest 95 [Suppl]:26–36
26. Hirsh J (1991) Heparin. N Engl J Med 324:1565–1574
27. Hirsh J (1991) Oral anticoagulant drugs. N Engl J Med 324:1865–1875
28. Van der Meer FJM, Rosendaal FR, Vandenbroucke JP, Briët E (1993) Bleeding complications in oral anticoagulant therapy. An analysis of risk factors. Arch Int Med 1993; 153: 1557–1562
29. The PIOPED Investigators (1990) Value of ventilation/perfusion scan in acute pulmonary embolism: results of the prospective investigation of pulmonary embolism diagnosis (PIOPED). JAMA 263:2753–2759
30. Biello DR, Mattar AG, McKnight RC, Siegel BA (1979) Ventilation-perfusion studies in suspected pulmonary embolism. Am J Roentgenol 133:1033–1037
31. McNeil BJ (1980) Ventilation-perfusion studies and the diagnosis of pulmonary embolism: concise communication. J Nucl Med 21:319–323
32. Hull RD, Raskob GE, Coates G, Panju AA, Gill GJ (1989) A new noninvasive management strategy for patients with suspected pulmonary embolism. Arch Intern Med 149:2549–2555
33. Moser KM (1990) Venous thromboembolism. Am Rev Respir Dis 141:235–249
34. Stein PD, Willis III PW, DeMets DL (1981) History and physical examination in acute pulmonary embolism in patients without preexisting cardiac or pulmonary disease. Am J Cardiol 47:218–223
35. Stein PD, Alavi A, Gottschalk A et al (1991) Usefulness of noninvasive diagnostic tools for diagnosis of acute pulmonary embolism in patients with a normal chest radiograph. Am J Cardiol 67:117–1120
36. Stein PD, Terrin ML, Hales CA et al (1991) Clinical, laboratory, roentgenographic, electrocardiographic findings in patients with acute pulmonary embolism and no pre-existing cardiac or pulmonary disease. Chest 100:598–603
37. Quinn MF, Lundell CJ, Klotz TA et al (1987) Reliability of selective pulmonary arteriography in the diagnosis of pulmonary embolism. Am J Radiol 149:469–471
38. Van Beek EJR, Bakker AJ, Reekers JA (1996) Interobserver variability of pulmonary angiography in patients with non-diagnostic lung scan results: conventional versus digital subtraction angiography. Radiology 198:721–724
39. Novelline RA, Galtarowich OH, Athanasoulis CA et al (1978) The clinical course of patients with suspected pulmonary embolism and a negat0ive pulmonary arteriogram. Radiology 126:561–567
40. Hull RD, Raskob GE, Carter CJ et al (1988) Pulmonary embolism in outpatients with pleuritic chest pain. Arch Intern Med 148:838–844

41. Stein PD, Athanasoulis CA, Alavi A et al (1992) Complications and validity of pulmonary angiography in acute pulmonary embolism. Circulation 85:462–468
42. Dalen JE, Brooks HL, Johnson LW et al (1971) Pulmonary angiography in acute pulmonary embolism: indications, techniques, and results in 367 patients. Am Heart J 81:175–185
43. Mills SR, Jackson DC, Older RA et al (1980) The incidence, etiologies, and avoidance of complications of pulmonary angiography in a large series. Radiology 136:299
44. Hudson ER, Smith RP, McDermott VG et al (1996) Pulmonary angiography performed with iopamidol: complications in 1434 patients. Radiology 198:61–65
45. Wallis JW, van Beek EJR, Reekers JA, van Rooy WJJ, Oudkerk M (1997) Terughoudendheid ten aanzien van pulmonalis angiografie bij longembolie niet terecht. Ned Tijdschr Geneesk 141:578–581
46. Kipper MS, Moser KM, Kortman KE, Ashburn WL (1982) Longterm follow-up of patients with suspected pulmonary embolism and a normal lung scan. Chest 82:411–415
47. Hull RD, Raskob GE, Coates G, Panju AA (1990) Clinical validity of a normal perfusion lung scan in patients with suspected pulmonary embolism. Chest 97:23–26
48. Hull RD, Hirsh J, Carter CJ et al (1983) Pulmonary angiography, ventilation lung scanning, and venography for clinically suspected pulmonary embolism with abnormal perfusion lung scan. Ann Intern Med 98:891–899
49. Van Beek EJR, Tiel-van Buul MMC, Büller HR, van Royen EA, ten Cate JW (1993) The value of lung scintigraphy in the diagnosis of pulmonary embolism. Eur J Nucl Med 20:173–181
50. Kruit WHJ, de Boer AC, Sing AK, van Roon F (1991) The significance of venography in the management of patients with clinically suspected pulmonary embolism. J Intern Med 230: 333–339
51. Ferris 13 (1983) Deep venous thrombosis and pulmonary embolism: correlative evaluation. Int Angiol 2:85–98
52. Heyboer H, Büller HR, Lensing AWA, Turpie AG, Colly LP, ten Cate JW (1993) A comparison of real-time compression ultrasonography with impedance plethysmography for the diagnosis of deep-vein thrombosis in symptomatic outpatients. N Engl J Med 329:1365–1369
53. Lensing AWA, Prandoni P, Brandjes DPM et al (1989) Detection of deep-vein thrombosis by real-time B-mode ultrasonography. N Engl J Med 320:342–345
54. Goodman LR et al (1995) Detection of pulmonary embolism in patients with unresolved clinical and scintigraphic diagnosis: helical CT vs angiography. Am J Roentgenol 164: 1369–1374
55. Remy Jardin M et al (1992) Central pulmonary thromboembolism: diagnosis with spiral volumetric CT with the single breath hold technique; comparison with pulmonary angiography. Radiology 185:381–387
56. Remy-Jardin M et al (1996) Diagnosis of pulmonary embolism with spiral CT: comparison with pulmonary angiography and scintigraphy. Radiology 200:699–706
57. Rossum AB van et al (1996) Pulmonary embolus: validation of spiral CTA in 149 patients. Radiology 201:467–470
58. Rossum AB van et al (1996) Role of spiral volumetric CT in the assessment of patients with clinical suspicion of pulmonary embolism and an abnormal VQ lung scan. Thorax 51:23–28
59. Mayo JR et al (1997) Pulmonary embolism: prospective comparison of helical CT with ventilation/perfusion scintigraphy. Radiology 205:447–452
60. Ferretti GR et al (1997) Acute pulmonary embolism: role of helical CT in 164 patients with intermediate probability at ventilation/perfusion scintigraphy and normal results and dvt-US. Radiology 205:453–458
61. Briët E, Beek EJR van, Oudkerk M (1993) Consensus diagnostiek longembolie. Ned Tijdschr Geneesk 137(5):225–259
62. Erkel AR van et al (1996) Spiral CT angiography for suspected pulmonary embolism: a cost-effectiveness analysis. Radiology 201:29–36

14 Helical CT in the Pediatric Chest

M. J. Siegel

14.1 Introduction

Helical computed tomography (CT) has a number of advantages in pediatric patients [1–4]. First, the retrospective reconstruction capabilities afforded by helical CT can improve lesion detection without increasing radiation exposure. Second, the relatively shorter scanning time has the potential to eliminate or at least minimize motion artifacts, decrease the need for sedation, and optimize contrast enhancement. Third, the absence or reduction of motion artifacts allows high-quality two- and three-dimensional reconstructions.

14.2 Technique

14.2.1 Sedation

Even though imaging time is shorter with helical CT, image degradation by patient motion still remains a problem in young children. Children under 5 years of age usually require parenteral sedation. The drugs most commonly used in this age-group are oral chloral hydrate and intravenous pentobarbital sodium [5]. Children under 18 months of age usually receive oral chloral hydrate, 50–100 mg/kg to a maximum dosage of 2000 mg. Patients 18 months of age and older are given intravenous pentobarbital sodium, 6 mg/kg up to a maximum dose of 200 mg, in small increments. Regardless of the choice of drug, the use of parenteral sedation necessitates continuous monitoring and maintaining adequate cardiorespiratory support during and after the procedure.

When sedation is needed, the child should receive no solid foods for 6 h and no liquids for 3 h prior to the study. Children who are not to be sedated should be given nothing by mouth for 3 h prior to the examination. This precaution is taken to reduce the risk of aspiration if nausea and vomiting occur during administration of intravenous contrast material.

Children older than 5 years of age usually will cooperate for CT studies after verbal reassurance and explanation of the procedure. The presence of a parent in the CT suite during the study is helpful to reassure and comfort the child.

14.2.2 Intravenous Contrast Medium

Nearly all CT examinations of the chest are performed with intravenous contrast material. If contrast material is to be given, an intravenous catheter should be in place when the child arrives in the CT suite. This avoids the agitation, and consequent patient motion, that would otherwise be associated with venipuncture performed immediately prior to administering contrast material. The gauge of butterfly needle or intravenous cannula will vary with patient size, but the largest possible one should be placed.

If intravenous access is through a butterfly needle or central venous catheter, hand injection of contrast medium is recommended. A power injector is used in children who have antecubital cannulas (22 gauge or larger) in place [2, 3, 6]. The rate of contrast injection is determined by the size of the catheter (Table 14.1). During the initial seconds of injection, the injection site should be carefully monitored for contrast extravasation. With appropriate selection of injection rates and patient monitoring, the use of a power injector is safe in children. Either low-osmolar (280–320 mgI/ml) or high-osmolar (282 mgI/ml) contrast media can be used for CT examinations. The usual dose of contrast medium is 2 ml/kg up to a maximum of 4 ml/kg or 150 ml.

Optimal enhancement is a result of the rate of contrast administration, the total volume of contrast, and the timing between the injection of contrast and the onset of scanning. In children who weigh less than 45 kg, the initiation of scanning should begin after 80% of the contrast medium has been administered, whether contrast agent is administered by hand or by power injection. Adult protocols can be used for larger children (>45 kg). Alternatively, an automated bolus tracking technique can be used to monitor contrast enhancement and initiate scanning.

14.2.3 Specific Technical Options

Helical CT scanning requires prescribing a number of parameters, including scan time duration, table feed speed (distance to be covered), slice thickness (resolution required), and reconstruction interval. These factors need to be selected according to patient size and clinical indication.

Two protocols usually suffice for most chest imaging. When a large area of the chest is to be scanned, such as a screening examination of the lungs or mediastinum, the following parameters are useful: 8–10 mm slice thickness, 8–10 mm/s table speed, pitch of 1–1.5, standard algorithm, and reconstruction of overlapping slices every 4–5 mm (Table 14.2).

Table 14.1. Rate of contrast injection versus needle size

Needle size (G)	Flow rate (ml/s)
22	1.2–1.5
20	1.5–2.0
18	2.0–3.0

Table 14.2. Protocol for pulmonary parenchymal disease

Indication	Survey examination of mediastinum and lungs (mediastinal tumor; vascular anomalies; trauma, suspected metastatic disease
Extent	Lung apices to caudal bases
Scanner settings	120 kVp, 170 mAs
Duration of exposure	Single helical scan: time dependent on patient size
Pitch	1.0–1.5
Collimation	4–8 mm
Patient instructions	Suspended inspiration
Contrast type	LOCM 280–320 mg iodine/ml or HOCM 282 mg iodine/ml (60% solution)
Contrast volume	2 ml/kg to maximum of 4 ml/kg (150 ml, maximum)
Contrast injection rate	Dependent on needle size and method of injection
Reconstruction interval	4–8 mm (contiguous scans)
Miscellaneous	1. If the child is sedated or uncooperative, CT scans are obtained at quite breathing 2. Contrast not required for evaluation of lung metastases 3. Slice thickness dependent on size of the patient; thinner 4 mm contiguous scans can be used in smaller patients 4. When both chest and abdomen are to be examined, the abdomen should be scanned first. Two-thirds of contrast volume should be given in the abdomen and one-third in the chest

When finer-detail and higher-resolution images are required over a smaller distance, such as the evaluation of lung masses or nodules or the tracheobronchial tree, the following parameters are suggested: 2–4 mm slice thickness, 2–4 mm/s table speed, pitch of 1, high-resolution algorithm, and reconstruction of overlapping slices every 1–2 mm (Table 14.3). Increasing the pitch (> 1) by the use of 2-mm-thick sections and a table feed of 4 mm/s may help to minimize motion artifacts in children who are unable to cooperate with breath-holding instructions. Two-dimensional and three-dimensional reconstructions are useful in the evaluation of airway abnormalities and peridiaphragmatic lesions.

CT sections are obtained with breath-holding at suspended inspiration in cooperative patients, usually children over 6 years of age. A single breath-hold technique is recommended over the multiple breath-hold technique (i.e., 10–15 s breath-holds with 10-s intergroup delays). The advantage of the multiple breath-holding technique is that it is more easily tolerated, but the disadvantage is the potential for anatomic misregistration between adjacent helical acquisitions. Scans are obtained during quiet respiration in children who are unable to cooperate with breath-holding instructions.

14.3 Applications of Thoracic Helical CT

Indications for helical CT of the chest in children include: (a) detection of occult pulmonary parenchymal disease, (b) characterization of focal parenchymal masses, (c) assessment of congenital or acquired tracheobronchial tree abnormalities, and (d) characterization of suspected or known mediastinal mass or great vessel anomalies.

Table 14.3. Protocol for focal mass characterization

Indication	Fine detailed technique (characterization of focal mass or abnormality of the tracheobronchial tree)
Extent	Through area of interest
Scanner settings	120 kVp, 170 mAs
Duration of exposure	Single helical scan: time dependent on patient size
Pitch	1.0–1.5
Collimation	2–4 mm
Patient instructions	Suspended inspiration
Contrast type	LOCM 280–320 mg iodine/ml or HOCM 282 mg iodine/ml (60% solution)
Contrast volume	2 ml/kg to maximum of 4 ml/kg (150 ml, maximum)
Reconstruction interval	1–2 mm
Miscellaneous	1. If the child is sedated or uncooperative, CT scans are obtained at quite breathing 2. High spatial resolution reconstruction (bone) algorithm useful in airway evaluation 3. Multiplanar reconstructions useful for evaluation of tracheobronchial tree and peridiaphragmatic area 4. Increased pitch (>1) may help to minimize staircasing artifacts 5. If bronchiectasis or other small airway disease is suspected on the screening CT, thinly collimated scans in inspiration and expiration should be obtained through the area of abnormality

14.3.1 Pulmonary Parenchymal Disease (Table 14.2)

CT scanning has become the established method for detecting and characterizing pulmonary nodules in children with known malignancies which have a high propensity for pulmonary dissemination. Demonstration of a pulmonary nodule or nodules may lead to additional treatment (surgery, chemotherapy, or radiation). Conventional CT has high sensitivity for identifying pulmonary nodules, but false-negative studies can result from variations in the depth of patient respiration or volume averaging. By enabling contiguous volumetric data acquisition and overlapping reconstructions, helical CT eliminates or minimizes these problems [7, 8], even in small children who are scanned during quiet breathing.

Small overlapping reconstructions (2–4 mm) should be used to confirm a nodule suspected on standard images and for cases requiring densitometry. To increase the accuracy of densitometry, the section thickness should be at least one half of the diameter of the nodule.

14.3.2 Focal Mass Characterization (Table 14.3)

The overlapping volumetric data and multiplanar images created during helical CT are useful to delineate the anatomy of complex congenital lesions (arteriovenous malformations and pulmonary sequestrations) and clarify the relationship of a lesion or nodule to the pleura or to the diaphragm [9]. Two- and

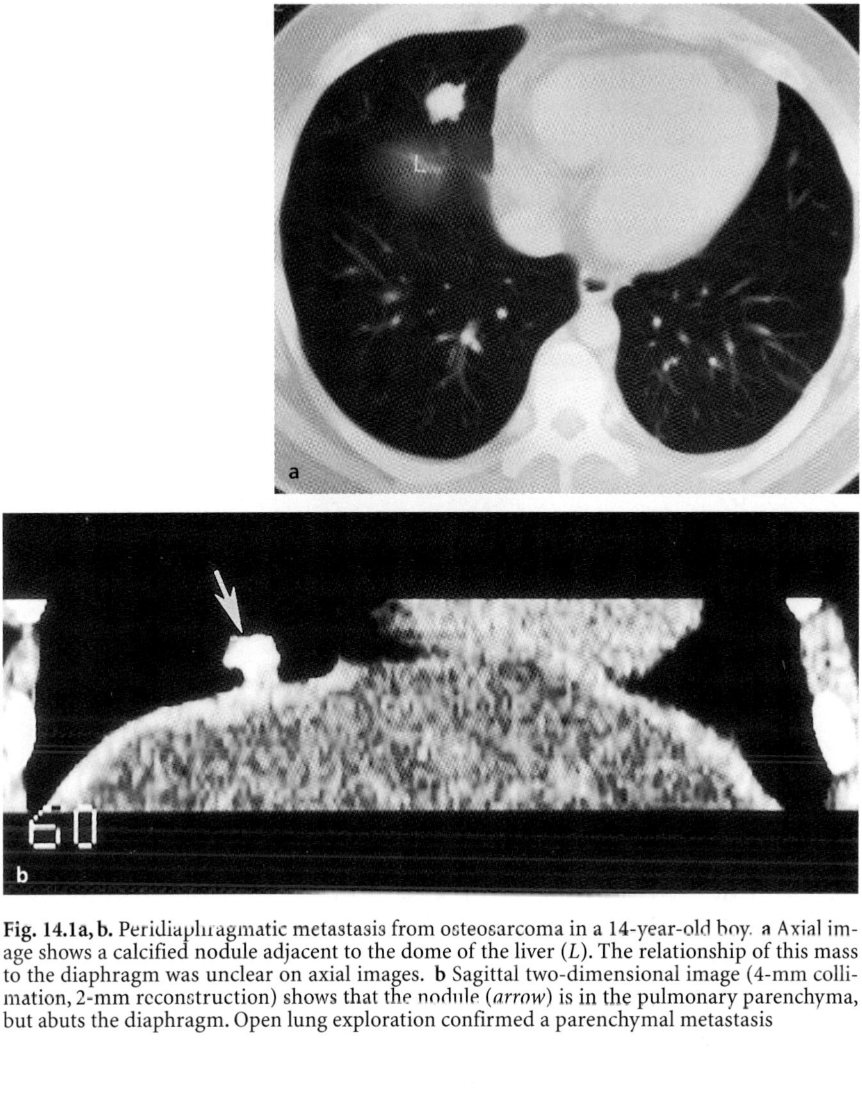

Fig. 14.1a, b. Peridiaphragmatic metastasis from osteosarcoma in a 14-year-old boy. **a** Axial image shows a calcified nodule adjacent to the dome of the liver (*L*). The relationship of this mass to the diaphragm was unclear on axial images. **b** Sagittal two-dimensional image (4-mm collimation, 2-mm reconstruction) shows that the nodule (*arrow*) is in the pulmonary parenchyma, but abuts the diaphragm. Open lung exploration confirmed a parenchymal metastasis

three-dimensional reconstructions in coronal and sagittal planes are particularly helpful in characterizing a lesion as intraparenchymal or pleural based (Fig. 14.1).

14.3.3 Tracheobronchial Tree Assessment (Table 14.3)

The tracheobronchial tree includes the trachea, carina, mainstem bronchi, and the lobar and segmental bronchi. These structures are easily definable with helical CT. Common indications prompting CT of the airway are: (a) evaluation of congenital anomalies, (b) detection of post-transplantation complications, and (c) identification of bronchiectasis and small airway disease [10, 11]. By comparison with adults, neoplasia is a rare indication for helical CT of the airway in children. Airway assessment requires a table speed sufficient to allow coverage of the entire trachea and proximal subsegmental bronchi.

The contiguous data set afforded by helical CT allows identification of virtually all normal segmental bronchi, especially when scans are obtained during suspended inspiration. As a result, detection of congenital anomalies is improved. Clinically important congenital anomalies include ectopic bronchi (tracheal

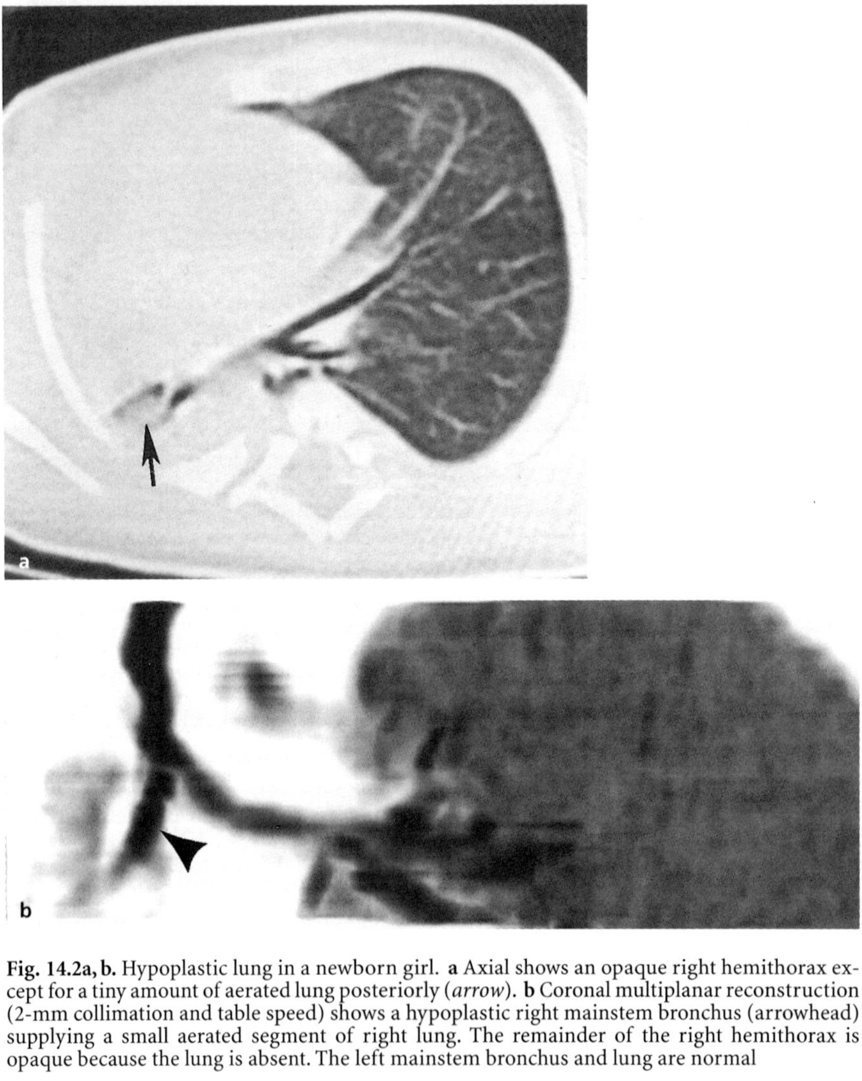

Fig. 14.2a, b. Hypoplastic lung in a newborn girl. **a** Axial shows an opaque right hemithorax except for a tiny amount of aerated lung posteriorly (*arrow*). **b** Coronal multiplanar reconstruction (2-mm collimation and table speed) shows a hypoplastic right mainstem bronchus (arrowhead) supplying a small aerated segment of right lung. The remainder of the right hemithorax is opaque because the lung is absent. The left mainstem bronchus and lung are normal

bronchus), supernumerary bronchi (cardiac bronchus), and hypoplastic or absent bronchi (Fig. 14.2).

Postoperative complications, such as small dehiscences and stenoses, which are not discernible on conventional CT, can be identified by helical CT. Thin-section axial and helical CT with multiplanar reconstructions each have a sensitivity of 90% for detecting stenoses. False-negative results are usually due to tracheomalacia. However, the extent of bronchial stenosis and extraluminal gas collections are shown best on two- or three-dimensional projections rotated to parallel the long axis of the trachea and bronchi (Fig. 14.3). Three-dimensional images can be viewed as a cine loop.

Dynamic imaging of the lungs with a series of helical CT scans during inhalation and exhalation is a useful technique to identify global or focal air-trapping associated with bronchiectasis and small airway abnormalities, such as bronchiolitis obliterans. It also has been used to quantitate the degree of tracheal collapse in patients with tracheomalacia. The faster scan times afforded by helical CT allow a comparison of identical levels without motion misregistration. When diffuse lung disease is suspected, scans are obtained with 1.5- to 2-mm collimation at three selected levels (the aortic arch, tracheal bifurcation, and lung bases) in forced inspiration and expiration. If focal disease (i.e., bronchiectasis, cystic disease) is suspected on the basis of the screening CT, thinly collimated scans in inspiration and expiration can be limited to the area of abnormality. Attenuation

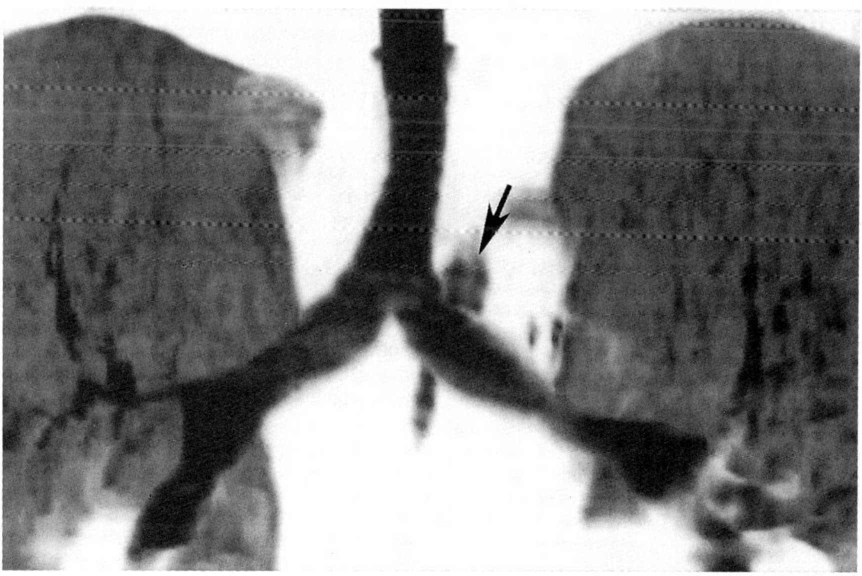

Fig. 14.3. Bronchial dehiscence in a 3-year-old recipient of a double lung transplant, non-breath-holder. Coronal multiplanar image (4-mm collimation and table speed, 2-mm reconstruction) shows an extraluminal gas collection (*arrow*) immediately adjacent to the anastomosis of the left mainstem bronchus with the trachea

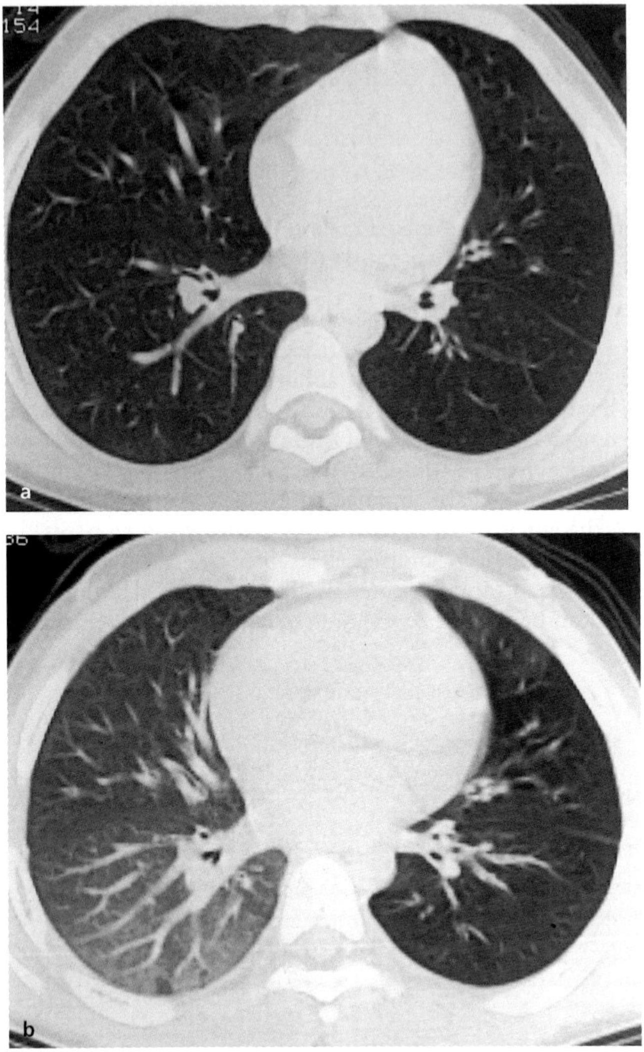

Fig. 14.4a, b. Swyer-James syndrome (acquired pulmonary hypoplasia) in a 9-year-old boy. **a** Inspiration CT through the lung bases shows a small left lung with attenuated vessels. **b** On expiration, the left lung is hypodense compared with the right lung, reflecting the presence of air trapping

values are then measured with region-of-interest cursors placed in the periphery of the lung. The mean attenuation value of normal lung increases homogeneously during exhalation, whereas in patients with air-trapping, mean lung attenuation value decreases with exhalation (Fig. 14.4). Air trapping is a better predictor of airway disease than either mosaic perfusion or bronchiectasis.

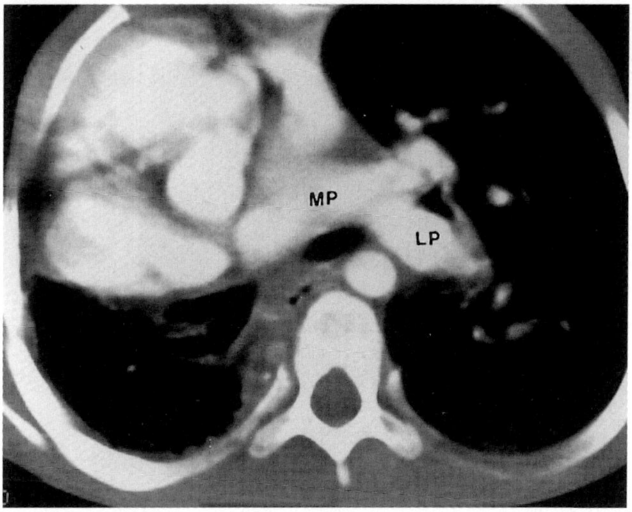

Fig. 14.5. Hypoplastic right lung and pulmonary artery in a 10-year-old boy. Contrast-enhanced scan (8-mm thickness and table speed) at the level of the pulmonary hila demonstrates excellent opacification of the main pulmonary artery (*MP*) and left pulmonary artery (*LP*). There is no right pulmonary artery seen

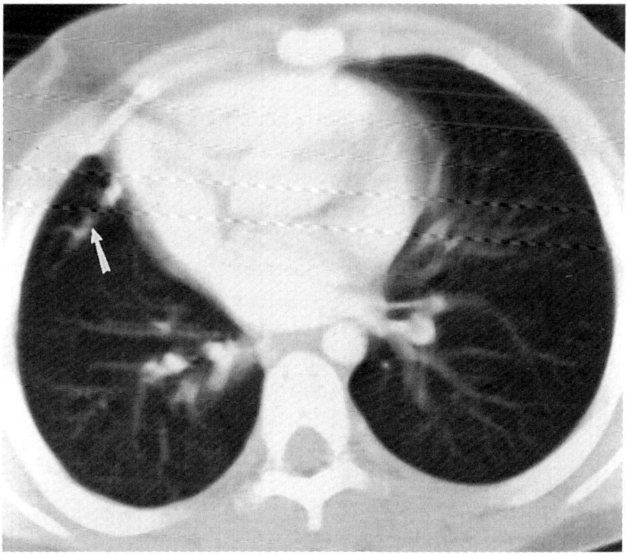

Fig. 14.6. Scimitar syndrome in a 2-year-old girl. Axial CT (4-mm thickness and table speed, 2-mm reconstruction) shows dextrocardia, a small right lung, and an anomalous right pulmonary vein (*arrow*) draining into the right atrium

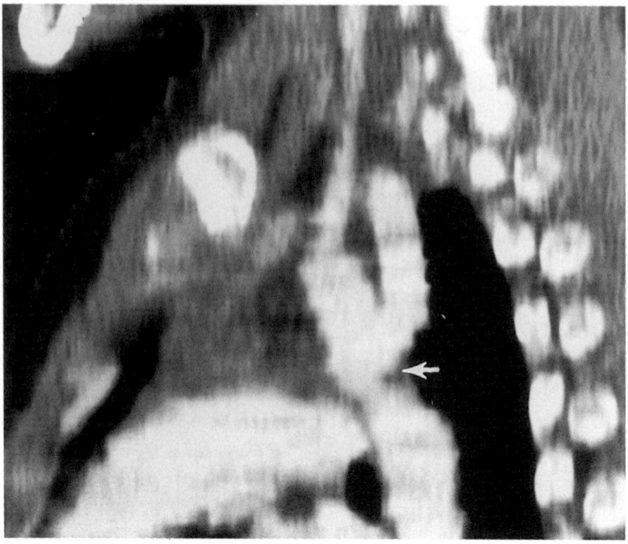

Fig. 14.7. Aortic coarctation in a 13-year-old boy. Sagittal two-dimensional reconstruction (4-mm thickness and table speed, reconstruction) shows a focal, high-grade constriction (*arrow*) in the descending aorta just below the level of the great vessels

14.3.4 Mediastinal Survey (Table 14.2)

Frequent indications for mediastinal and hilar CT include (a) identification of vascular anomalies and (b) determination of tumor extent. Axial images provide most of the pertinent information, but multiplanar images are occasionally helpful for clarifying the anatomy of complex vascular lesions.

A number of congenital abnormalities can affect the aorta, superior vena cava, and pulmonary arteries. Absence, hypoplasia, and abnormal position and origin of the great vessels are easily identified with helical CT following administration of intravenous contrast medium (Figs. 14.5–14.7).

The capabilities for retrospective reconstructions and more consistent precise delivery of contrast medium improve detection of mediastinal infiltration, vascular occlusion or encasement, and lymph node enlargement. Helical CT is particularly valuable in detecting nodal enlargement which otherwise might be missed by conventional CT. The resultant information can facilitate surgical planning or radiation therapy.

References

1. Frush DP, Siegel MJ, Bisset GS (1997) Challenges of pediatric spiral CT. RadioGraphics 17: 939–959
2. Siegel MJ, Luker GD (1995) Pediatric applications of helical (helical) CT. Radiol Clin North Am 33:997–1022

3. Siegel MJ (1998) Pediatric helical techniques. In: Silverman P (ed) Helical (spiral) computed tomography: a practical approach to clinical practice. Lippincott-Raven, Philadelphia (in press)
4. White KS (1996) Helical/helical CT scanning: a pediatric radiology perspective. Pediatr Radiol 26:5–14
5. Frush DP, Bisset GS III, Hall SC (1996) Pediatric sedation in radiology: the practice of safe sleep. AJR 167:1381–1387
6. Kaste SC, Young CW (1995) Safe use of power injectors with central and peripheral venous access devices for pediatric CT. Pediatr Radiol 26:499–501
7. Remy-Jardin M, Remy J, Giraud F, Marquette CH (1993) Pulmonary nodules: detection with thick-section helical CT versus conventional CT. Radiology 187:513–520
8. Wright AR, Collie DA, Williams JR, Hasemi-Malayeri B, Stevenson AJM, Turnbull CM (1996) Pulmonary nodules: effect on detection of helical CT pitch. Radiology 199:837–841
9. Brink JA, Heiken JP, Semenkovich J, Teefey SA, McClennan BL, Sagel SS (1994) Abnormalities of the diaphragm and adjacent structures; findings on multiplanar helical CT scans. AJR 163 :307–310
10. Lucidarme O, Greneir P, Cocke E, Lenoir S, Aubert B, Beigelman C (1996) Bronchiectasis: comparative assessment with thin-section CT and helical CT. Radiology 200:673–679
11. Quint LE, Whyte RI, Kaserooni EA et al (1995) Stenosis of the central airways: evaluation by using helical CT with multiplanar reconstructions. Radiology 194:871–877

15 Cardiac CT with Prospective Cardiac Gating

R. A. Coulden, M. P. Hayball

15.1 Introduction

CT has revolutionised body imaging over the past 20 years but has had surprisingly little impact on cardiac diagnosis. Acquisition times are long relative to the length of the cardiac cycle, with motion reconstruction artefacts severely degrading image quality. Despite progressive reductions in exposure time and the development of slip ring technology, the potential for anatomical and functional imaging of the heart has never been fully realised.

Recognising that faster data acquisition was the key to cardiac CT, Boyd et al. developed an electron beam CT (EBCT) scanner specifically designed for cardiac imaging [1].

To overcome the limitations of conventional third-generation systems the rotating X-ray tube and detector array are replaced with fixed target and detector rings encircling the patient. With no moving parts, images can be acquired in as little as 50 ms with up to 17 images per second at one location. Combining rapid imaging with ECG triggering makes three operating modes possible: (a) sequential scanning to give a series of contiguous slices all obtained at the same point in the cardiac cycle, (b) multiple images at one level throughout the cardiac cycle (cine imaging), and (c) repeated imaging at the same level at the same point in the cardiac cycle. The three modes are used to assess cardiac anatomy, ventricular wall motion and myocardial perfusion, respectively.

Since its development 10 years ago a substantial body of literature has grown up around the use of EBCT in the heart. It has been widely used in assessing coronary artery and valve calcification [2], delineating pericardial and intra-cardiac masses, and measuring ventricular function [3], muscle mass [4], intra-cardiac shunts and myocardial perfusion [5]. EBCT is a powerful investigative tool, but it also has serious drawbacks. Poor contrast resolution and non-uniform slice width across the field of view make it inferior to conventional CT for applications outside the heart. It has therefore never been widely adopted. The case for faster scanning and cardiac CT in general, however, has been established.

Cardiac motion for the purposes of transaxial imaging can be considered in two planes, in-plane and through-plane. In-plane motion causes streak artefact and blurring on the reconstructed image whereas through-plane motion leads to misregistration. Through-plane motion is generally an order of magnitude greater than in-plane motion. Figure 15.1 shows the relationship between left ventricular wall motion as demonstrated by M mode echocardiography and the ECG. Following early diastole when there is rapid ventricular dilatation, there is a peri-

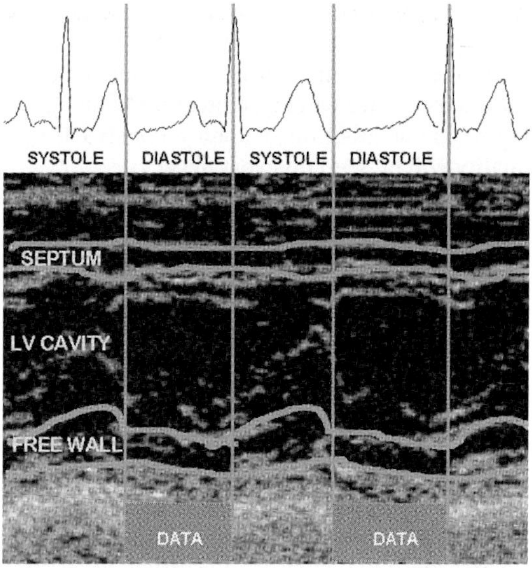

Fig. 15.1. M-mode echocardiogram showing relationship between ECG, systole and diastole. *Grey*, highlighted myocardial borders. There is relatively little motion of the endocardium during diastole compared with systole

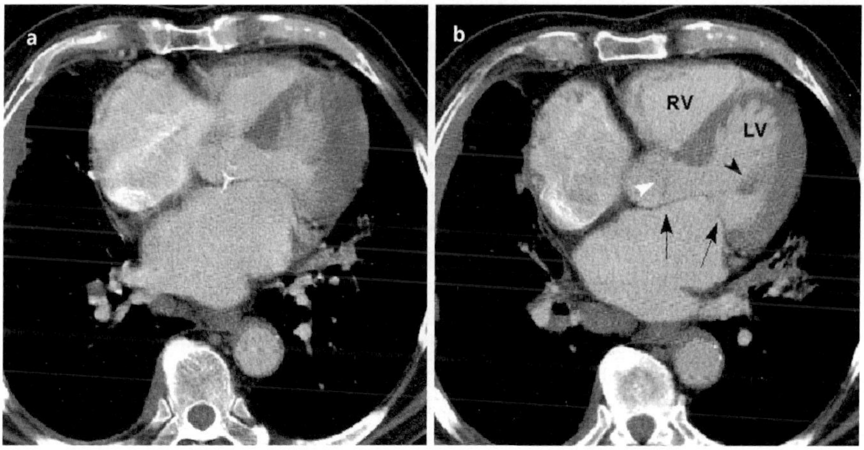

Fig. 15.2a, b. Two consecutive 750 ms slices through the left ventricle in a patient with a heart rate of 50 bpm. **a** Systolic acquisition. **b** Diastolic acquisition. Timing was by chance. **b** Improvement in delineation of the endocardium and subvalvar apparatus (*black arrowhead*). Aortic valve (*white arrowhead*) and mitral valve leaflets (*black arrows*) are also shown

od of slow filling with relatively little motion. While this is of variable length and can alter substantially with heart rate, it does offer a data acquisition window relatively free from motion.

The development of conventional CT systems with sub-second rotation times has renewed interest in cardiac CT, giving us the chance to exploit this 'quiet' period for the first time. Considering subjects with a bradycardia (i.e. heart rate 50 bpm) the R-R interval or cardiac cycle length is 1200 ms; a 750 ms acquisition is far shorter than the cardiac cycle length and occasionally chances into this quiet period. Figure 15.2 presents an example of such an occurrence where marked improvement in intra-cardiac detail can be seen when compared with the adjacent slice which was acquired during systole. By applying cardiac triggering to the acquisition or data reconstruction the same improvement in image quality will be seen on every slice.

Many manufacturers have developed reconstruction algorithms which use data from a partial rotation allowing an even shorter data acquisition time. The minimum rotation required to reconstruct a single slice depends on the fan beam geometry of the individual scanner. For the SOMATOM Plus 4A this represents a 240° arc equivalent to an exposure time of 500 ms. We describe our experience of partial rotation reconstruction and diastolic image acquisition to the heart.

15.2 Principles of ECG-Triggered CT

The two main approaches to cardiac imaging using conventional CT are prospective triggering and retrospective reconstruction. Both aim to use data acquired during the 'quiet' part of the cardiac cycle. Prospective triggering involves data acquisition during a predetermined window in the cardiac cycle whereas retrospective reconstruction entails selective reconstruction of diastolic data from a continuous stream of data acquired in the normal way. For prospective triggering the subjects ECG is monitored and after a pre-defined delay following the onset of systole (as indicated by the R wave) the X-ray beam is switched on. Data acquisition must be complete before the next R wave. Success depends entirely on the accurate initiation of X-ray 'beam on' from an external signal. With this in place, implementation for single slice or sequential imaging is simple.

Retrospective triggering applies only to image reconstruction and requires no hardware modifications to control X-ray 'beam on'. Data acquisition is performed as normal but the subjects ECG is recorded throughout. Timing information from the ECG is then used to select appropriate 240° datasets collected during diastole. Systolic data is not used in the reconstructions representing unnecessary irradiation. Without prospective triggering data acquisition can start by chance at any time in the cardiac cycle. To ensure that sufficient diastolic data is available for reconstruction more than one rotation per slice is needed when cardiac cycle length is greater than 750 ms.

Application of both approaches is simplest for single-slice or sequential techniques but spiral imaging is also possible. As Fig. 15.3 shows, triggering leaves gaps in the data helix, which require complex interpolation before reconstruction can take place. The data gaps limit minimum reconstruction intervals, and a pitch of 1 or less is needed to reduce this effect.

15.3 Methods for ECG-Triggered CT

The following account relates to our experience of cardiac triggered CT using a SOMATOM Plus 4A (Siemens, Erlangen, Germany).

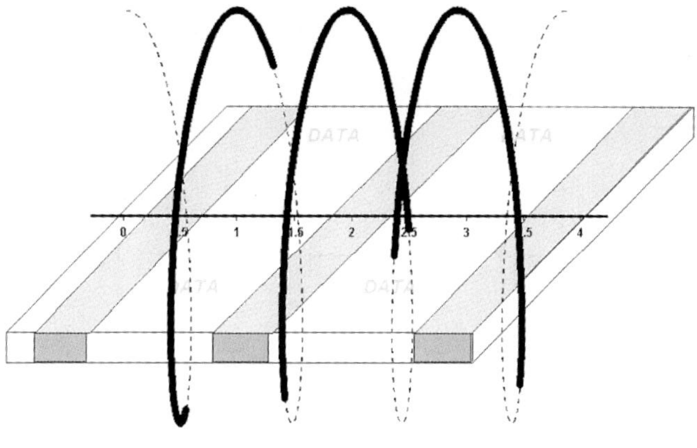

Fig. 15.3. Spiral data acquisition with ECG triggering showing data gaps occurring as a result of eliminated systolic data. This effect limits the minimum reconstruction interval to be equal to the table travel associated with one cardiac cycle

15.3.1 Prospective ECG Triggering

A 3-lead bedside ECG monitor with an analog output is attached to the patient. The ECG monitor output signal is digitised and processed in real time on a PC using custom-written 'in-house' software. The R wave peak is detected using a falling slope with magnitude threshold and applying a minimum R-R interval to avoid premature detection of large T-wave peaks. Following the detection of the R wave peak the PC waits for a user defined delay (t_{del}) before sending the trigger signal to the scanner. The CT scanner has been modified to respond to an external signal and switches the X-ray beam on within 20–50 ms of receiving the trigger. The time delay is selected to acquire the image during the phase of least cardiac motion, i.e. between the end of the T-wave and the start of the next R-wave (Fig. 15.4). Once the trigger delay has been selected, the ECG triggered option is

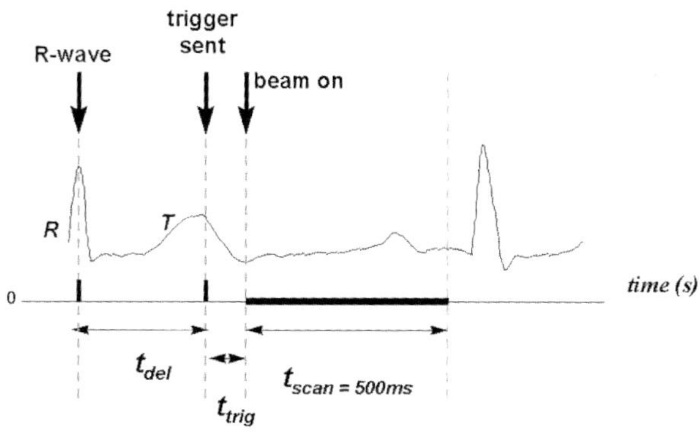

Fig. 15.4. ECG monitoring software detects the R wave and sends a trigger to the scanner to start acquisition after a predefined delay (t_{del}). This is chosen to coincide with diastole. There is a short systematic delay (t_{trig}) before the X-ray beam is switched on. Data acquisition is complete within 500 ms

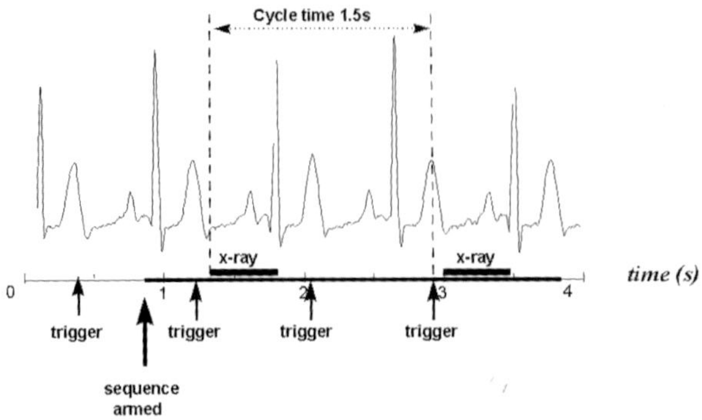

Fig. 15.5. The prospective triggering system sends a trigger signal to the scanner on every heart beat at the pre-set delay. The scanner, however, ignores this signal until 'armed' and then triggers on the first signal received after arming. In this sequence the table moves after each slice introducing a refractory period of 1.5 s before the scanner can respond to the next trigger. This results in data acquisition on alternate beats

selected on the CT console. A 750-ms rotation time with a 240° acquisition (500 ms exposure) is used with other imaging parameters selected to suit the application. Once the sequence is configured and the trigger mode is armed, exposures only occur in connection with the PC trigger signal. A light detector circuit positioned next to the 'beam on' warning light is fed back to the PC to verify acquisition timing

The minimum cycle time (start of image to start of next image) is 1.5 s with table motion between scans or 0.8 s without table motion. Figure 15.5 shows the trigger signal sent by the PC for every cardiac cycle. Before the sequence start, i.e. before the ECG trigger mode is armed, the trigger (a) is ignored. The first acquisition commences after the first trigger following the sequence start (b). Once the image is complete, the table moves and the scanner is refractory to further trigger signals for 1.5 s after the initial trigger. Hence in this example the trigger (c) after sequence start is ignored during the refractory period, and the second acquisition follows the trigger (d). With a heart rate of 75 bpm or less this results in imaging on every other beat. Without table motion the refractory period is 0.8 s, and imaging occurs on every beat.

15.3.2 Retrospective ECG Triggering

Using the same ECG monitoring system and PC processing as described above, the subject's ECG is recorded during conventional data acquisition. Retrospective partial rotation reconstruction is then applied to the resulting dataset. For a single slice this can be done arbitrarily by performing multiple 240° reconstructions at 0.1 s intervals and selecting the best, or by using cross-registration with the ECG and selecting a 240° dataset acquired during diastole. Partial rotation spiral reconstruction algorithms are available, but we have had little success to date in using them.

15.4 Applications

The value of ECG triggered conventional CT has yet to be established, but previous published experience with EBCT is an indication of its potential. Using sequential scanning and prospective triggering, we have already seen marked improvement in the demonstration of cardiac structure although intravenous contrast is needed to visualise cardiac chambers and subvalvar apparatus (Fig. 15.6). Using our current system, demonstration of normal valve leaflets is still often impossible, but diseased and immobile valves may be shown. Echocardiography, however, with its substantially faster imaging rate, is better suited to the investigation of valve disease; therefore CT is unlikely to have a significant role.

Diastolic chamber size and ventricular muscle thickness are well shown, but with present limitations on minimum exposure time there are no means for cine imaging. Ventricular function cannot be assessed. As prospective triggering allows for acquisition of contiguous slices in the same phase of the cardiac cycle, it may be possible to use a contrast enhanced block of data, covering the whole ventricle, to calculate muscle mass. This would entail planimetry of muscle area on each slice and the use of Simpson's rule as has been described for EBCT and MRI [6]. The use of ECG-triggered conventional CT in this way, however, has yet to be validated.

Conventional CT is already used in the assessment of masses involving the heart, but one would expect improvements in image quality with ECG triggered acquisition. Other modalities such as echocardiography and MRI, however, may be more appropriate. Some improvement should also be expected in imaging the pericardium in patients with suspected pericardial constriction.

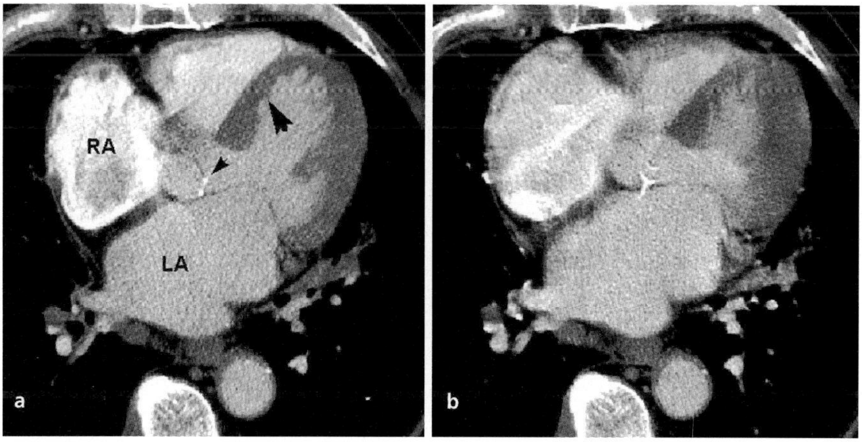

Fig. 15.6a, b. Two images through the left ventricle at the same slice position during intravenous contrast enhancement. **a** Prospectively ECG triggered. **b** Not prospectively ECG triggered. *Small arrow*, an area of aortic valve calcification; *large arrow*, improved endocardial definition

Coronary calcification is always associated with atheroma. Numerous reports using EBCT have shown that the total amount of coronary calcium (calcium score as proposed by Agaston et al. [7]) correlates well with the extent of the atheroma [8]. This in turn is a reliable indicator of risk for future cardiac ischaemic events. The presence of calcification irrespective of its severity at any one site is not correlated with the severity of stenosis at that site [9] and is not a predictor of future plaque rupture at that site.

The absence of coronary calcium is also important. In subjects with suspected ischaemic heart disease the absence of coronary calcification excludes significant disease. The evidence clearly shows coronary calcification to be an important indicator of disease, but only EBCT has been found to be a reliable and reproducible tool for quantification. A recent report using twin spiral CT suggests that conventional CT may be semi-quantitative [10], although accurate quantification requires shorter exposure times than used in that study. Our preliminary experience with prospective triggered CT is encouraging. Not only is coronary calcification reliably shown, but compared with non-triggered acquisitions, motion-related star and streak artefacts can be virtually eliminated (Fig. 15.7). Formal trials of the reproducibility of quantification have yet to be completed. If accurate quantification is possible using ECG triggered conventional CT, this is likely to become an important indication.

Transmitted cardiac pulsation is a well-recognised cause of motion artefact on high-resolution CT images of the lung, particularly in the left lower lobe and lingula. Pseudo-bronchiectasis and artefactual bronchial wall thickening are common. Early results with ECG triggered CT show substantial improvement in these artefacts with no resulting loss of diagnostic information from the reduction in exposure time from 750 to 500 ms (Fig. 15.8). Due to the ease of implementation prospective triggering is likely to become a routine part of all HRCT if not all CT in the chest.

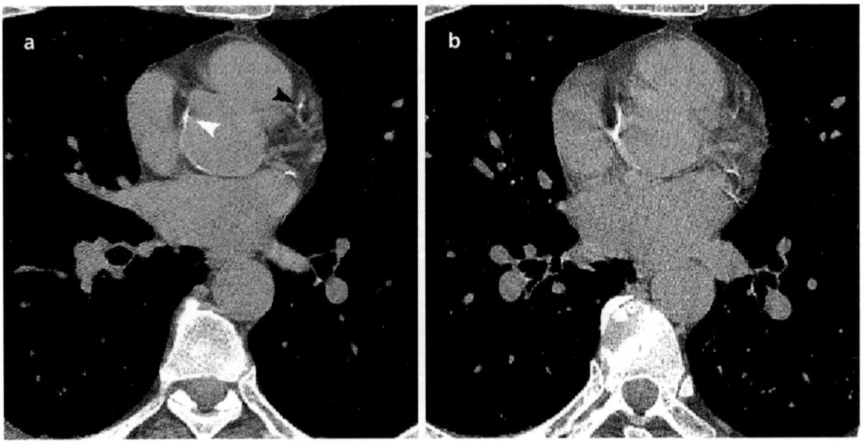

Fig. 15.7a, b. Two 3-mm sections through the aortic root showing improved resolution of aortic (*white arrow*) and left anterior descending coronary artery calcification (*black arrow*) with prospective ECG triggering. **a** Triggered. **b** Not triggered

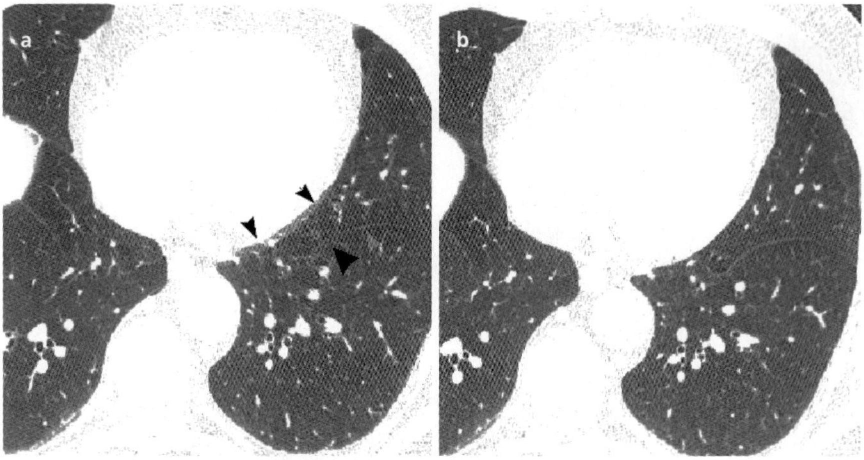

Fig. 15.8a, b. Two 1-mm high-resolution CT images of the lung at the same slice position reconstructed with a high definition algorithm. **a** Performed without prospective triggering, showing cardiac motion artefact (*small arrows*) and blurring of the oblique fissure (*large arrow*). **b** ECG triggered

Repeated scanning at a single level during the passage of a bolus of contrast medium is a well-described method for calculating solid organ perfusion. Applying dye dilution theory to the distribution of the contrast bolus, the peak rate of change of attenuation value within a tissue can be used to calculate absolute tissue perfusion in milliliters per minute per gram of tissue. This has been reported and validated in the liver, spleen [11] and kidney [12]. Cardiac motion artefact has always precluded its use with conventional CT in the heart although the same approach has been used for measuring myocardial perfusion with EBCT [13]. Our initial experience with prospective ECG triggered CT shows promise, as illustrated in Fig. 15.9; however, validation by comparison with other methods has not yet been carried out. Myocardial scintigraphy is the mainstay of clinical myocardial perfusion imaging (^{201}Tl or ^{99m}Tc isonitrile scanning), but this is only qualitative. There is no non-invasive technique for measuring myocardial perfusion in man. Given the prevalence of ischaemic heart disease in the Western world, this is perhaps the most exciting potential application for the technique.

We have little experience of retrospective triggered reconstruction and then only with spiral datasets. Multiplanar and 3D reconstructions of mediastinal structures in the long axis are often marred by ripple artefact which is a direct consequence of cardiac motion (Fig. 15.10). Experience with EBCT and early reports using retrospective triggered reconstruction show that this can be improved. Processing, however can be very time consuming, as was shown in a recent report describing retrospective triggered reconstruction to assess coronary calcification [14]; in this study 3–4 h of processing was common. This may reduced by registration with simultaneous ECG recording, but numerous problems remain. Not least is the unnecessary irradiation incurred by discarding the systolic data. A prospectively triggered spiral acquisition is still awaited.

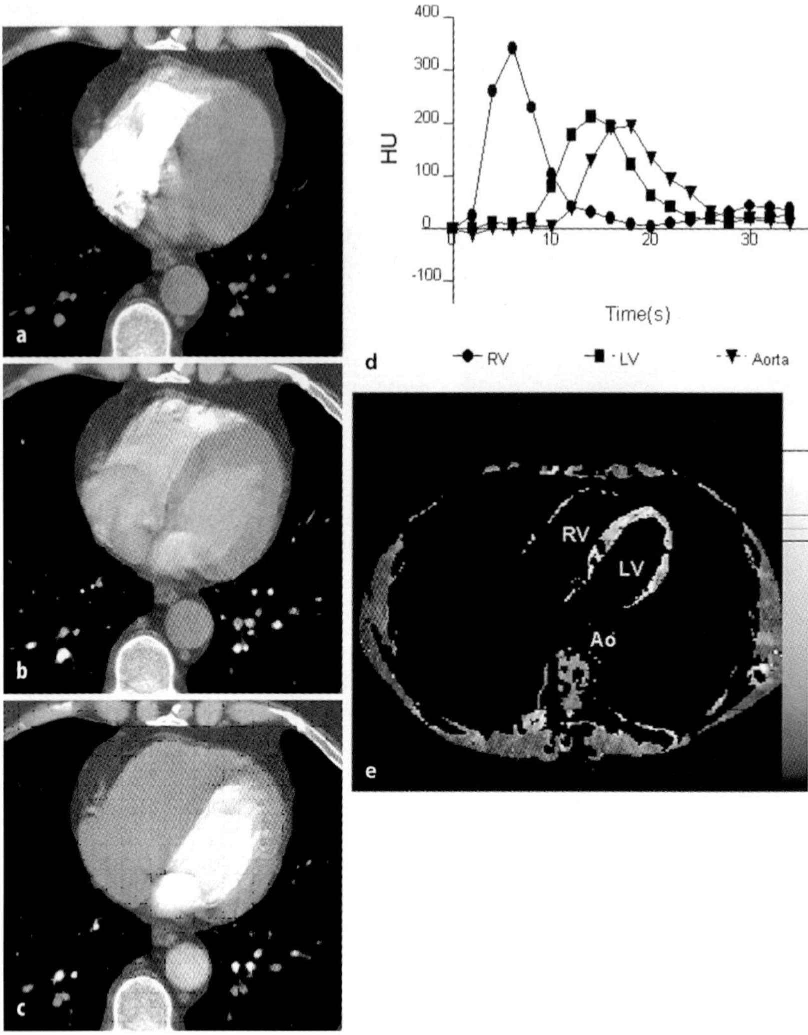

Fig. 15.9. a–e Repeated prospectively triggered sections through the heart during the passage of a bolus of intravenous contrast medium. Contrast passes from the right ventricle (**a**), to both ventricles (**b**) and then to the left ventricle (**c**). ECG triggering reduces cardiac motion artefact between slices and allows time/attenuation curves to be drawn for regions of interest (**d**) or on a pixel-by-pixel basis. (**e**) Relating time-intensity curves to the aortic input function for each pixel a map of absolute tissue perfusion can be created. Left ventricular myocardial perfusion is homogeneous in normal subjects and is higher (*light grey*, 1.5 ml/min/g) than voluntary muscle in the chest wall (*dark grey*, 0.6 ml/min/g)

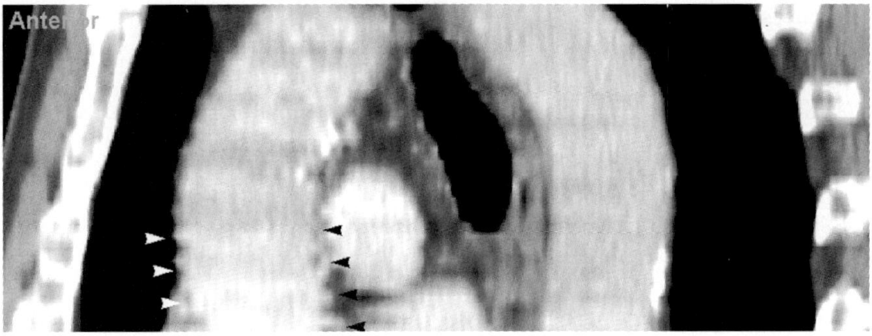

Fig. 15.10. Oblique sagittal reconstruction of the aortic arch showing ripple artefact (*black, white arrows*) related to cardiac motion. This is most marked in the aortic root where transmitted cardiac motion is greatest. There is no ripple on the surface of the descending aorta

15.5 Conclusion

Prospective and retrospective ECG triggered CT are now available using conventional scanners. Our early work with a SOMATOM Plus 4A shows that substantial improvements in image quality can be made and a number of applications are envisaged. These will include routine application of ECG triggering to CT of the heart and in particular to high resolution CT of the lung. Coronary calcification quantification and myocardial perfusion imaging will require further development work but are likely to be important. The role of triggering in spiral image acquisitions is more speculative. There will be some improvement in transaxial imaging, but the greatest benefit will be seen when triggered datasets are used for Z axis reconstructions. Despite the enormous potential of the technique, problems remain. The most significant is that a 500-ms acquisition is still too long. The advantages of triggering are negligible at heart rates greater than 75 bpm. When partial reconstruction is used, the asymmetric acquisition geometry can lead to beam-hardening artefacts on the reconstructed image. This may be unimportant in anatomical imaging but is definitely not so when accurate attenuation measurement is needed.

As with all evolving technologies, ECG triggered conventional CT (prospective or otherwise) should be openly embraced, but its real value will not be established for some time to come.

Acknowledgments. We are grateful for the assistance and ECG triggering modifications provided by S. Brown (Papworth Hospital) and by J. Regn, M. Kirchgorg and M. Fluhrer (Siemens Medical Engineering, Erlangen, Germany). M.H. is partly supported by a grant from Merck.

References

1. Boyd DP, Lipton MJ (1983) Cardiac computed tomography. Proc IEEE 71:305–320
2. Kaufman RB, Sheedy PF II, Breen JF et al (1994) Detection of heart calcification with electron beam CT, intraobserver and interobserver reliability for scoring quantification. Radiology 190:347–351
3. Reiter SJ, Rumberger JA, Feiring AJ et al (1986) Precision of right and left ventricular stroke volume measurements by rapid acquisition cine computed tomography. Circulation 74: 890–900
4. Feiring A, Rumberger JA, Reiter SJ et al (1985) Determination of left ventricular mass in dogs with rapid acquisition cardiac computed tomographic scanning. Circulation 6:1355–1361
5. Rumberger JA, Feiring AJ, Lipton MJ (1987) Use of ultrafast computed tomography to quantitate regional myocardial perfusion: a preliminary report. J Am Coll Cardiol 9:59–72
6. Lipton MJ, Rumberger AJ (1991) The assessment of left ventricular systolic and diastolic function by ultrafast computed tomography. Am J Cardiac Imag 5:318–327
7. Agatston AS, Janowitz WR, Hildner FJ et al (1990) Quantification of coronary artery calcium using ultrafast computed tomography. J Am Coll Cardiol 15:827–832
8. Tanenbaum SR, Dandos GT, Veselik KE et al (1989) Detection of calcific deposits in coronary arteries by ultrafast computed tomography and correlation with coronary angiography. Am J Cardiol 63:870–872
9. Bormann J, Stanford W, Stenberg R et al (1990) Ultrafast CT detection of coronary artery stenosis. Circulation 82:111-162
10. Shemesh J, Apter S, Rozenamn J et al (1995) Calcification of coronary arteries, detection with double helix CT. Radiology 197:779–783
11. Blomley MJK, Coulden RA, Dawson P et al (1995) Liver perfusion studied with ultrafast CT. J Comput Asssist Tomogr 19:424–429
12. Miles KA, Hayball MP, Dixon AK (1994) Functional imaging of changes in human intrarenal perfusion using quantitative dynamic computed tomography. Invest Radiol 29:911–915
13. Ludman PF, Coats AJS, Burger P et al (1993) Validation of measurement of regional myocardial perfusion in humans by ultrafast X-ray computed tomography. Am J Card Imag, 7:267–279
14. Woodhouse CE, Janowitz WR, Viamonte M Jr (1997) Coronary arteries: retrospective cardiac gating technique to reduce cardiac motion artefact at spiral CT. Radiology 204:566–569

16 Imaging of the Heart by ECG-Oriented Reconstruction from Subsecond Spiral CT Scans

M. KACHELRIESS, W. A. KALENDER, M. KARAKAYA, S. ACHENBACH, J. NOSSEN, W. MOSHAGE, W. A. BAUTZ

16.1 Introduction

Coronary artery desease is one of the most important causes of death in western countries. This explains the high demand for noninvasive imaging techniques for the heart. X-ray based techniques, in addition to magnetic resonance and ultrasound imaging, remain important as only they are able to image and, potentially, to quantify coronary calcification. Fluoroscopy, conventional computed tomography (CT), spiral CT, and electron-beam CT have not yet become fully established; fluoroscopy fails to detect small amounts of calcium, conventional CT is not able to scan the volume of interest adequately during a single breathhold, and electron-beam CT systems are seldom available due to their high cost.

The development of continuously rotating scanners followed by the introduction of spiral CT [1, 2] has led to a renaissance of CT. Its volume-scanning capability together with the increase in rotation speed (subsecond scans are available on many scanners today) has made volume scans of whole anatomical regions during a single breathhold a clinical reality. The use of standard spiral reconstruction techniques in cardiac imaging is not satisfactory because the scanning time, although subsecond, is in the order of one heart cycle, and motion artifacts are thus introduced. The widespread 180°LI algorithm, for example, involves a data range of $2 \times (180° + \Phi)$, where the fan angle Φ is 52° in our case, which yields a temporal resolution of approximately 1 s for a 0.75 s scanner. This is the time for one heart cycle, assuming a typical heart rate of 60 bpm.

To achieve high image quality in cardiac imaging effective scan times shorter than 100 ms are desirable. This can be achieved by electron-beam CT but not by conventional CT scanners. Therefore we have developed two specific cardiac spiral algorithms: 180°CI (Cardio-Interpolation), a modified z-interpolation with electrocardiogram (ECG) gated selection of corresponding heart phases (stepwise linear interpolation between successive spiral data segments in the same heart phase) and 180°CD (Cardio-Delta), a partial scan reconstruction. Both approaches should significantly improve the quality of cardiac imaging. Here we present the new algorithms 180°CI and 180°CD and processed patient data, comparing them with the standard spiral algorithm 180°LI.

16.2 Materials and Methods

Ten patients with heart rates from 53 to 93 bpm underwent single-breathhold spiral CT scanning for 30–40 s with 0.75 s per 360° rotation. All scans were performed on a Somatom PLUS 4 (Siemens Medical Systems, Erlangen, Germany) using a table increment d = 3 mm per 360° rotation and a nominal slice thickness S = 3 mm. The ECG was simultaneously recorded during the scan. We used customized software to detect automatically the R peaks from the ECG signal and to synchronize this information with the projection numbers.

Windows of allowed projections are navigated relative to the R-R interval by two user selectable parameters: offset and width (Fig. 16.1). The offset determines the start position of the window (first allowed projection) within a heart cycle, and the width determines its size (number of allowed projections). For example, offset = 30% and width = 50% means that data lying in the first 30% and the last 20% of the cardiac cycle are unacceptable (forbidden) data and data from 30% to 80% are allowed for use in reconstruction. Offset and width are used to select primarily a heart phase with relatively little cardiac motion.

16.2.1 Algorithm 180°CI

The algorithm 180°CI is a modification of the most commonly used z-interpolation algorithm 180°LI. The ECG information is utilized to skip data points falling into forbidden data ranges and to choose the next allowed data points for interpolation (Fig. 16.1). The search is limited to a maximum range which can be selected by the user. In the cases presented below, we chose a maximum distance of 6 mm (which is twice the table feed d) on each side of the reconstruction plane

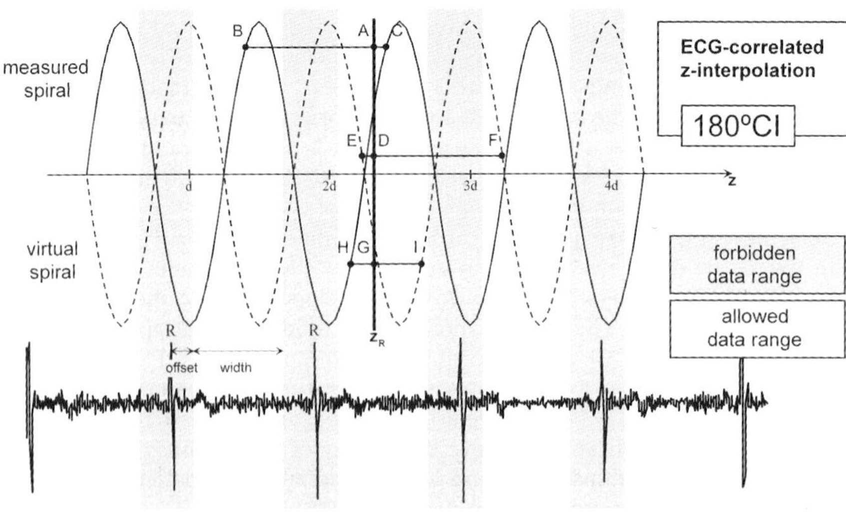

Fig. 16.1. Algorithm 180°CI. Only allowed data are used for reconstruction. The allowed data ranges are determined by selecting the width (here 65%) and offset (here 20%) relative to the cardiac cycle. Three examples for interpolation at position z_R are shown: the value at *A* cannot be obtained between directly neighboring, measured and virtual spiral segments but must be taken from *B* and *C*, which are separated by 360°. A similar situation occurs for *D*, which is interpolated from *E* and *F* with a distance of 360°. *G*: direct interpolation as in 180°LI

z_R. Having found two allowed data points – one on either side of the reconstruction plane – linear interpolation is carried out to obtain the corresponding projection value in the reconstruction plane at $z=z_R$. (Obviously, when choosing width = 100%, the algorithm 180°CI results in 180°LI.) The synthesized projections then undergo the standard image reconstruction process, for example, filtered backprojection. The reconstruction position z_R can be chosen arbitrarily and retrospectively, as is customary in spiral CT.

16.2.2 Algorithm 180°CD

A partial scan reconstruction of spiral data centered about z_R results by the algorithm 180°CD. It uses only data closest to the reconstruction plane, and no z-interpolation is performed (Fig. 16.2). The data range needed for reconstruction is $180° + \delta$, with $\delta < \Phi$ (standard z-interpolation algorithms involve a data range of $2 \times (180° + \Phi)$ or more). Effective scan time and therefore artifacts due to cardiac motion are reduced when the data range is as low as possible, i.e., when δ is as small as possible.

It can be shown that δ depends on the object dimensions [3] and, as long as the object is not a cylinder centered on the axis of rotation, on the reconstruction position z_R. For typical dimensions of a thoracic cross-section of 25 cm × 40 cm, δ varies between 26° and 42° with $\Phi = 52°$ and a field of measurement of 50 cm. This means that the effective scan time ranges from 430 ms to 463 ms for a 0.75 s

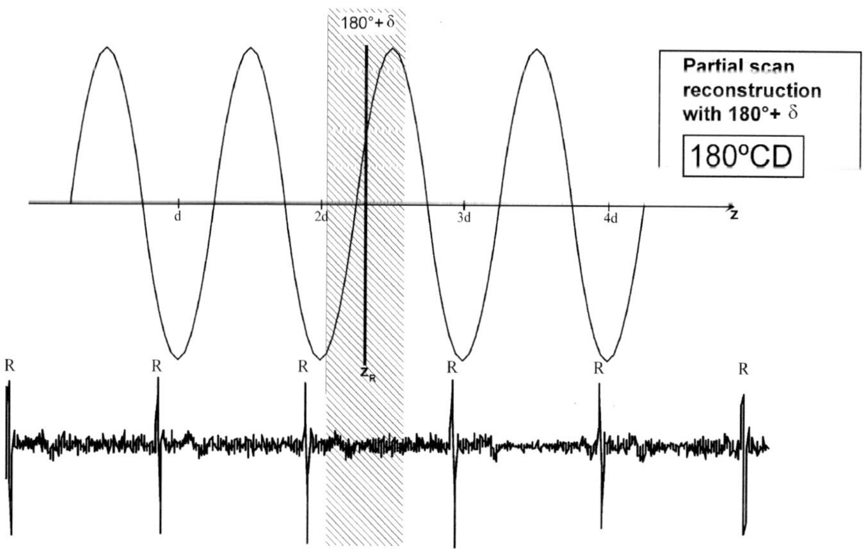

Fig. 16.2. Algorithm 180°CD. Only nearest neighboring data are used to reconstruct at position z_R. The data range is $180° + \delta$ where δ depends on the object dimensions and reconstruction position. Typically $\delta = 10°$ to $40°$ resulting in effective scan times of 395 ms to 408 ms

rotation. If we consider only the moving heart, assuming 10 cm × 15 cm for the heart's dimension, $\delta = 10°$ to $16°$ and effective scan times from 395 ms to 408 ms result.

16.3 Results

Figure 16.3 presents typical results, comparing the three algorithms: three columns with five images each that are reconstructed at successive z-positions with an increment of 1 mm. The left column shows 180°LI, the middle 180°CI, and the right 180°CD reconstructed images. The standard reconstruction 180°LI suffers from motion artifacts. Especially at $z_R = -2$ mm and $z_R = -1$ mm the edges of the anatomic structures seem to overlap. The calcifications are blurred in all reconstructions. These artifacts are corrected to a great extent by 180°CI, especially the calcifications show an improved contiguity throughout the slices and they are depicted more sharply (arrow). The partial scan reconstruction 180°CD improves the motion artifacts only slightly and only in those phases where the heart is in relatively slow motion: $z_R = -1$ mm and $z_R = 2$ mm. Unfortunately, it does not improve overall image quality, since it introduces new streaking artifacts. From Fig. 16.3 we see that the artifact content of the new algorithms is increased, mostly by parallel streaks. The reasons are not yet fully clarified; the selection of data segments may introduce discontinuities in 180°CI and yield parallel streaks. The partial scan reconstruction 180°CD produces even more pronounced streaks than 180°CI; this is the typical behavior of reconstructed spiral data without z-interpolation [1, 4].

Multiplanar reformations provide a very good impression of the value of 180°CI. While the transaxial views show some new artifacts, the multiplanar reformations are definitely of improved quality (Fig. 16.4). Since the cardiac interpolation images always represent the same cardiac phase, they provide smooth continuous contours in multiplanar reformations images.

16.4 Discussion

The new algorithms 180°CI and 180°CD show promising results in cardiac imaging. Especially promising is 180°CI; motion artifacts are largely corrected, and the anatomy is depicted consistently throughout the whole scan volume. Furthermore, calcifications, which cannot be detected at all or which are imaged twice by the standard method, are depicted sharply by 180°CI. This is very important for quantifying coronary calcium, which is usually carried out via a thresholding process [5] because calcifications in images that suffer from motion artifacts are more likely to remain below the chosen threshold (typically 130 HU). Moreover, 180°CI is well suited for volume representations, such as multiplanar reformations and 3D displays.

Successive images from 180°CD do not necessarily contain data from corresponding heart phases since the partial scan reconstruction depicts the momentary position of the heart. Therefore this algorithm is not suitable for volume representations. Nevertheless, there is the possibility of prospective selection of the reconstruction position based on the ECG information: reconstructing at a cer-

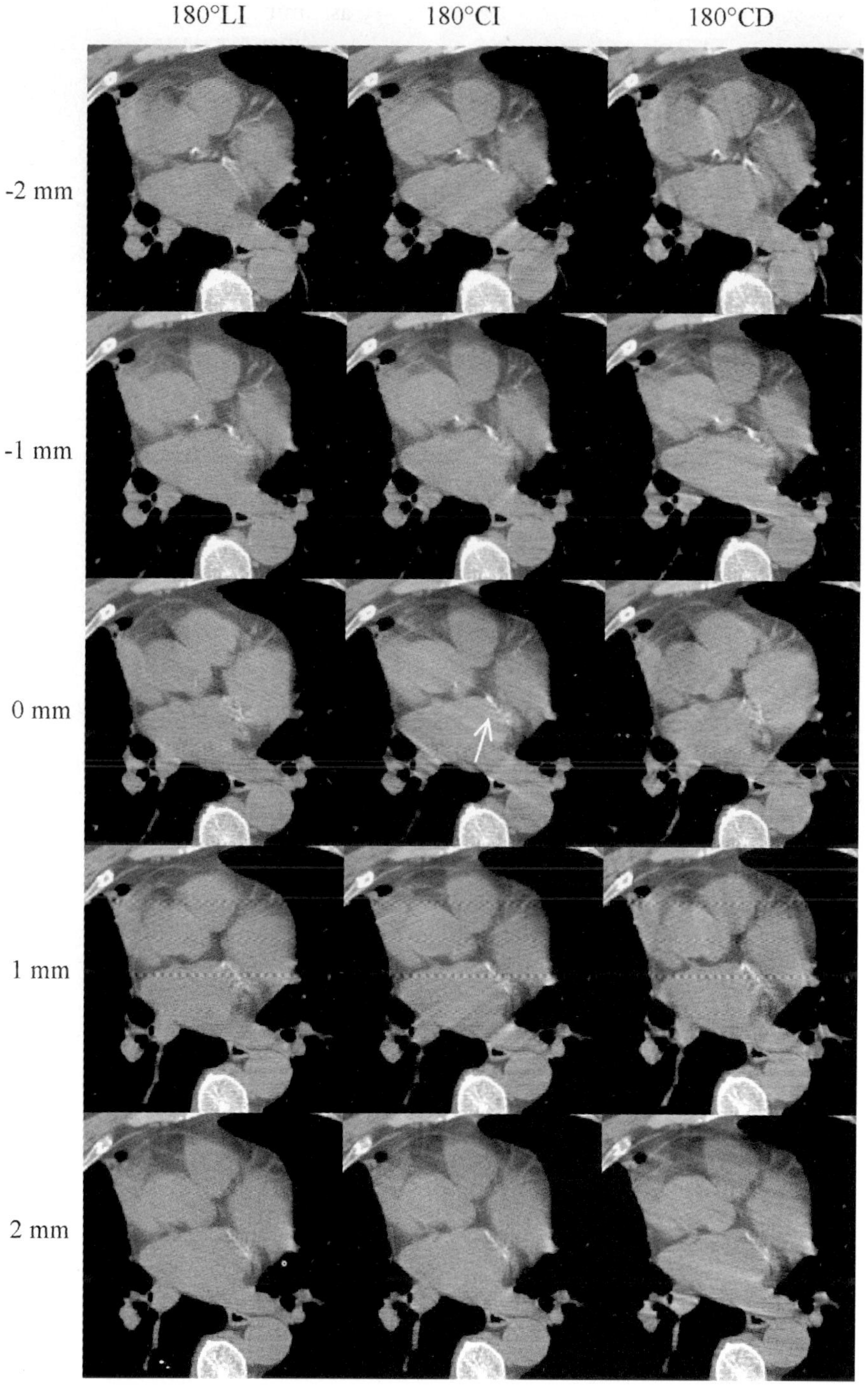

Fig. 16.3. Comparison of algorithms. *Left*, 180°LI; *middle*, 180°CI; *right*, 180°CD. Images are reconstruced at successive positions with an increment of 1 mm. Only 180°CI depicts calcifications clearly throughout the volume. (Patient's heart rate: 81 bpm, offset = 20%, width = 70%)

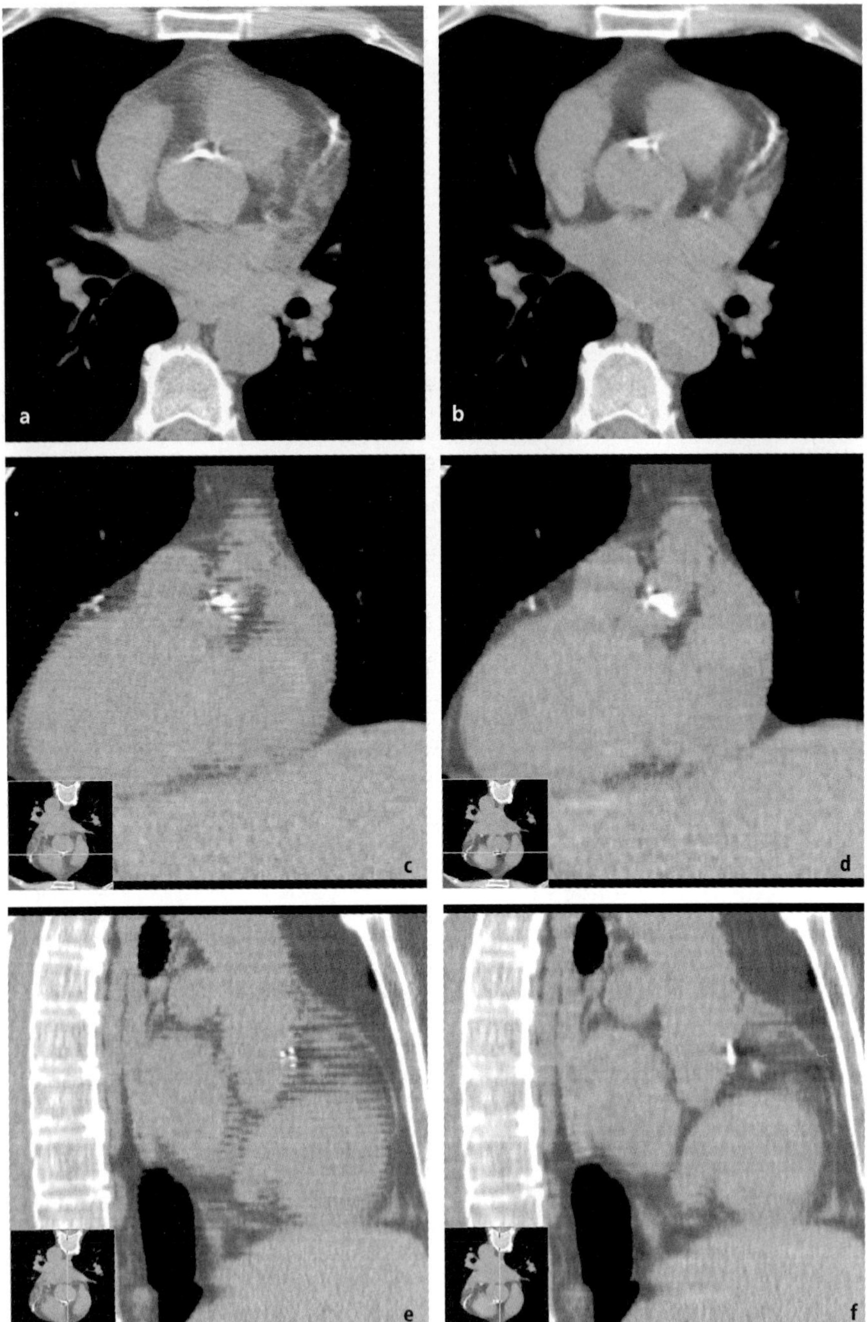

Fig. 16.4. Comparison of algorithms 180°LI (**a**, **c**, **e**) and 180°CI (**b**, **d**, **f**). **a**, **b** Transaxial images. **c**, **d** Coronal reformations. **e**, **f** Sagittal reformations. The 180°CI interpolation shows the anatomy best in its contiguity and motion artifacts (*stepping artifacts*) are effectively reduced. (Patient's heart rate: 78 bpm, offset = 20%, width = 70%)

tain offset from the R peak yields images for the same heart phase, but with varying z-increments (since the heart rate varies during the scan). This approach may become more important with faster scanners or with prospective ECG gating.

Unfortunately, the new algorithms suffer from new artifacts in the image plane, due either to selecting data from different spiral segments (180°CI) or to not interpolating the spiral data (180°CD). These discontinuities in the algorithms result in parallel streaks in the images. Further efforts must be taken to reduce these artifacts. For example, modifications in our algorithms which produce smooth transitions from data segment to data segment are under development.

Future CT systems with higher and adjustable rotation speeds and with multirow detector systems might overcome these problems. Higher rotation speeds will result in a higher temporal resolution and therefore reduce motion artifacts in a natural way. Adjustable rotation speed is important to avoid the resonance problem whenever the heart rate is close to the rotation frequency. The 180°CI slice sensitivity profiles depend on the z-position (or, equivalently, on the chosen offset), as was shown elsewhere [3]. Multirow data acquisition could be used to sample the complete volume without data gaps (forbidden data) and would also yield slice sensitivity profiles independent of z-position.

References

1. Kalender WA, Seissler W, Klotz E, Vock P (1990) Spiral volumetric CT with single-breath-hold technique, continuous transport, and continuous scanner rotation. Radiology 176:181–183
2. Kalender WA, Polacin A (1991) Physical performance characteristics of spiral CT scanning. Med Phys 18:910–915
3. Kachelrieß M, Kalender WA (1998) ECG-correlated image reconstruction from subsecond spiral CT scans of the heart. Med Phys (submitted)
4. Kalender WA (1995) Principles and performance of spiral CT. In: Medical CT and ultrasound: current technology and applications. Advanced Medical, Madison, pp 379–410
5. Agatston AS, Janowitz WR, Hildner FJ, Zusmer NR, Viamonte M, Detrano R (1990) Quantification of coronary artery calcium using ultrafast computed tomography. J Am Coll Cardiol 15:827–832

17 CT-Guided Diagnostic Punctures of the Chest

D. Hahn, G. Schultz

17.1 Introduction

CT-guided diagnostic punctures are very well established in diagnostic radiology since many years. Percutaneous biopsies are accepted as a minimal invasive procedure for obtaining a histological diagnosis of various chest abnormalities. Success rate and complications depend on a number of parameters such as needle size, number of biopsies taken, path length through the lung, and location of the abnormality. The shift from performing biopsies with fluoroscopy to CT guidance has become routine. Many diagnostic interventions are still carried out using conventional CT systems. In recent years technology has changed, and in many institutions spiral CT systems are now available. The purpose of this study was to evaluate the diagnostic efficacy of CT-guided biopsies of chest lesions using different techniques.

17.2 Material and Methods

From September 1994 to December 1997 171 CT-guided biopsies of the chest were performed in 171 patients. The study included 125 males and 46 females with the a mean age of 58.7 years. The youngest patient was 13 years old, the oldest patient 83 years. 63 chest biopsies were done using a Somatom plus S (Siemens AG, Erlangen) and 108 chest-biopsies using a Somatom plus 4A (Siemens AG, Erlangen). There were 132 pleural, subpleural, or pulmonary lesions, 37 mediastinal lesions, and 2 lesions of the chest wall. An automatic cutting needle (Bip system) was used in all patients. Needle size and length varied depending on the size and localization of the lesion: 14, 16, or 18 G and 59, 89, or 119 mm. The size of the biopsied lesions ranged from 8 to 132 mm, with a mean of 40.2 mm. The path length through the lung varied between 2 and 80 mm with a mean of 29.2 mm.

17.3 Results

The overall complication rate of the 171 CT-guided biopsies was 21.8%. Pneumothorax occurred in 17% of patients, pneumothorax requiring chest tube placement in 3%, hematopericardium in 0.6%, and hematothorax with drainage in 0.6%. One patient (0.6%) died directly after the intervention due to myocardial infarction unrelated to the biopsy. In 37 mediastinal biopsies the complication rate was 3% for hematopericardium and 8% for pneumothorax, all without chest tube placement. In 132 pleural, subpleural and pulmonary biopsies in 22% a pneumothorax without chest tube placement occurred and in 4% a pneumothorax requiring chest tube placement.

The final histological diagnosis was until now available in 146 of 171 biopsies. It was called positive when there was a definitive histological diagnosis of a malignant tumor. The classification negative was chosen when there was a final histological diagnosis of a benigne lesion, inflammatory changes or when follow up examinations were available for more than six month. The 146 final diagnosis included 127 malignant tumors and 19 benign lesions. 25 patients, which were examined during the last few month, could not be evaluated until now because of a negative biopsy and the missing follow up study after six month. In 124 patients a malignant tumor was found in the biopsy which means a true positive finding in 83%. In 19 patients the final diagnosis of a benign or inflammatory lesion was found which means a true negative rate of 13%. There were now false positive findings. In six patients (4%) the first biopsy was called false negative because no malignant histology could be found. All 6 patients however had a malignant lesion proven by second biopsy (3 patients), surgery or follow up examinations (3 patients). The positive predictive value of this study was 100%, the negative predictive value 76%. Including the second biopsy of the 3 patients who were false negative in the first examination, the negative predictive value is going up to 84%.

17.4 Conclusion

CT-guided diagnostic punctures of the chest are very well established today. They have a very high diagnostic accuracy and in most cases provide a final histological diagnosis. CT-guided biopsies can avoid many invasive surgical procedures such as mediastinoscopy, thoracoscopy, and thoracotomy. The complication rate in CT-guided interventions is similar to or lower than that in surgical interventions, but they are less invasive even than minimal invasive surgical procedures. For a genuine histological diagnosis core biopsies should be carried out. Fine-needle aspirations are seldom sufficient for a definitive histological diagnosis. Because of the relatively low complication rate and the high diagnostic accuracy only automatic cutting needle systems should be used.

18 Three-Dimensional Imaging and Virtual Reality Applications of Spiral CT

R. B. Jeffrey

18.1 Introduction

Three-dimensional imaging (3DI) is at the intersection of a number of emerging technologies. First, is the unprecedented price-performance ratio of current computers that have increased enormously in computational speed, at the same time that costs for computer hardware have plummeted. Second, is the rapid development of interactive 3-D graphics software to provide optimal 3-D visualization. The final factor has been the development of breathheld spiral CT as a mature technology. The rapid scan acquisition of spiral CT affords volumetric data sets free of motion and respiratory artifacts to be utilized for 3-D imaging.

Musculoskeletal applications of 3DI have been in clinical practice for nearly 15 years and have relied largely upon shaded surface display as the primary visualized method. However, the recent development spiral CT has made possible 3-D CT angiography (CTA) and virtual endoscopic imaging using a combination of rendering methods such as maximal intensity projections, curved planar reformations, and perspective volume rendering.

18.2 CT Angiography

CTA has gained widespread acceptance as a minimally invasive technique to image vascular disorders [1–3]. CTA and magnetic resonance angiography (MRA) are currently highly competitive techniques. The development of ultrafast gradients and the use of contrast agents have greatly facilitated abdominal and peripheral vascular MRA. With the use of maximum intensity projections (MIP) the editing of MRA data sets is often far less complex than with CTA. Unlike MRA, CTA is readily able to visualize calcifications and stent grafts. Our current approach is to use MRA in patients with comprised renal function, pediatric patients, and in patients in whom a large anatomic region of interest is to be evaluated such as the aortoiliac and peripheral vascular system. CTA is used to evaluate limited anatomic regions and in particular is ideal for the planning and follow-up of vascular intervention such as stent grafts.

There are several key elements for success with CTA. Chief among these is patient education to sustain a breathhold for at least 30 s and accurate timing of the contrast bolus to maximize the arterial opacification of the targeted volume to be scanned. We prefer to use a minitest bolus of approximately 15 cc and to scan periodically just above the target volume to determine the precise time delay curve for each individual patient. For most abdominal and peripheral vascular applications, 3 mm collimation is used with a pitch of 2. A collimation of 3 mm is utilized in the upper abdominal aorta to visualize the splanchnic vessels and 5 mm collimation to visualize the iliac circulation. This combination works well to visualize the entire aortoiliac circulation. A rapid bolus injection is utilized on the order of 5 ml/s with nonionic contrast. Typical contrast volumes include 150–200 ml for most aortoiliac studies. Following data acquisition, overlapping reconstructions are performed normally at 2 mm. The scanned data is then reconstructed with a targeted field of view of 20 cm to maximize resolution.

It is essential to view axial source images in addition to 3-D reformations of CTA data as they are often important incidental findings noted only on the axial images. In the past 2 years we have diagnosed unsuspected renal cell carcinoma in five patients. In addition, we have diagnosed mesenteric lymphadenopathy, common duct stones, hepatic and splenic metastases, and other important findings on the axial source images. Standard reformations for the aortoiliac circulation include: shaded surface display, MIP, curved planar reformations of the splanchnic vessels as well as quantitative measurement of aneurysms. Curved planar reformations are essential for evaluations of stents and stent graphs to view the lumen in cross-section.

18.3 Virtual Reality Applications of Spiral CT Data

Commonly employed 3-D rendering methods include either ray-tracing projectional techniques (maximum intensity or ray sum) or thresholding techniques (shaded surface display). These orthographic techniques perform rendering without perspective. The resulting images are as if viewed by magnification from an infinite distance. Perspective volume rendering, although computationally more demanding and complex, has the distinct advantage of viewing structures or interfaces within the data set with the perspective of the human eye at a fixed distance. Thus, structures closer to the viewpoint appears larger than structures further away. Perspective volume rendering permits visualization of body cavities and hollow viscoses from a unique internal view that can be used to endoscopic or "fly-through" images (Figs. 18.1–18.4).

With perspective volume rendering all the voxels in the dataset are assigned both opacity and color based on attenuation values. It is possible to manipulate the opacity and lighting curves to "shine a light source into the data set" to create unique 3-D images that simulate virtual endoscopy. In order to visualize surface interfaces an attenuation difference of about 200 HU units is required. Thus distention of the air-filled colon following a cleansing routine makes possible virtual colonoscopy when a light source is projected into the 3-D data-set along the course of the colon. The development of automatic path plans and rapid endoscopic movies has for the first time made it possible to perform endoscopic imaging that may play a role in colon cancer screening.

Initial reported sensitivities of detecting polyps greater than 1 cm are in the range of 75%–90% [4, 5]. Errors may be due to problems related to fluid or residual stool within the colon and segments of the colon that are poorly distended.

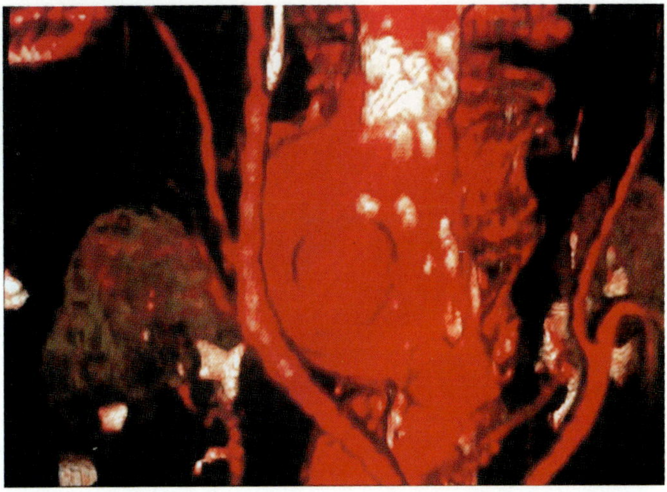

Fig. 18.1. Fly-around view of abdominal aorta. In this perspective volume rendered CT angiogram of the abdominal aorta, the intra and extraperitoneal fat is rendered translucent, allowing a "fly around" view of an abdominal aorta aneurysm

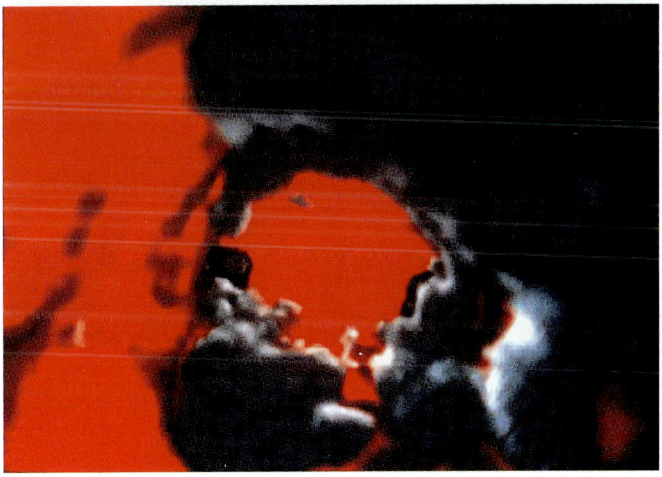

Fig. 18.2. Fly-through view of the abdominal aorta. An angioscopic view of the abdominal aorta demonstrates marked calcific plaque formation in the midaorta

These frequently occur in the sigmoid colon, and thus we have used as a standard routine in addition to supine air-filled views, additional limited second spiral acquisition through the sigmoid colon. Future developments include highly automated endoscopic movies and potential use of neural networks to and in interpretation.

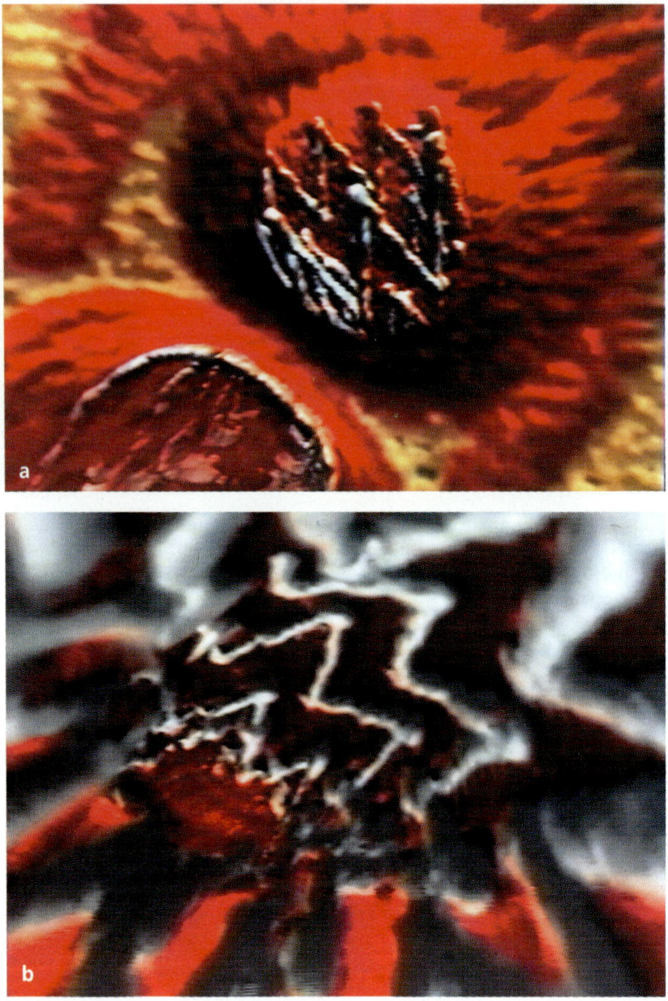

Fig. 18.3A, B. Perspective volume rendering of thoracic aortic CT angiogram. **A** Note a fly-around view of a thoracic aorta stent graph. **B** Note the angioscopic view internally within the stent

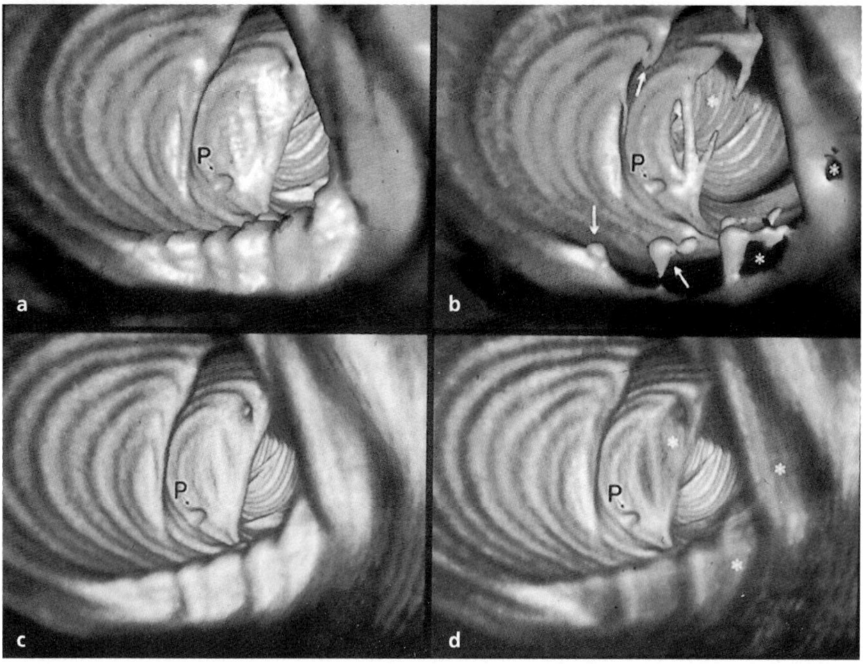

Fig. 18.4a–d. Comparison of perspective volume rendering and perspective surface display. **a** Note perspective shaded surface display using a threshold of –980 HU optimal to display into small polyps (*P*) within the colon. **b** The threshold is set too high (–930) and portions of the colonic wall not rendered, and appears as gaps (*) or distorted folds (*arrows*). **c** A perspective volume rendered image, with an opacity curve that renders all the voxels. Note the lack of artifacts. **d** A perspective volume rendering is performed with different opacity curve making the lower areas of attenuation more transparent, creating a more translucent appearance of thinner structures (*). However, there are no discontinuities as seen with the surface display. (From [7])

References

1. Rubin GD, Dake MD, Napel S et al (1994) Spiral CT of renal artery stenosis: comparison of three-dimensional rendering techniques. Radiology 190:181–189
2. Galanski M, Prokop M, Chavan A, Schaefer CM, Jandeleit K, Nischelsky JE (1993) Renal arterial stenoses: spiral CT angiography. Radiology 189:185–192
3. Rubin GD, Dake MD, Napel SA, McDonnell CH, Jeffrey RBJ (1993) Abdominal spiral CT angiography: initial clinical experience. Radiology 186:147–152
4. Hara AK, Johnson CD, Reed JE, Ahlquist DA et al (1997) Detection of colorectal polyps with CT colography: initial assessment of sensitivity and specificity. Radiology 205:59–65
5. Royster AP, Fenlon HM, Clarke PD et al (1997) CT colonoscopy of colorectal neoplasms: two-dimensional and three-dimensional virtual-reality techniques with colonoscopic correlation. AJR 169:1237–1242
6. Rubin GD, Beaulieu CF, Argiro V et al (1996) Perspective volume rendering of CT and MR Images: applications for endoscopic imaging. Radiology 199:321–330
7. Rubin GD et al (1996) Preoperative volume rendering of CT and MR images: application for endoscopic imaging. Radiology 199:325–330

19 Automatic Bolus Tracking for Spiral CT of the Liver

C. CLAUSSEN, F. MEHNERT, P. PEREIRA, P. HUPPERT

19.1 Introduction

Intravenously administered contrast material has proven essential in computed tomography (CT) examinations of the liver. It is needed to improve tissue contrast and to detect and characterize liver lesions. Even early dynamic CT studies with single-slice technique revealed a unique contrast perfusion curve of the liver parenchyma and various patterns of liver lesion enhancement depending on their blood supply and degree of vascularity [4].

The major problem was that incremental CT enabled dynamic examinations only at a single slice level. The present availability of fast CT scanners with spiral acquisition and large heat capacity tubes now permits routine scanning of the whole liver in 10–20 s during one breathhold. With this technique hepatic spiral CT scans can even be performed twice during one bolus of contrast material, allowing the liver to be imaged separately in the hepatic-arterial phase and the portal-venous phase. This so-called biphasic contrast-enhanced CT of the liver has been shown to improve detection and characterization of liver lesions [2, 3, 14, 15, 20, 23].

With the shorter scanning times it is particularly important to optimize the timing between contrast bolus and initiation of the spiral scans. Differences in blood circulation time and various contrast material transit times in patients can affect accuracy of imaging of perfusion phases [5, 13, 18]. Therefore methods are desirable that permit automatic initiation of diagnostic scanning depending on the arrival of the contrast material bolus in the liver. This chapter presents our initial experience with an automatic bolus tracking technique for biphasic and monophasic spiral CT of the liver that enables individual bolus-triggered scanning delays.

19.2 Principle of Automatic Bolus Tracking

Bolus tracking is performed in our institution using a software program (C.A.R.E. Bolus) implemented on a Somatom Plus 4 scanner (version B30B, Siemens, Erlangen). The procedure is based on repetitive monitoring scans at one slice level during respiration and analysis of the time-density curve in a chosen region of interest (ROI) to determine the optimal individual scanning time. The ROI is chosen on a reference scan. The monitoring scans are performed at 50 mA to minimize additional radiation exposure. The delay of the monitoring scans and the time between the repetitions can be set before the examination. The reconstruction of these scans and the time-density curve in the ROI is displayed at the operator's monitor within 1 s, enabling fast manual interaction if necessary. As soon as a predefined contrast enhancement threshold within the ROI is reached, spiral scanning is initiated and begins after a delay of about 7 s. This delay is technically required but is also used for reposition of the table at the start position and to give a breathing command to the patient.

19.3 Material and Methods

Six patients who were admitted routinely for evaluation of an unknown liver lesion ($n=3$), a hepatocellular carcinoma ($n=2$), or suspected hypervascular liver metastases ($n=1$) were examined with dual-phase spiral CT of the liver. One patient with suspected liver metastases due to rectal carcinoma was evaluated with portal-venous spiral CT of the liver.

For biphasic spiral CT we used the following examination protocol: Before contrast administration patients routinely received an unenhanced spiral CT of the liver, which is considered to further improve detectability [7, 25]. The reference scan that defines the level of the monitoring scans is placed at the diaphragm level. The monitoring scans are started with a delay of 8 s after beginning of intravenous contrast material administration and repeated every 2 s. The ROI is positioned in the descending aorta with a contrast enhancement threshold of 60 HU for initiation. The 7-s delay for table repositioning and breathing commands creates a time window for the contrast material to enhance hepatic arteries and hypervascular liver lesions. For the portal-venous phase we use an delay of 15 s after completion of the arterial phase, which seems the appropriate interscan delay to image the liver at its maximal parenchymal enhancement [18]. The spiral CT scans in all three phases (unenhanced, arterial, and portal-venous phase) are performed with a collimation of 8 mm, a pitch of 1.5, and a reconstruction interval of 7 mm. For biphasic spiral CT the patients receive 120 ml nonionic contrast material at a iodine concentration of 300 mg/ml. The contrast bolus is administered with power injection at a flow of 4 ml/s.

For the monophasic portal-venous spiral CT of the liver we use the following parameters: For optimization of liver enhancement the ROI is placed within the liver parenchyma at a slice level where it stays in the liver even during quiet breathing. Care must been taken to avoid large vessels and hepatic lesions when positioning the ROI. We choose a slice level for the monitoring scans about 3 cm below the diaphragm as shown on the inspiratory measured topogram. During breathing this reference slice cuts the liver halfway between the diaphragm and the caudal liver margin. The monitoring scans are started with a delay of 40 s after contrast injection, the scans are repeated every 5 s. The threshold for initiation of diagnostic scanning we choose at a parenchymal enhancement of 40 HU. We perform the monophasic spiral CT of the liver with a collimation of 8 mm, a pitch of 1.5, and reconstruction interval of 7 mm. The injection protocol includes a flow of 3.0 ml/s and a volume of 120 ml contrast material (300 mg/ml iodine concentration).

19.4 Results

All examinations have been completed without technical or patient-related problems. Fig. 19.1 presents an example of the reference scan with the ROI in the descending aorta and the following low dose monitoring scans. The arrival of the contrast material bolus triggers scan initiation, when the threshold value of 60 HU is reached. In Fig. 19.2a the increase in density values within the ROI is illustrated as it is displayed on the monitor during the examination. After the examination a list of the increasing density values are printed on an additional image

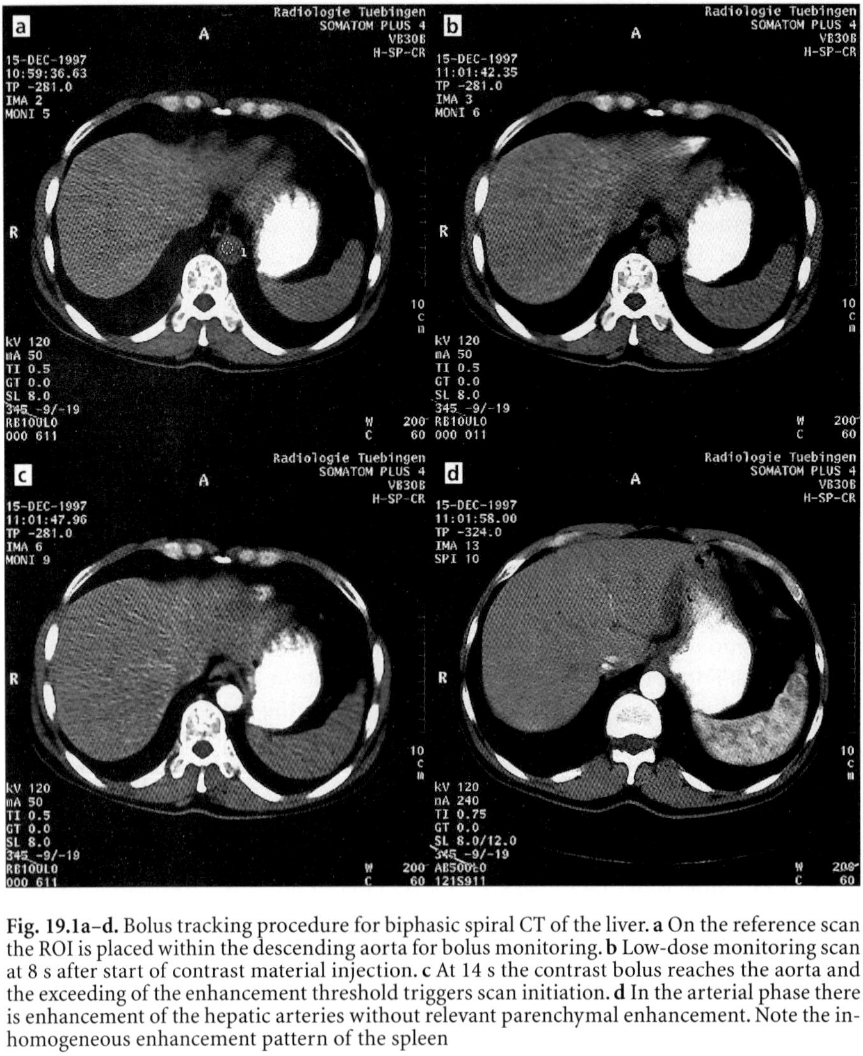

Fig. 19.1a–d. Bolus tracking procedure for biphasic spiral CT of the liver. **a** On the reference scan the ROI is placed within the descending aorta for bolus monitoring. **b** Low-dose monitoring scan at 8 s after start of contrast material injection. **c** At 14 s the contrast bolus reaches the aorta and the exceeding of the enhancement threshold triggers scan initiation. **d** In the arterial phase there is enhancement of the hepatic arteries without relevant parenchymal enhancement. Note the inhomogeneous enhancement pattern of the spleen

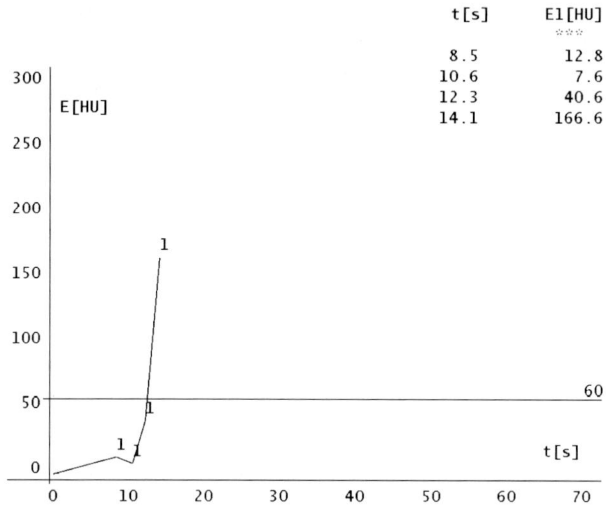

Fig. 19.2a, b. a Curve of the aortic enhancement values that are plotted at operator's monitor during monitoring phase until the threshold level of 60 HU is reached. **b** List of delay times of the monitoring scans and the according increase of the attenuation values

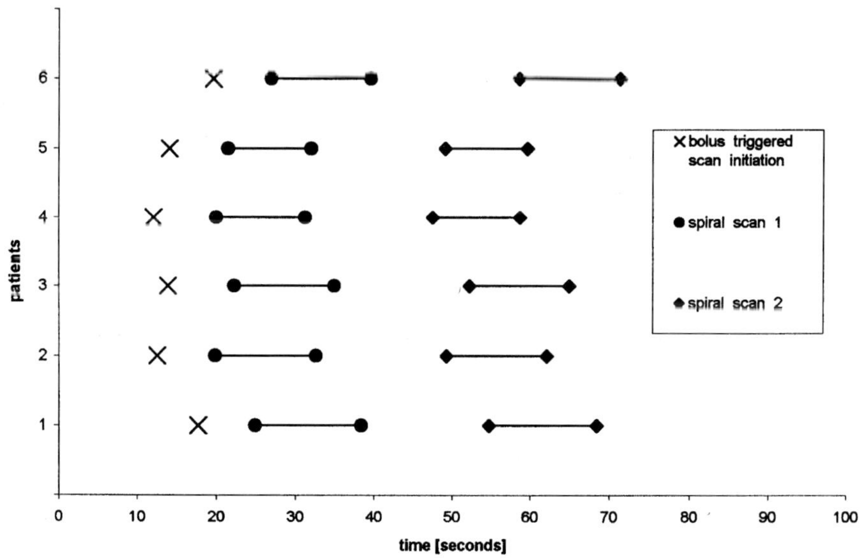

Fig. 19.3. The time course of bolus-triggered scan initiation, arterial phase spiral scan, and portal-venous spiral scan of six patients shows variability of the aortic contrast material transit times between 12 and 20 s

(Fig. 19.2b). Despite the patient's breathing during the low-dose scans no dislocations of the ROI out of the aorta occurred.

The time relations of bolus-triggered scan initiation, first spiral scan, and second spiral scan for the six patients are demonstrated in Fig. 19.3. The contrast enhancement threshold (60 HU) in the aorta was reached between 12 and 20 s (mean 15 s) after the start of contrast material injection. The spiral scans in the arterial phase began between 20 and 27 s (mean 22.5 s) with an average delay of 7.5 s after bolus-triggered scan initiation. The duration of the arterial phase spiral scans was between 10.5 and 13.6 s which was determined by the size of the liver at the topogram. The arterial spiral scans were completed 31.2–39.6 s after initiation of injection. The interval between completion of the first spiral scan and start of the portal-venous spiral scan ranged between 15.7 and 18.0 s, resulting in starting times between 48.3 and 58.6 s after beginning of contrast bolus administration.

In all six patients the contrast enhancement of liver parenchyma during the arterial phase spiral scans was still below 20 HU. On all images the spleen presented an inhomogenous uptake of contrast material of at least 10 HU, indicating imaging of an arterial parenchymal phase. In most cases a slight enhancement of the portal vein was seen by contrast material having already passed the spleen. This seldom affect the diagnostic value of the arterial phase scan because the portal-venous contrast material flow does not yet contribute to parenchymal enhancement.

In the portal-venous phase three patients reached a minimum enhancement of the parenchyma of more than 50 HU, while the three other (one with fatty liver degeneration, two with severe liver cirrhosis) presented a mean parenchymal enhancement between only 30 and 40 HU. Intraindividually, however, the parenchymal enhancement was very constant through the portal-venous scans, showing differences in parenchymal density below 10 HU.

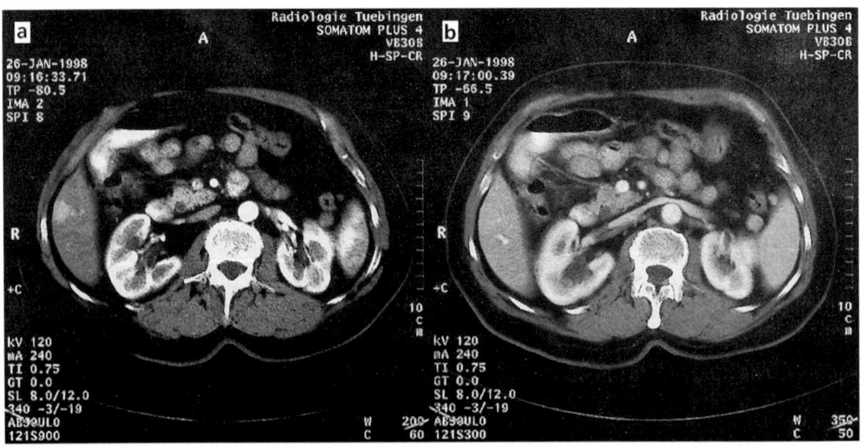

Fig. 19.4a, b. Bolus-triggered biphasic spiral CT of a patient with hepatic adenoma. **a** In the arterial phase the tumor is hyperdense to the surrounding liver parenchyma. **b** In the portal-venous phase the tumor is masked presenting an equivalent density to the enhanced liver parenchyma

Figure 19.4 gives an illustration of bolus-triggered CT images of a patient with a hepatic adenoma, a liver lesion, that is hyperdense in arterial phase and can be masked in portal-venous phase.

For the patient who received a monophasic portal-venous spiral CT Fig. 19.5 shows the reference scan and the following monitoring scans until the threshold of 40 HU is reached. The curve of enhancement and the enhancement values that are displayed at the monitor during the tracking phase are illustrated in Fig. 19.6.

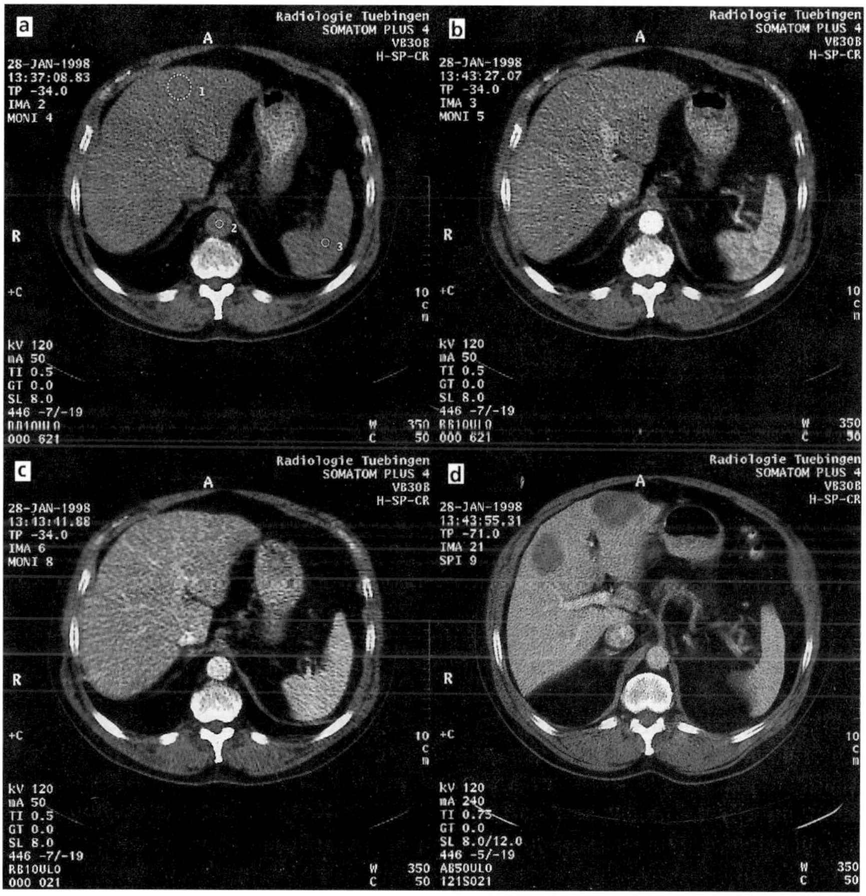

Fig. 19.5a–d. Bolus tracking technique for monophasic portal-venous spiral CT of the liver in a patient with liver metastases due to rectal carcinoma. **a** The ROI for bolus monitoring is placed in the liver parenchyma, additional ROIs are set in the aorta and the spleen. **b** Low-dose scan at 40 s after start of contrast material administration shows a strongly enhanced aorta and an inhomogeneously enhanced spleen. **c** At 55 s the enhancement threshold of 40 HU is reached in the liver parenchyma, triggering automatic scan initiation. **d** Portal-venous scans show good enhancement of the portal vein and the liver parenchyma demarcating hypodense metastatic lesions

patic structures. Certainly at least half of all patients receive accurate timed examinations with a standard delay of 20–25 s, but how can these patients be identified in advance? According to Kopka et al. [19] up to 40% of patients receiving biphasic spiral CT of the liver can profit from low-dose bolus tracking technique.

19.5.2 Monophasic Spiral CT of the Liver

The appropriate time window of monophasic spiral scanning of the liver has been of great controversy. The injection protocols and guidelines for time delay change as rapidly as the speed of the scanners increases [6, 8, 12, 26, 29]. Nowadays the best time of monophasic liver CT is considered the portal-venous perfusion phase at peak of parenchymal enhancement. During this time the contrast between hypovascular liver lesions and the normal parenchyma is thought to be maximized. In general, a parenchymal density enhancement of at least 40–50 HU should be achieved for best assessment of these lesions. Scanning of the liver should be completed before onset of the equilibrium phase [1, 8].

Several studies have shown that peak of hepatic enhancement is elevated with increasing volume of contrast material [13, 27]. Using more rapid injection rates, peak enhancement of the liver is reached sooner, but this does not affect maximum values of parenchymal enhancement significantly [11, 29]. This means that if a fixed volume of contrast material is used, the optimal delay of the portal-venous scanning depends on the injection rate.

Reported delay times ranged from 50 to 70 s between the beginning of injection and the beginning of scanning. Some authors recommend injection protocols with two different flow rates [12]. It has been realized that peak hepatic enhancement takes place about 25–32 s after the end of contrast material injection irrespective of the injection rate and the volume [16, 29]. A contrast material delivery nomogram for hepatic spiral CT has been established [29]. Still there is a variability of hepatic enhancement due to patient-related factors. As shown in our example, bolus tracking technique can be used to optimize liver enhancement during portal-venous phase scanning [17, 27].

Studies comparing this technique with constant time delay show significantly higher mean parenchymal enhancement with bolus tracking [17, 28]. It has been demonstrated that with a flow of 4.0 ml/s and 100 ml contrast material 100% of patients exceed 40 HU for mean parenchymal enhancement, compared to only 70% of patients with a fixed scanning delay of 40 s [17]. With a flow of 3.0 ml/s and 150 ml contrast material the liver attenuation of 100% of patients was more than 50 HU above baseline [28]. This study found that mean parenchymal enhancement using 125 ml contrast material and bolus tracking technique is comparable to the mean enhancement with 150 ml and fixed time delay of 60 s. This shows that for equivalent hepatic enhancement the automated bolus tracking technique can help to reduce contrast material load.

A problem that can occur is that the ROI becomes dislocated during the process of bolus monitoring due to patient motion. Therefore the appropriate level for monitoring must be chosen, as noted above. The position of the ROI, however, can be controlled visually at the operator's monitor, and diagnostic scanning can be started manually by the visual impression of enhancement if necessary. In very few patients, for instance, those with cirrhosis, fatty changes, or extensive metastases that would compromise blood flow of the portal vein, the initiation threshold may not be reached during the portal perfusion phase of the contrast material. For this reason a certain default time (for example, 70 s with a flow of 3.0 ml/s) should be determined to prevent any prolonged delays in scanning [28].

19.6 Conclusion

The use of automatic bolus tracking technique to individualize the delay between injection of contrast material and initiation of the diagnostic scans has proven to be advantageous in hepatic spiral CT. It is useful to optimize timing for the short arterial perfusion phase of the liver and leads to a higher and more consistent mean parenchymal enhancement in the portal-venous phase. For an equal degree of hepatic enhancement the volume of contrast material can be reduced compared to examinations with fixed time delays. We expect that this bolus tracking technique could be equally effective in dynamic studies of other parenchymal organs and in CT angiography.

References

1. Baron RL (1994) Understanding and optimizing use of contrast material for CT of the liver. Am J Roentgenol 163 (2):323–331
2. Baron RL, Oliver JH, Dodd GD, Nalesnik M, Holbert BL, Carr BI (1996) Hepatocellular carcinoma: evaluation with biphasic, contrast-enhanced, helical CT. Radiology 199 (2): 505–511
3. Bonaldi VM, Bret PM, Reinhold C, Atri M (1995) Helical CT of the liver: value of an early hepatic arterial phase. Radiology 197 (2):357–363
4. Claussen CD, Lochner B (1983) Dynamische Computertomographie. Springer, Berlin Heidelberg New York Tokyo
5. Claussen CD, Banzer D, Pfretschner C, Kalender WA, Schörner W (1984) Bolus geometry and dynamics after intravenous contrast medium injection. Radiology 153 (2):365–368
6. Cox IH, Foley WD, Hoffmann RG (1991) Right window for dynamic hepatic CT. Radiology 181 (1):18–21
7. Feuerbach S, Lorenz W, Klose KJ, Gmeinwieser J, Lackner KJ, Landwehr P, Grabbe E, Klöppel R (1996) Kontrastmittelapplikation bei der Spiral-Computertomographie: Ergebnisse einer Konsensuskonferenz. Fortschr Röntgenstr 164 (2):158–165
8. Foley WD, Hoffmann RG, Quiroz FA, Kahn CE, Perret RS (1994) Hepatic helical CT: contrast meterial injection protocol. Radiology 192 (2):367–371
9. Frederick MG, McElaney BL, Singer A, Park KS, Paulson EK, McGee SG, Nelson RC (1996) Timing of parenchymal enhancement on dual-phase dynamic helical CT of the liver: how long does the hepatic arterial phase predominate? Am J Roentgenol 166 (6):1305–1310
10. Funke M, Kopka L, Vosshenrich R, Oestmann JW, Grabbe E (1995) Bolusgetriggerte Spiral-CT: Ein neues programmgesteuertes Verfahren zur Kontrastoptimierung. Fortschr Röntgenstr 162 (4):335–337
11. Garcia PA, Bonaldi VM, Bret FM, Liang L, Reinhold C, Atri M (1996) Effect of rate of contrast medium injection on hepatic enhancement at CT. Radiology 199 (1):185–189
12. Heiken JP, Brink JA, McClennan BL, Sagel SS, Forman HP, DiCroce J (1993) Dynamic contrast-enhanced CT of the liver: comparison of contrast medium injection rates and uniphasic and biphasic injection protocols. Radiology 187 (2):327–331
13. Harmon BH, Berland LL, Lee JY (1992) Effect of varying rates of low-osmolarity contrast media injection for hepatic CT: correlation with indocyanine green transit time. Radiology 184 (2):379–382

14. van Hoe L, Baert AL, Gryspeerdt S, Vandenbosh G, Nevens F, van Steenbergen W, Marchal G (1997) Dual-phase helical CT of the liver: value of an early-phase acquisition in the differential diagnosis of noncystic focal lesions. Am J Roentgenol 168 (5): 1185–1192
15. Hollett MD, Jeffrey RB Jr, Nino-Murcia M, Jorgensen MJ, Harris DP (1995) Dual-phase helical CT of the liver: value of arterial phase scans in the detection of small (< or = 1.5 cm) malignant hepatic neoplasms. Am J Roentgenol 164 (4): 879–884
16. Irie T, Kusano S (1996) Contrast-enhanced spiral CT of the liver: effect of injection time on time to peak hepatic enhancement. J Comput Assist Tomogr 20 (4): 633–637
17. Kopka L, Funke M, Fischer U, Vosshenrich R, Oestmann JW, Grabbe E (1995) Parenchymal liver enhancement with bolus-triggered helical CT: preliminary clinical results. Radiology 195 (1): 282–284
18. Kopka L, Rodenwaldt J, Fischer U, Mueller DW, Oestmann JW, Grabbe E (1996) Dual-phase helical CT of the liver: effects of bolus tracking and different volumes of contrast material. Radiology 201 (2): 321–326
19. Kopka L, Rodenwaldt J, Grabbe E (1997) Dual phase helical CT of the liver: is a contrast material bolus tracking device necessary for all patients (abstract)? Radiology 205 (P): 338
20. Lee HM, Lu DS, Krasny RM, Busuttil R, Kadell B, Lucas J (1997) Hepatic lesion charcterization in cirrhosis: significance of arterial hypervascularity on dual-phase helical CT. Am J Roentgenol 169 (1): 125–130
21. van Leeuwen MS, Noordzij J, Feldberg MA, Hennipman AH, Doornewaard H (1996) Focal liver lesions: characterization with triphasic spiral CT. Radiology 201 (2): 327–336
22. Mitsuzaki K, Yamashita Y, Ogata I, Nishiharu T, Urata J, Takahashi M (1996) Multiple-phase helical CT of the liver for detecting small hepatomas in patients with liver cirrhosis: contrast-injection protocol and optimal timing. Am J Roentgenol 167 (3): 753–757
23. Oliver JH 3rd, Baron RL, Federle MP, Rockette HE Jr (1996) Detecting hepatocellular carcinoma: value of unenhanced or arterial phase CT imaging or both used in conjunction with conventional portal venous phase contrast-enhanced CT imaging. Am J Roentgenol 167 (1): 71–77
24. Oliver JH 3rd, Baron RL (1996) Helical biphasic contrst-enhanced CT of the liver: technique, indications, interpretation and pitfalls. Radiology 201 (1): 1–14
25. Oliver JH 3rd, Baron RL, Federle MP, Jones BC, Sheng R (1997) Hypervascular liver metastases: do unenhanced and hepatic arterial phase CT images affect tumor detection? Radiology 205 (3): 709–715
26. Silverman PM, Cooper C, Trock B, Garra BS, Davros WJ, Zeman R (1995) Establishing the optimal temporal window for liver CT using a time density analysis: implication for helical (spiral) CT. J Comput Assist Tomogr 19 (1): 73–79
27. Silverman PM, Brown B, Wray H, Fox SH, Cooper C, Roberts S, Zeman RK (1995) Optimal contrast enhancement of the liver using helical (spiral) CT: value of SmartPrep. Am J Roentgenol 164 (5): 1169–1171
28. Silverman PM, Roberts SC, Ducic I, Tefft MC, Olson MC, Cooper C, Zeman RK (1996) Assessment of a technology that permits individualized scan delays on helical hepatic CT: a technique to improve efficiency in use of contrast material. Am J Roentgenol 167 (1): 79–84
29. Tello R, Seltzer SE, Polger M, Spaulding S, Savci G (1997) A contrast agent delivery nomogram for hepatic spiral CT. J Comput Assist Tomogr 21 (2): 236–245

20 Dual-Phase Spiral CT of Pancreatic Neoplasms

R. B. Jeffrey

20.1
Introduction

Biphasic spiral CT of the pancreas is an extremely valuable technique for diagnosing and staging patients with suspected pancreatic carcinoma [1–7]. During the arterial phase of the injection the normal pancreatic parenchyma enhances intensely. This improves the conspicuity of hypoattenuating lesions such as adenocarcinoma. The arterial phase is also excellent for identifying vascular lesions such as neuroendocrine tumors and arterial encasement. The portal venous phase, however, is essential for a complete assessment of resectability for pancreatic carcinoma as hepatic metastasis are often best demonstrated during this portion of the injection. In addition, splenic vein occlusion and the development of perisplenic varices are optimally imaged during the venous phase.

20.2
Technique

Initial noncontrast scans of the pancreas are obtained using 5- to 10-mm slice collimation during a breathhold to localize the superior and inferior extent of the pancreatic parenchyma. A 20-gauge angiocath is inserted into an antecubital vein. Nonionic (150 ml) contrast is injected at a rate of 5 ml/s. Arterial phase images are obtained after 25-s delay. Scanning is initiated with a breathheld technique through the pancreas using a 3-mm collimation and a pitch of 1.5. The arterial phase images are reconstructed every 2 mm and a separate set of images are photographed with a 20-cm field of view to evaluate for subtle vascular abnormalities.

Following the completion of the arterial phase images the patient is then repositioned and instructed to take multiple deep breaths prior to beginning the portal venous phase scan. The liver is scanned at a 5-mm collimation using a pitch of 1.5 to encompass the entire liver. The images are reconstructed every 5 mm.

20.3
Evaluation of Pancreatic Carcinoma

The main indication for biphasic spiral CT of the pancreas is to diagnose and stage patients with suspected pancreatic carcinoma (Figs. 20.1–20.4). These patients often present with jaundice and have a pancreatic mass detected first on ultrasonography. In other patients the referring clinician may have a very high

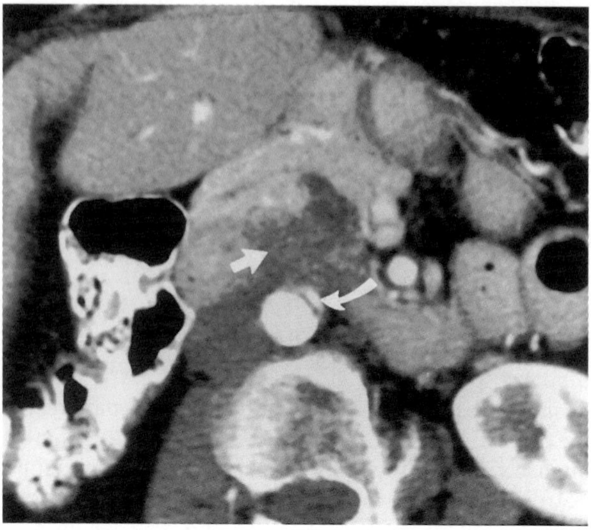

Fig. 20.1. Arterial phase image of pancreatic carcinoma. Note the sharp demarcation between the hypodense tumor and the normal pancreas (*arrow*, pancreatic carcinoma). The tumor extends posteriorly to involve the abdominal aorta and encases the origin of the inferior mesenteric artery (*curved arrow*)

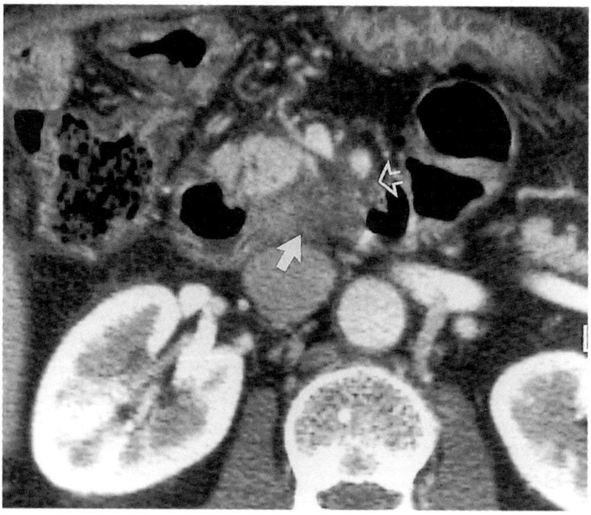

Fig. 20.2. Arterial phase image demonstrating arterial encasement. Note the clearly defined hypodense tumor of the uncinate process carcinoma (*arrow*) with invasion of the root of the mesentery and encasement of the superior mesentery artery (*open arrow*)

suspicion for pancreatic carcinoma based on clinical or laboratory findings and may proceed directly to biphasic spiral CT. Because our institution is a referral center, outside scans performed during only the portal venous phase are not infrequently felt inadequate for local staging of pancreatic carcinoma and the examination is repeated for that reason (Figs. 20.5, 20.6).

The normal pancreatic parenchyma enhances intensely during the arterial phase when a high-volume contrast injection (5 ml/s) is utilized. Hollett et al. noted that the mean pancreatic enhancement during the arterial phase was 82 HU and only 62 HU during the portal venous phase [1]. This represents a

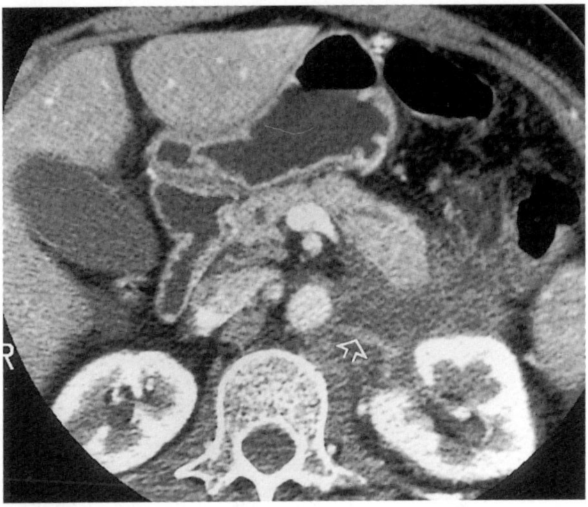

Fig. 20.3. Arterial phase image demonstrating arterial encasement. Note the hypodense tumor arising from the tail of the pancreas invading the perirenal space and encasing the left renal artery (*open arrow*)

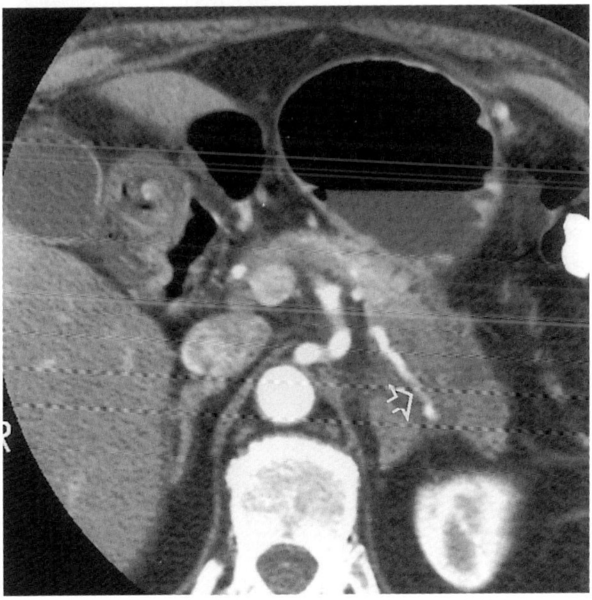

Fig. 20.4. Arterial encasement of splenic artery. Note hypodense tail of pancreas tumor invading the perirenal space and encasing the splenic artery (*arrow*, splenic artery)

highly significant difference as there is nearly a 25% diminution in the pancreatic parenchymal enhancement during the portal venous phase. The avid enhancement of the normal pancreas helps to increase the conspicuity of ductal adenocarcinoma due to its hypovascular nature. Lu et al. evaluated dual-phase spiral CT for pancreatic tumors and found that the contrast differences between adenocarcinoma and normal pancreas was significantly greater during the early arterial

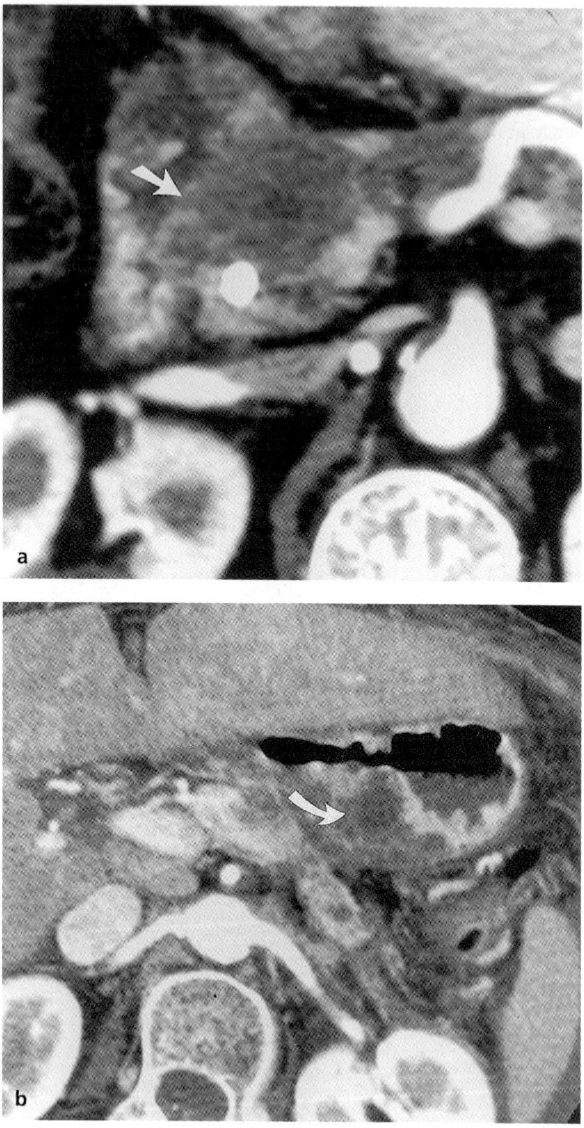

Fig. 20.5a, b. Gastrointestinal invasion of pancreatic carcinoma. **a** Note invasion of medial wall of duodenum (*arrow*). **b** Note invasion of posterior wall to stomach (*arrow*)

phase images than in the later portal venous phase of enhancement [2]. In our experience, not only are small ductal adenocarcinomas identified with greater confidence on arterial phase images, but subtle alterations in the dimension of the main pancreatic duct are also better appreciated using thin collimation (3 mm/s) and rapid injection arterial phase images.

One important clue to an underlying pancreatic parenchymal mass is the "interrupted duct sign." In some lesions of the body and tail of the pancreas this may be the most conspicuous feature of an underlying pancreatic carcinoma. Dil-

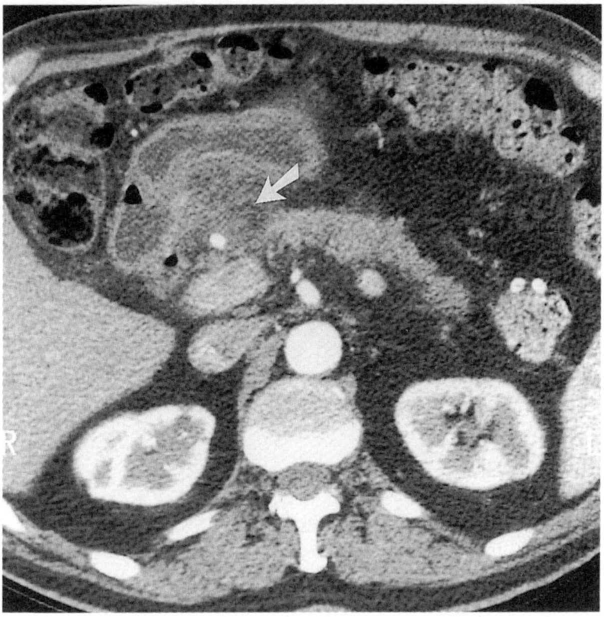

Fig. 20.6. Perivascular infiltration due to pancreatitis, not tumor. Following ERCP, note perivascular soft tissue infiltration surrounding gastroduodenal artery (*arrow*). This was due to recent ERCP and not tumor

atation and discontinuity of the pancreatic duct should always raise the possibility of pancreatic mass rather than chronic pancreatitis. Chronic pancreatitis should only be diagnosed with confidence if there is dilatation of the pancreatic duct throughout the entire pancreas with visualization of intraductal calculi.

In addition to improving detection of the primary pancreatic lesion, arterial phase images are of considerable value in assessing for resectability. Arterial encasement of the splanchnic vasculature is an unequivocal sign indicating unresectability. Subtle soft tissue thickening and "cloaking" of the splenic, hepatic, celiac or superior mesenteric arteries is often the major finding indicative of an unresectable lesion. Dense opacification of the celiac axis and splanchnic vasculature greatly facilitates diagnosis of subtle vascular encasement. Tumor infiltration around very tiny mesenteric vessels, such as branches of the jejunal arteries may also be diagnosed with this technique.

Although portal venous phase images are essential for detection of metastatic lesions from pancreatic carcinoma, arterial phase images may be of value in improving the specificity of hepatic metastases by demonstrating peripheral rim enhancement around the lesion. Often small (less than 1.5 cm) hypodense lesions seen on the portal venous phase are nonspecific and, particularly when necrotic, may mimic benign hepatic cysts. The demonstration of peripheral enhancement around the hypodense lesion is strongly correlated with underlying malignancy in the absence of clinical signs suggesting an abscess. Hepatic cysts do not demonstrate this peripheral rim enhancement.

Arterial phase images of the pancreas may also greatly aid in the diagnosis of hypervascular pancreatic neoplasms such as neuroendocrine tumors and hypervascular pancreatic metastasis (chiefly renal cell carcinoma and sarcomas). Although most functioning islet cell tumors are clinically discovered due to laboratory abnormalities and specific symptoms, many nonfunctioning islet cell tumors present with only vague symptoms due to mass effect. The prognosis of most neuroendocrine tumors of the pancreas is significantly better than ductal adenocarcinoma; therefore an attempt should be made to resect the lesion whenever possible. Our current evaluation for both functioning and nonfunctioning islet cell tumors is to perform biphasic spiral CT of the pancreas followed by careful intraoperative sonography. Selective angiography and venous sampling are no longer part of the diagnostic work up. In patients who are not able to receive intravenous contrast, MRI, particularly using fat-suppressed T1-weighted images and gadolinium-enhanced gradient recalled images are also of clear value in identifying these small tumors.

References

1. Hollett MD, Jorgensen MJ, Jeffrey RB Jr (1995) Quantitative evaluation of pancreatic enhancement during dual-phase helical CT. Radiology 195:359–361
2. Lu DS, Vedantham S, Krasny RM, Kadell B, Berger WL, Reber HA (1996) Two-phase helical CT for pancreatic tumors: pancreatic versus hepatic phase enhancement of tumor, pancreas, and vascular structures. Radiology 199:697–701
3. Bonaldi VM, Bret PM, Atri M, Garcia P, Reinhold C (1996) A comparison of two injection protocols using helical and dynamic acquisitions in CT examinations of the pancreas. AJR 167: 49–55
4. Freeny PC, Traverso LW, Ryan JA (1993) Diagnosis and staging of pancreatic adenocarcinoma with dynamic computed tomography. Am J Surg 165:600–606
5. Thoeni RF, Blankenberg F (1993) Pancreatic imaging: computed tomography and magnetic resonance imaging. Radiol Clin North Am 31:1085–1113
6. Hosoki T (1983) Dynamic CT of pancreatic tumors. AJR 959–965
7. Bluemke DA, Cameron JL, Hruban RH (1995) Potentially resectable pancreatic adenocarcinoma: spiral CT assessment with surgical and pathologic correlation. Radiology 197:381–385

21 Contribution of Fast and Spiral CT to Diagnostic Punctures of Abdominal Lesions

J. de Mey, B. Op de Beeck, M. Osteaux

21.1 Introduction

The breakthrough in using computed tomography (CT) to guide diagnostic puncture occurred in the 1980s, with the development of body CT. Further progress continues to made in CT-guided diagnostic puncture as a result of recent technological advances (fast scan, spiral scan, CT-scopy), new puncture material, and the development of less aggressive surgical techniques.

21.2 Material

Fine-Needle Aspiration. The advantage of this technique is the diameter of the needle (up to 29 G), which provides safe passage to all tissues without important complications. New cytological techniques permit a more accurate diagnosis. This technique is used mainly in the echographically guided thyroid and breast puncture. For abdominal pathology the results of fine-needle aspirations are less satisfactory than real tissue biopsy needles [1–3].

The Hybrid Needles. These needles also have a reduced diameter. In most cases cytological examination is possible only on the collected material. For this reason real tissue biopsy needles often replace these needles.

Tissue Biopsy Needles

- Side-notch biopsy, manual or automatic: The advantage of these is to provide a real tissue cylinder so that the pathologist can perform a histological examination. A diameter of up to 21 G [2, 3] yields excellent diagnostic results. Automatic needles are much easier to use than manual ones. A larger notch can provide more tissue; however, needles with a large notch have reduced stability, particularly when the diameter is under 18 G, so that one can obtain zero biopsies in soft tissue.
- Side-notch biopsy gun: The tissue cylinder is usually of better quality than that provided by automatic or manual biopsy. However, this needle has the disadvantages of requiring sterilization and of a difficult use of the gantry due to its weight and dimensions.
- Biopsy gun end notch: This system seems the perfect combination between the fine-needle aspiration and real tissue biopsy. However, tests with this material have shown many zero biopsies [4].

Bone Biopsy. Bone biopsy consists of two techniques. The first is the technique used to obtain cortical bone; specific bone biopsy needles are used. Secondly, we can (through this bone biopsy needles) perform a soft tissue biopsy of interosseous material with a simple side-notch biopsy needle coaxial.

Coaxial Puncture. This technique is somewhat more complex. One must use two separate needles; however, this ensures that tract metastasis is avoided. Multiple biopsies can also be performed more easily in the same region [5, 6].

21.3 Technique

21.3.1 Puncture Tract

Tissues to avoid are veins with a large diameter, the choledocus, the Wirsung duct, and the urether. Other structures can be passed throughout with smaller needle diameter – the aorta, pulmonary tissue, stomach, small intestine, and colon. Organic tissue such as liver, spleen, and kidneys can be passed throughout with a moderate risk. In looking for a tract to perform the puncture we prefer to have a safe passage, which means only through muscle, fat tissue, or fibrotic tissue.

21.3.2 The Puncture

Localization. First the patient is laid in a stable position, which should not be changed during the entire intervention. The next step is to scan the patient and look for a safe passage throughout the lesion. In this way spiral CT can be useful if a safe passage is to be executed in a plane other than the axial one. We look preferentially for a safe passage in the axial plane or in the plane of the gantry with gantry tilt. An angle of 90° or 180 ° is preferred for easy puncture; certainly when fast scanning, spiral CT or CT-scopy is not possible. Some surgeons use a small metal grid [14] as skin marker; however a simple metal marker (e.g., paperclip) is also convenient.

Anesthetics and Preparation. After disinfecting the region, local anesthetic can be administered with xylocaine 2%, using a 5-cm 21 G intramuscular needle. Larger lumbar puncture needles can also be used if necessary. Control CT with the small needle in place is recommended, resulting in a good image of the needle tract and the lesion.

Puncture and Biopsy. Needle depth can be calculated on the scan. Some needles have centimeter markers to help in guaging needle depth. Other needles are provided with a plastic marker. Alternatively, one can merely mark the needle with an alcohol pen. Biopsy must be taken in a nonnecrotic part of the mass. Tissue biopsy can be transported in Bouin (for anatomopathology); in physiological serum (for lymphoma suspicion) we can also transport the tissue in the needle itself for microbiological examinations.

With the new scan techniques there are the following workout:

Outside of the Gantry. Scanning can be performed, and on the scan images we can mark the tract and measure the depth and the angle. When the patient is outside the gantry, puncture can be carried out from the skin in the calculated depth with the calculated angle. This method has several disadvantages. First, we are working with a patient who is breathing and moving. The lesion can be displaced. Also, when we insert the needle, some lesions are very fibrotic and can be pushed away by the needle. The method without needle control in the gantry is certainly not first choice.

Mixed Method. Procedure inside and outside the gantry. The needle can be manipulated when the patient is outside the gantry. After the needle is placed, scan controls can be carried out to determined whether it is in the correct position. Spiral control is sometimes more accurate for an exact needle tip localization [7]. Manipulating the needle outside the gantry has the advantage that the operator can work in a comfortable position. Operations in the gantry are often more difficult and require a skilled operator.

Puncture in the Gantry. This method is used mainly when CT-scopy is possible. It is the most accurate method for smaller lesions. When possible, CT-scopy should be used when the puncture is performed in a plane other than the axial one. To minimize irradiation on the surgeon's hand CT-scopy can be be stopped occasionally during needle manipulations. When working in the gantry, it is not necessary to measure the depth or the angle. Without CT-scopy, gantry tilt and working in the gantry plane following the laser beam can be the solution to obtaining more accurate nonaxial punctures.

21.4 Complications

Bleeding. A small hematoma can be seen along the tract and depend on the size of the needle. However, this is rare when the procedure is followed accurately, and a good tract is chosen. If possible, for liver and spleen punctures passage should be through healthy organic tissue and thus avoid a subcapsullar bleeding.

Pneumothorax. There is always the possibility of a pneumothorax. However, passage through 1 cm of the costodiaphragmatic sinus can be performed without high risk [8] for liver biopsies.

Pancreatitis. Pancreatitis is a normal complication when carrying out a puncture of the pancreas,. However, this is often limited; the risk is greater when the needle diameter is above 18 G.

Peritonitis, Fistulisation, Tract Metastasis. The risk of major complications is very low, even after passage of bowel with needle not higher than 18 G.

21.5 Conclusion

Recent developments in CT have had an important impact on today's procedures of diagnostic punctures. Ten years ago a well-marked place on the patient's skin and angle and depth measurements were the most important features in performing diagnostic punctures on CT. With today's new techniques we can start a puncture very quickly while the patient is in the gantry. During the procedure the depth and angle can be changed while the needle is placed under CT guidance. In this way a biopsy of smaller lesions can be easily performed in more difficult regions. A spiral acquisition improves the choice of the tract in planes other than the axial and improves visualization of the needle tip. Based on the spiral acquisition, angle measurements can be executed on the reconstruction maps. CT-scopy certainly has many advantages for smaller lesions; however, the image does not have the same resolution as the scan one, and manipulation of the needle in the gantry is more difficult for nonskilled radiologists.

References

1. Welch TJ, Sheedy PF, Johnson CD, Johnson CM, Stephens DH (1989) CT-guided biopsy: prospective analysis of 1000 procedures. Radiology 171:493–496
2. Noppen MMP, de Mey J, Meysman M et al (1995) Percutaneous needle biopsy of localized pulmonary, mediastinal, and pleural diseased tissue with an automatic disposable guillotine soft-tissue needle. Chest 107:1615–20
3. Dodd LG, Mooney EE, Layfield LJ, Nelson RC (1997) Fine-needle aspiration of the lever and pancreas: a cytology primer for radiologists. Radiology 203 (1):1–9
4. Hopper KD, Abendroth CS, Sturtz KW et al (1995) CT percutaneous biopsy guns: comparison of end-cut and side-notch devices in cadaveric specimens. AJR 164:195–199
5. Kudryck BT, Martinez CR, Gunasekeran S et al (1995) CT-guided renal biopsy using a coaxial technique and an automated biopsy gun. Southern Med J 88:543–546
6. Swerdlow DR, Thaete FL (1994) CT-guided core biopsy of difficult lesions: a modified coaxial approach. AJR 163:195–196
7. Silverman SG, Bloom DA Seltzer SE et al (1992) Needle-tip localization during CT-guided abdominal biopsy: comparison of conventional and spiral CT. AJR 159:1095–1097
8. Gervais DA, Gazelle GS, Lu DSK et al (1996) Percutaneous transpulmonary CT-guided liver biopsy: a safe and technically easy approach for lesions near the diaphragm. AJR 167:482–483

22 Spiral CT of the Musculoskeletal System

E.K. FISHMAN

22.1
Introduction

Although the role of computed tomography (CT) as a primary study for the evaluation of musculoskeletal pathology diminished with the advent of clinical magnetic resonance imaging (MRI), the recent developments in spiral CT has again increased the interest in these applications [1–4]. This is in great part related to the capabilities of spiral CT to rapidly scan patients with optimization of the delivery of contrast and data acquisition and to create volume data sets which can be used for highly detailed three-dimensional (3D) reconstructions. The impact of 3D imaging is felt especially in orthopedic applications, where clinical decision making is complex and treatment options vary.

The role of CT in evaluation of the musculoskeletal system can be divided into trauma, infection/inflammatory disease, oncologic applications, and miscellaneous conditions. The two most common applications in our clinical practice are trauma and inflammatory disease [5–8]. Trauma imaging, not surprisingly, is closely tied to multiplanar and 3D imaging. The number of cases with inflammatory/infectious disease is because our population is heavily weighted toward immunosuppressed patients, whether due to bone marrow transplants or AIDS.

The advent of spiral CT is making substantial changes in our referring physicians' selection of radiologic examinations. In the musculoskeletal system the importance of a rapid diagnosis as well as a complete understanding and definition of extent of disease is something that spiral CT can routinely provide. Spiral CT can also provide this information in a very cost-effective manner in even the most uncooperative patients. The information obtained through CT is classically a critical part of patient management decisions.

22.2
Clinical Applications

22.2.1
Trauma

Regardless of the anatomic area of involvement, be it the acetabulum, pelvis or wrist, CT plays a major role in patient diagnosis, triage and management [9–12]. The role of CT can typically be divided into cases in which on plain film evaluation the presence of a fracture is somewhat in doubt, and those cases in which the diagnosis is made, but CT is performed to better define the extent of injury to help plan surgery or decide between surgery and a more conservative management. The uncertainty on plain radiography could be because of poor positioning of the patient, indeterminate radiographs, or disagreement between the patient's symptoms and the radiographic findings. In these cases CT can be performed to determine whether there is indeed a fracture.

When performing musculoskeletal CT it is important to optimize the technical aspects of the examination (Table 22.1). We routinely use spiral CT with narrow collimation in the 2- to 3-mm range, although this varies depending on the body part studied. The reconstruction interval is typically 3 mm but can be 1 mm, particularly in areas such as the wrist, where thin-section and narrow-incremental reconstruction is mandatory. One of the obvious advantages of volume data sets with spiral CT is the creation of additional scans without additional radiation exposure to the patient.

When evaluating musculoskeletal trauma we have found that reconstruction of images with the bone or high-resolution algorithm is most valuable. This algorithm varies from scanner to scanner as well as between scanners from the same manufacturer. It is important that one become familiar with his own system and choose the bone reconstruction algorithm that works best for him. The technical support staff of the equipment vendor should provide the parameters that are available and from these one can select that which is most appropriate.

Although in most cases intravenous contrast is not necessary when evaluating bony trauma, there are situations in which it can become extremely important. For example, in pelvic trauma if vascular injury is suspected, a spiral CT using CT angiographic technique would be ideal. In this process we can evaluate the lower abdominal aorta, iliac vessels, and their branches as well as the bony pelvis in a single examination. Similarly, in patients with sternal or sternoclavicular joint injury it is important to not only evaluate the bony structures to define the extent of fracture and dislocation but also to obtain a vascular study to exclude injury to

Table 22.1. Parameters of spiral CT by application

	Skeletal trauma with 3D imaging	Acetabulum and hip joint (trauma)	Muscle infection, abscess
Scan parameters			
kVp	120	120	120
mAs	280	280	280
s	0.75	0.75	0.75
Phase of respiration	Patient must remain motionless	Inspiration or shallow breathing	Suspended respiration
Slice thickness	3 mm	3 mm	5 mm
Pitch	1–1.5	1–1.5	1–1.5
Spiral exposure time	30–40 s	Usually around 30 s	30–40 s
Reconstruction interval	2 mm	2 mm	3–5 mm
Superior extent	2 cm above area in question	Mid-bony pelvis	2–4 cm above suspected lesion
Inferior extent	2 cm below area in question	Inferior aspect of symphysis pubis	2–4 cm below suspected lesion
IV contrast	Use depends on clinical situation	None unless CT angiogram is needed	120 ml Omnipaque-350

the aorta or great vessels. One of the advantages of this combined study technique is that in many cases angiography can be avoided.

In choosing the specific scan parameters for a anatomic area several variables must be considered. The first is the area or volume that needs to be covered. For scanning the wrist narrow collimation in the range of 2 mm can be used with data reconstructions at 1-mm intervals. The pitch can be in a range of 1–1.5. If, however, we need to scan a larger area such as the femur or an area from the knee to the ankle, we must make several compromises. In some cases we can use narrow collimation such as 3 mm but increase the pitch to 2 and cover a reasonable distance with the newer subsecond scanners. In other cases wider slice collimation of 5 mm can be performed in order to cover a longer distance. Initially our experience was somewhat disappointing with using higher pitch in musculoskeletal imaging. Images were not very sharp, were very noisy, and were generally unsatisfactory. With our newest Plus 4 scanners and their higher mAs settings as well as new bone reconstruction filters this problem has apparently been resolved.

An important aspect of musculoskeletal trauma imaging is the use of reformated images. These typically are categorized as multiplanar reconstruction (MPR) and 3D imaging. MPR is the reformating of data typically along the sagittal and coronal plane, although any off-axis can also be obtained. This is available on all scanners and typically takes several seconds to several minutes to perform. The advantage of spiral CT with MPR is that it is cost-effective and provides the clinician with images in any plane or perspective chosen. This is particularly valuable in supplementing the information provided by routine transaxial CT images.

The second process revolves around 3D imaging. Much has been written about the various techniques used for 3D imaging, including volume-rendering technique, shaded surface technique, and maximum intensity projection [13–16]. Except for those cases with secondary vascular imaging the key reconstruction algorithms used in musculoskeletal imaging are shaded-surface display and volume rendering. We exclusively use volume rendering as implemented on the Siemens 3D Virtuoso (Figs. 22.1, 22.2, 22.3).

Our experience over the past dozen or so years is that 3D reconstructions are especially valuable to the referring physician in understanding the "personality of the injury." Orthopedic surgeons are advocates of this technique and find that it provides information that simple transaxial images do not. It is our feeling that the best way of looking at 3D imaging is interactively in "real-time" on a workstation (Silicon Graphics Infinite Reality or O2), and we have found this to be helpful in clinical practice.

22.2.2 Musculoskeletal Inflammation

With the ever-increasing numbers of immunosuppressed patients, be it due to bone marrow transplant, high-dose steroid patients for treatment of renal disease, or AIDS patients, increasing numbers of patients present with possible musculoskeletal infection [17]. Our experience has been that spiral CT is a rapid and

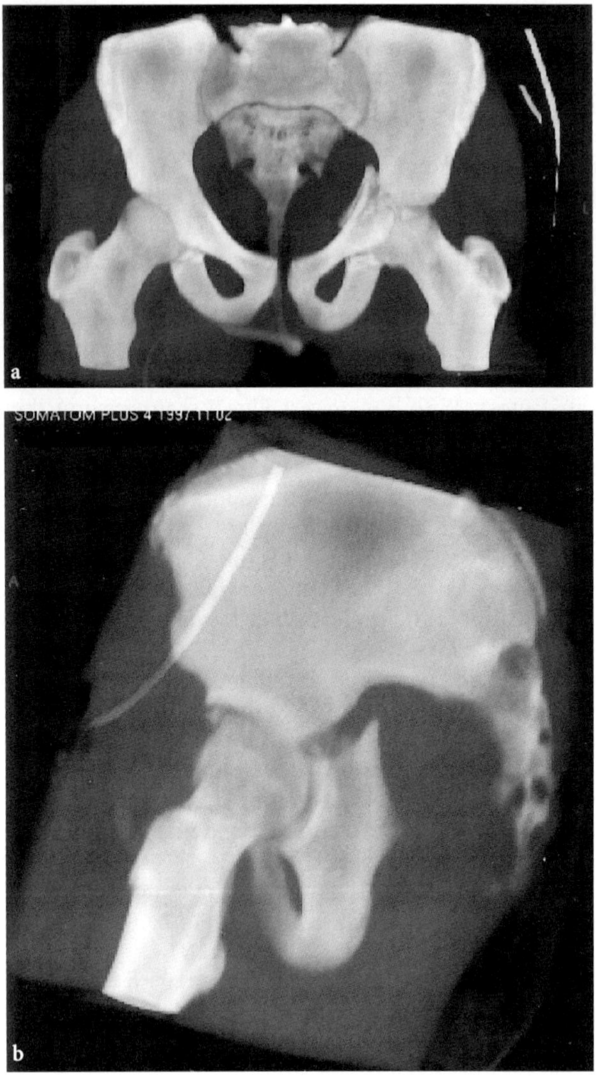

Fig. 22.1a, b. Acetabular fracture. 3D volumetric reconstruction demonstrates left acetabular fracture with displacement of posterior acetabular component requiring a posterior approach for repair

accurate technique for evaluating suspected or known musculoskeletal infection. The key advantages in these cases are related to the ability for timed contrast delivery and data acquisition, which helps accentuate the difference between normal and abnormal structures such as in muscle (Fig. 22.4; Table 22.1).

In cases when IV contrast is not used, but substantial inflammation is present we can still usually detect the pathologic process. However, information regarding extent of inflammation and level of involvement may be suboptimal. With intravenous contrast we find that the normal musculature enhances up to 50–70 HU, making detection of pathology easier. Our protocols for contrast-enhanced studies require injection of 120 ml Omnipaque-350 (Nycomed, Prince-

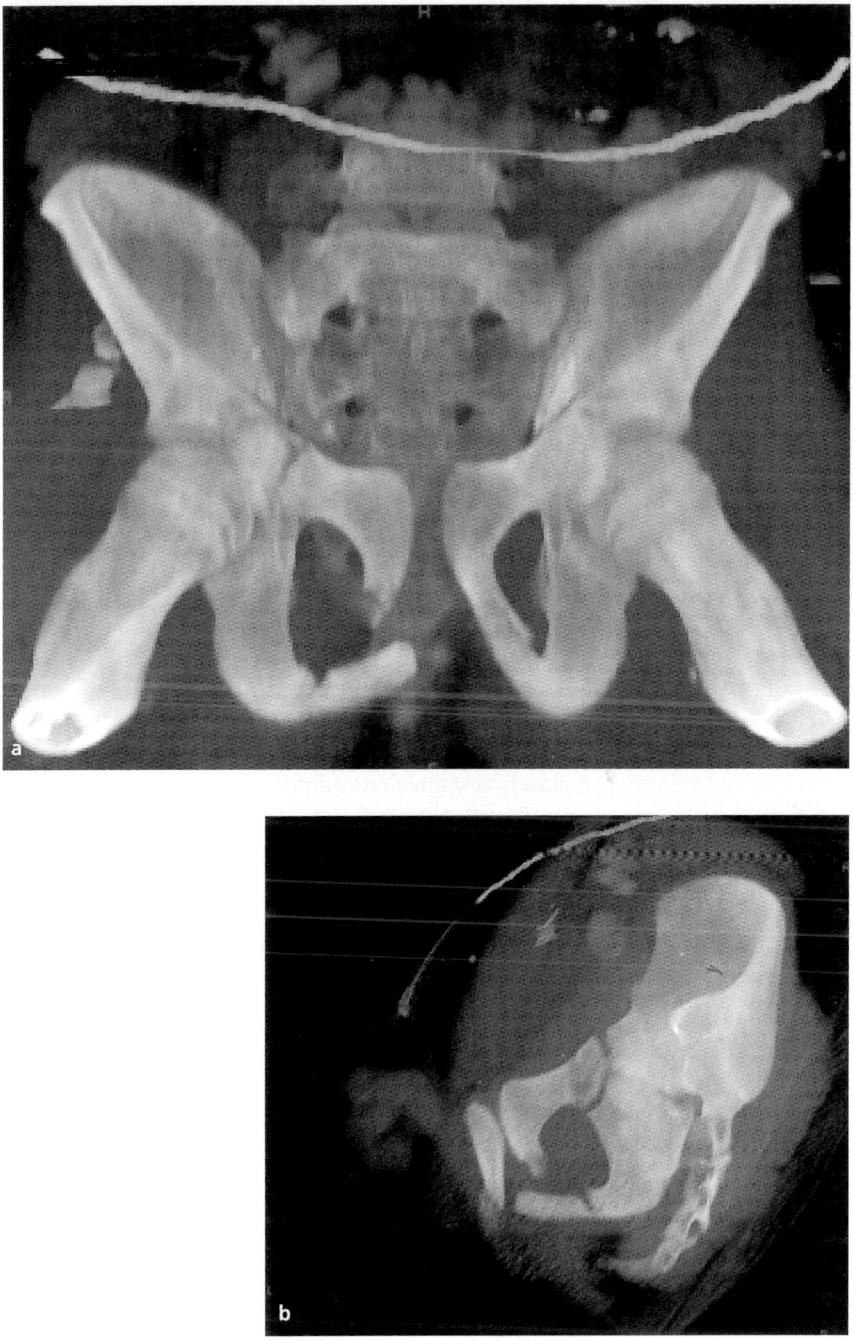

Fig. 22.2A, B. Fracture of acetabulum and symphysis pubis. Select views demonstrate how complex injuries can be viewed from any plane or perspective using 3D volume rendering

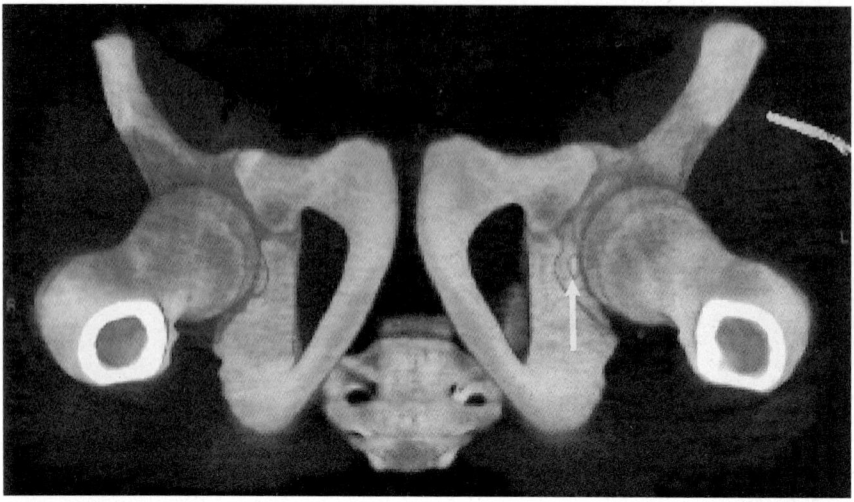

Fig. 22.3. Intra-articular fragment in left hip joint. The patient had persistent pain following fracture dislocation of left hip with reduction. *Arrow*, 3-mm bone fragment is seen in the left hip joint

ton, NJ) and data acquisition beginning at 30–40 s after initiation of injection of contrast (Table 22.1). We have found this to be ideal time to optimize differentiation between normal and abnormal muscle. It should be noted that one of the potential limitations at least from a theoretical perspective is that enhancing muscle abscesses and tumors can closely resemble one another. However, in most cases the clinical history is obviously different, and the case is typically not problematic.

Fig. 22.4. Intramuscular abscess. Spiral CT demonstrates a low-density lesion with rim enhancement compatible with an intramuscular abscess

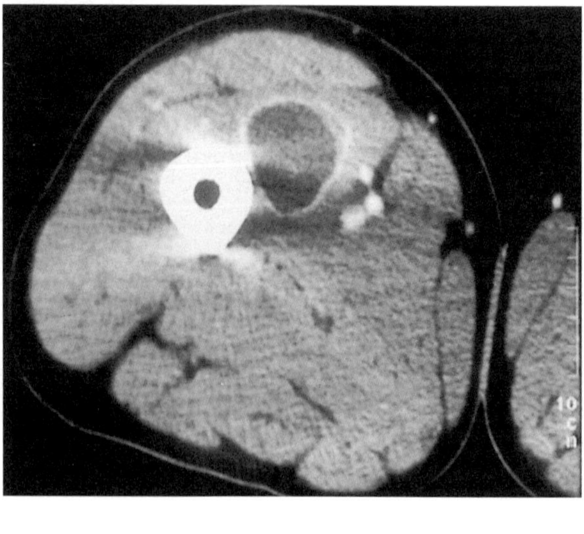

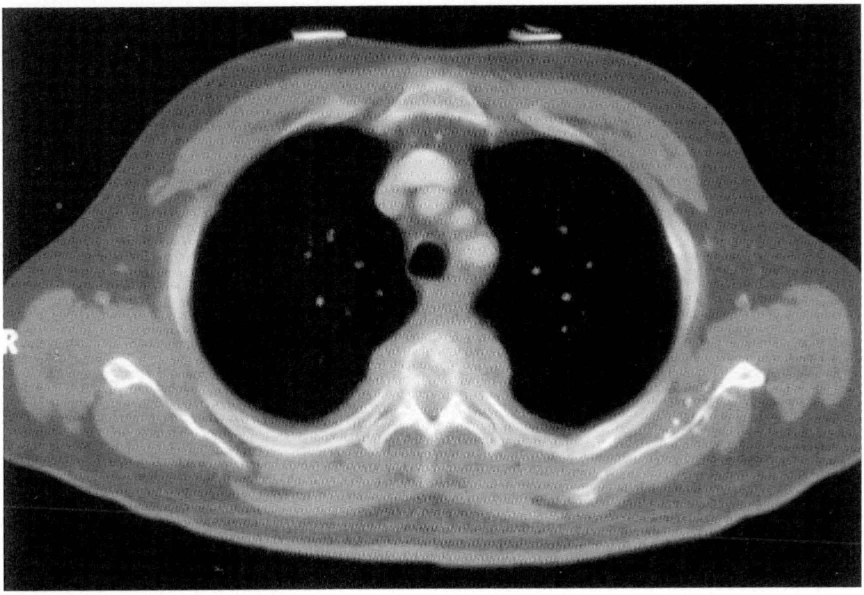

Fig. 22.5. Osteomyelitis thoracic spine with paraspinal abscess. Axial view demonstrates destruction of the thoracic vertebral body with a paraspinal abscess

When evaluating muscle inflammation, it is also important to review bone windows through the scan volume (Fig. 22.5). Often bony involvement is a primary source of an inflammatory process; it may also become involved secondarily. This is particularly true of infection in the chest wall (especially around the sternoclavicular joint) and the sacrum. To save time and filming costs images can be reviewed in cine mode on a workstation.

In the evaluation of musculoskeletal infection we typically reconstruct the data with a standard algorithm. The high-resolution algorithm or bone algorithms create substantial noise, which is suboptimal for viewing the soft tissues. In cases in which high-resolution images of bone are desired, reconstruction of the data with both algorithms is ideal.

In most cases of musculoskeletal inflammation 3D or multiplanar imaging is not needed. However, in select cases it may be very valuable, particularly in determining the extent of inflammation, which may be helpful to the surgeon in preoperative planning. This is especially true in processes that involve bone such as osteomyelitis of the spine or other complex anatomic zones such as the sacroiliac joint or hip joint.

22.2.3 Musculoskeletal Tumors

Although MRI is the accepted study of choice for musculoskeletal tumors, the recent Radiology Diagnostic Oncology Group report showed no statistical differ-

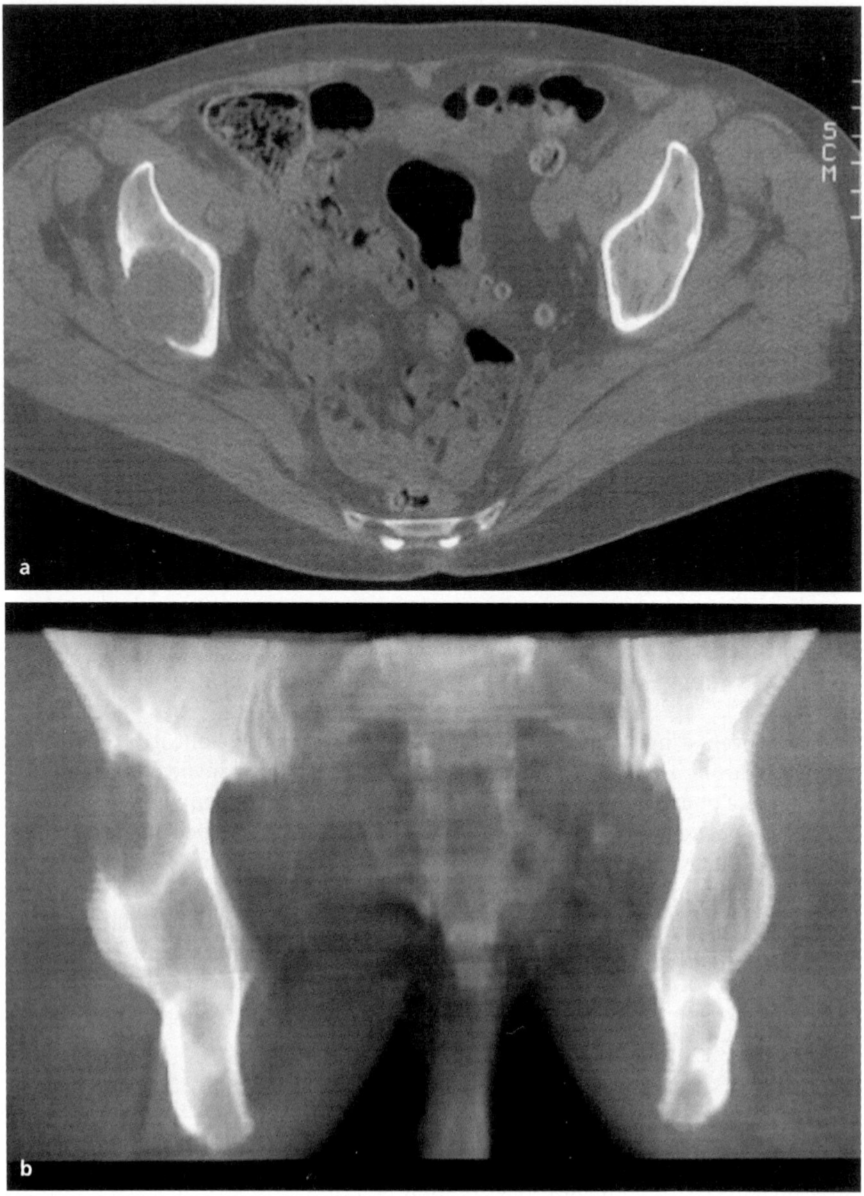

Fig. 22.6a, b. Lytic metastases to bone. Spiral CT with 3D reconstruction demonstrate a lytic lesion in the right acetabulum well defined on the 3D views. The 3D views can be used for radiation therapy planning

ence in staging between CT and MRI in the evaluation of musculoskeletal tumors [18]. We have always found CT to be valuable in looking at soft tissue masses, particularly by determining attenuation values [19]. With CT it is very easy to determine whether a lesion is a lipoma, and whether it is hemorrhagic. Similarly, in looking at bony tumors CT can clearly detect and define the presence and type of matrix present (Fig. 22.5). The extent of tumor can be well documented with CT, and as noted there is little difference statistically between it and MRI.

One of the most common oncologic uses for CT is as a problem-solving tool in cases where there is suspected bony metastasis and discordance between clinical examination, radiographs, and bone scans. In these cases focused high-resolution CT can be carried out to determine whether there is any bony involvement. In these cases thin collimation with narrow interscan spacing is very valuable. We also find that MPR and 3D imaging is very valuable when lesions involve areas near a joint space, and one is trying to determine whether the patient is in danger of pathologic fracture (Fig. 22.6). MPR is very valuable in the sagittal plane when looking at the acetabulum and lumbar spine and in determining the extent of pathology in these regions.

The role of CT in the evaluation of primary musculoskeletal tumors varies from institution to institution. CT is excellent at defining the presence and type of matrix (Fig. 22.7) within a lesion as well as determining the extent of bony destruction. IV contrast and spiral CT provide a good assessment of tumor involvement in soft tissue. However, MRI does appear to be superior because of its direct multiplanar capabilities.

One interesting finding related to spiral CT is the frequency of incidental detection of musculoskeletal metastasis (Fig. 22.8). We have seen many cases of metastasis to muscle presenting as hypervascular lesions ranging in size from 5 to

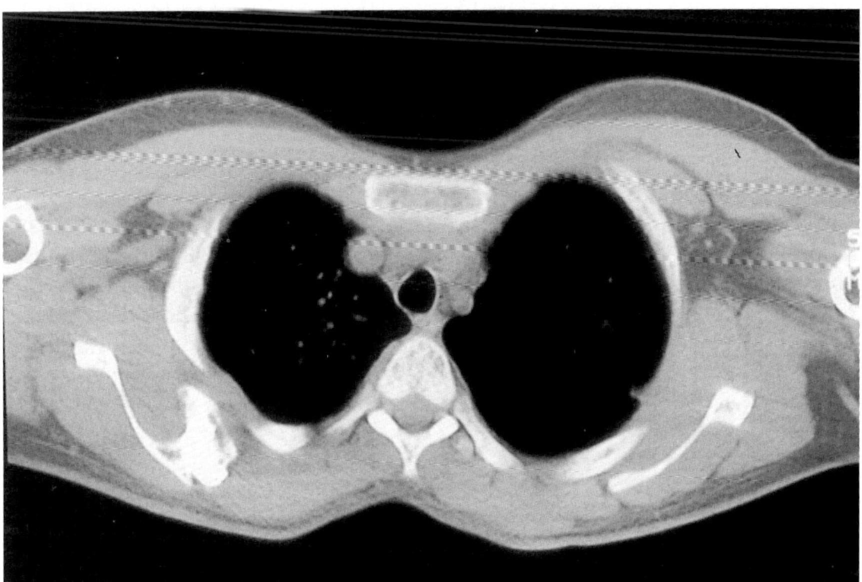

Fig. 22.7. Osteochondroma of the right scapula. Spiral CT demonstrates an osteochondroma arising from the right scapula. No evidence of malignant degeneration of the lesion is seen

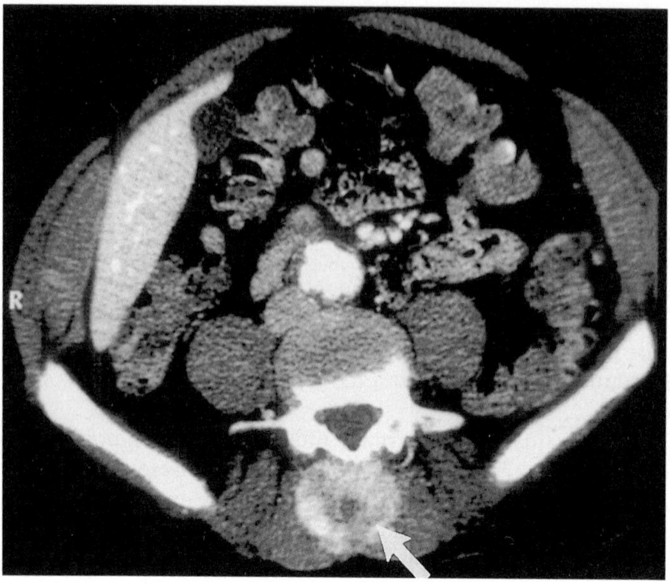

Fig. 22.8. Metastatic lung cancer to paraspinal muscle. The patient presented with acute abdominal pain which clinically was thought to be abdominal aortic aneurysm. Spiral CT was performed which demonstrated an enhancing mass (*arrow*) in the paraspinal muscles which was subsequently proven to be metastatic lung cancer

20 mm. In most cases the patients have not been symptomatic due to these lesions. The common tumors in which we have found this to occur have been lung cancer, renal cancer, and lymphoma.

22.3 Conclusion

Spiral CT provides unique opportunities for imaging the musculoskeletal system by providing the capabilities of high-quality volume data sets and the optimal ability for time contrast infusion and data acquisition. The continued development of 3D imaging and multidimensional displays provide substantial advantages in musculoskeletal imaging. With the continued development of both CT technology and computer software the role of CT in musculoskeletal imaging will continue to expand in the near future.

References

1. Pretorius ES, Fishman EK (1995) Helical (spiral) CT of the musculoskeletal system. Radiol Clin North Am 33 (5):949–979
2. Fishman EK (1995) Spiral CT evaluation of the musculoskeletal system (IN) Fishman EK, Jeffrey RB (eds) Spiral CT: principles, techniques and clinical applications, Raven, New York
3. Fishman EK, Wyatt SH, Bluemke DA, Urban BA (1993) Spiral CT of musculoskeletal pathology: preliminary observations. Skeletal Radiol 22:253–256

4. Ney DR, Fishman EK, Kawashima A, Robertson DD Jr, Scott WW (1992) Comparison of helical and serial CT with regard to three-dimensional imaging of musculoskeletal anatomy. Radiology 185 (3):865–869
5. Fishman EK (1995) Oncologic applications of spiral CT. In: Fishman EK, Jeffrey RB (eds) Spiral CT: principles, techniques and clinical applications, Raven, New York
6. Kuszyk BS, Fishman EK (1996) Direct coronal CT of the wrist: helical acquisition with simplified patient positioning. AJR 166:419–420
7. Tecce PM, Fishman EK (1995) Spiral CT with multiplanar reconstruction in the diagnosis of sternoclavicular osteomyelitis. Skeletal Radiol 24:275–281
8. Beauchamp NJ, Scott WW Jr, Gottlieb LM, Fishman EK (1995) CT evaluation of soft tissue muscle infection and inflammation: a systematic compartmental approach. Skeletal Radiol 24:317–324
9. Scott WW Jr, Fishman EK, Magid D (1987) Acetabular fractures: optimal imaging. Radiology 165:537–539
10. Pretorius ES, Scott WW Jr, Fishman EK (1995) Acute trauma of the shoulder: role of spiral CT imaging. Emerg Radiol 2 (1):13–17
11. Kode L, Lieberman JM, Motta AO, Wilber JH, Vasen A, Yagan R (1994) Evaluation of tibial plateau fractures: efficacy of MR imaging compared with CT. AJR 163:141–147
12. Kuhlman JE, Fishman EK, Ney DR, Magid D (1988) Complex shoulder trauma: three-dimensional CT imaging. Orthopedics 11:1561–1563
13. Fishman EK, Magid D, Ney D et al (1991) Three-dimensional imaging. Radiology 181: 321–327
14. Kuszyk BS, Ney DR, Fishman EK (1995) The current state of the art in three-dimensional oncologic imaging: an overview. Int J Radiat Oncol Biol Phys 33 (5):1029–1039
15. Kuszyk BS, Heath DG, Bliss DF, Fishman EK (1996) Skeletal 3D CT: advantages of volume rendering over surface rendering. Skeletal Radiol 25:207–214
16. McEnery KW, Wilson AJ, Pilgram TK, Murphy Jr WA, Marushack MM (1994) Fractures of the tibial plateau: value of spiral CT coronal plane reconstructions for detecting displacement in vitro. AJR 163:1177–1181
17. Magid D, Fishman EK (1992) Musculoskeletal infections in patients with AIDS: CT findings. AJR 158:603–607
18. Panicek DM, Gatsonis C, Rosenthal DI et al (1997) CT and MR imaging in the local staging of primary malignant musculoskeletal neoplasms: report of the Radiology Diagnostic Oncology Group. Radiology 202:237–246
19. Ma LD, Frassica FJ, Scott WW Jr, Fishman EK, Zerhouni EA (1995) Differentiation of benign and malignant musculoskeletal tumors: potential pitfalls with MR imaging. Radiographics 15:349–366

Part V
Technical Developments, Postprocessing

Moderators: G. M. Glazer, W. A. Kalender

23 Spiral CT: How New Technology Has Improved Scanner Utilization and Productivity

M.E. Baker

23.1 Introduction

Over the past 15–20 years medical equipment manufacturers have consistently promised that technological improvements in their machines would not only enhance disease detection but would also improve patient examination throughput and technologist's efficiency. The dramatic improvements in CT technology over the years serve as an example of these promises fulfilled. Although one could argue that quantitative data is absent for confirmation, all of the improvements in CT since the days of the slow, first-generation scanners have in fact improved both diagnostic accuracy and scanner efficiency.

However, as improvements in CT have become increasingly less dramatic, it may be more difficult to document true gains. It is very difficult to demonstrate improvements in cost-effectiveness with any new features on CT, especially as it relates to disease detection. Nonetheless, if we believe that improvements provide us true advantages, we must quantify the promised improvements in order to justify their acquisition. With spiral examinations of the liver retrospective reconstruction using narrower z-axis intervals detects more, smaller lesions. However, it remains to be seen whether detecting smaller lesions in fact alters patient management, as confirming that these lesions represent tumor is often impossible.

Spirally acquired images, however, produce higher quality postprocessed multiplanar, and 3-D images than discrete or sequential images. Further, using spiral technique, higher intravascular contrast enhancement is possible over more extended z-axis. If one chooses to replace standard diagnostic angiography with CT angiography (CTA), acquiring spiral technology clearly leads to savings in costs. Cost cutting therefore is another method of justifying new technology acquisition.

In the past 3 years my Division Chairman has constantly challenged me to show how new technology is advantageous. Anecdotal promises of improved image quality or diagnostic accuracy are insufficient evidence to convince him to acquire new technology. Therefore I have chosen to measure improvements in scanner and technologist efficiency with new technology and to use this quantitative data to justify new product acquisition.

The purpose of this chapter is show how we can measure improved scanner productivity and efficiency. I demonstrate how a change from the Siemens Plus Classic CT platform (used both in nonspiral and spiral modes) with gas detectors to an all Plus 4 CT platform dramatically changed the way in which CT is performed at the Cleveland Clinic Foundation (CCF) over the years 1994–1997. In mid-1994 we had three CT scanners (all Somatom Plus Classic platforms). Currently we have five CT scanners (four in the main department, all of which are Plus 4 devices, (one of which has the solid detector with rapid reconstruction, one rapid reconstruction with CT fluoroscopy, and two the Plus 4 level only). I present the following information:

- Three-year historical data documenting the changes in total number of examinations and the resultant effect on technologist staffing.
- Prospective data recently published in the *American Journal of Roentgenol* documenting the real time savings in examinations when moving from the Plus Classic platform to the Plus 4 platform.
- Noncontrolled historical data documenting the decreased room time for intervention when using CARE Vision CT fluoroscopy vis-à-vis room time using standard CT technique for interventions. To date our prospective study has not enrolled sufficient patients to be meaningful.
- Noncontrolled data showing the improved room time for examinations for the Plus 4 with solid detector and rapid reconstruction vis-à-vis the Plus 4 without the above improvements (data which convinced our Division Chairman, and then the Capital Equipment Committee, that adding these two improvements to our preexisting Plus 4 machines without these options was in the best interest of patient throughput).

23.2 Historical Data

In 1993 at CCF there were the following CT scanners:

- Somatom Plus (installed 1988)
- Somatom Plus Classic (×2) (installed 1992 and 1993)
- Total 1993 examinations = 25,550

In 1994 at CCF there were the following CT scanners:

- Somatom Plus
- Somatom Plus Classic (×2)
- Somatom AR HP (installed Nov. 1994)
- Somatom Plus Classic 4 (Installed Nov. 1994)
- Total 1994 examinations = 29,083

In 1995 at CCF there were the following CT scanners:

- Somatom Plus (replaced by Somatom Plus 4, Oct. 1995)
- Somatom Plus Classic (×2)
- Somatom AR HP
- Somatom Plus 4
- Total 1995 examinations = 29,881

In 1996 at CCF there were the following CT scanners:

- Somatom Plus 4 (installed Apr. 1996; replaced Somatom Plus Classic)
- Somatom Plus 4 (installed Oct. 1996; replaced Somatom Plus Classic)
- Somatom Plus 4 (×2)
- Somatom AR HP
- Total 1996 examinations = 32,569

In 1997 there were the following CT scanners:
- Somatom Plus 4 (× 4)
- Two machines without solid detector or rapid reconstruction (used 2 shifts/day with 2 RTs per scanner during 1 first shift)
- One machine without the solid detector but with rapid reconstruction (used primarily for interventions 4/8 h 1 first shift and then used occasionally for any examination during second shift)
- One machine with both the solid detector and rapid reconstruction (used only first shift with only one technologist)
- Somatom AR HP
- Total 1997 examinations = 41,601 (estimated)

While the overall number of our examinations has dramatically increased since the introduction of the Plus 4 systems (63% from 1993), the most significant increase has been in body examinations (abdomen and/or pelvis), which are scanner intensive (120–150 image examinations). In 1995, 14,811 examations were performed whereas in 1997, 19,682 were performed.

In terms of the impact on scheduling, in 1995 we scanned an average of 15 outpatients Saturdays and 10 Sundays. We performed these examinations because our Monday through Friday schedule could not accommodate the needs of our medical center. Most of these patients would have preferred to have their scans during the week, on the same day as their clinic appointment. Soon after installing two Plus 4 scanners the total number of outpatients scanned on either day dropped to one or two (performed for patient convenience and not due to an overbooked schedule).

This change in weekend outpatient examination performance allowed us to reduce our technical staff on the weekends. Technical staffing in 1995 was 33 FTEs/week; in 1996 this dropped to 27.5 FTEs/week. Thus we were able to scan the same number of patients (slightly more) with fewer technologists between Monday and Friday, rather than over the full 7 day week. In 1997 there were 27.24 FTEs/week budgeted; actual FTEs were 25.94.

This expanded schedule also led to improved patient and referring clinician–customer relationships. More oncology patients could be scanned on the same day as their clinic visit, rather than at separate the visits (scan one day, seen another day). Further, more examinations on these patients were performed in the clinic rather than at outside institutions.

Thus changing from Plus Classic to Plus 4 technology vastly improved productivity and customer service, utilizing fewer technologist hours during the routine work week.

23.3 Prospective Evaluation of Scanner Efficiency: Plus Classic vs. Plus 4

Data from 1049 CT examinations were recorded prospectively over a 5-week period. During the study period we used two Somatom Plus 4 scanners and two Somatom Plus Classic scanners. The patients were not randomized to the scanners. We measured the following parameters with respect to scanner type, examination protocol, patient age, gender, number of technologists, inpatient/outpatient status, and occurrence and type of problem: (a) room time (total time patient occupied the CT scanner room), (b) scanner time (specific time scanner dedicated to a specific patient; the longer of either time that image processing was complete minus time patient entered room or total time patient spent in room).

Both times were calculated for the ten most common examination protocols ($n = 769$) and compared between the Plus Classic and the Plus 4 scanners. Analysis of covariance was performed to adjust for the differences between the patients scanned on the two scanners.

The examination types were primarily nonspiral on the Plus Classic scanner and both spiral and nonspiral on the Plus 4 scanner. We did not use the spiral mode on the Plus Classic because this scanner platform could not perform two sequential spiral scans with adequate mAs. Further combining sequential and spiral scans together on the same patient created sorting problems for filming and for our digital review station.

23.4 CT Examination Protocols

The overall mean room time and the overall mean scanner time, both adjusted for covariates, were significantly less for the Plus 4 ($p = 0.0001$ and 0.0014, respectively). The examination protocol also significantly affected the differences in time ($p = 0.0001$ for both mean room and scanner time). The difference in room time was significant for 6/10 examination protocols (641 patients and 84% of the examinations). The difference in scanner time was significant for 4/10 examination protocols (519 patients and 68% of the examinations).

Sinus, skull, facial bones, spine performed at 2, 3, or 5 mm collimation; kidney examinations both pre- and postcontrast performed at 5 mm collimation; chest, abdomen, and pelvis examinations performed at 8 mm collimation. Z-axis reconstruction = collimation for all examinations except perihilar area of chest, livers and kidneys which are reconstructed at 1/2 = collimation (Tables 23.1–23.4).

Table. 23.1. Plus Classic vs. Plus 4 (from [1])

	Z-axis (est.)	Plus Classic		Plus 4	
Examination		Tech.	No. of images	Tech.	No. of images
A/P	50 cm	NS	63	Sx2	94
Head (+c or −c)	–	NS	19	NS	19
Sinus	–	NS	6	NS	6
Chest	45 cm	Sx1	75	Sx1	75
Chest, A/P	95 cm	S chest NS A/P	138	Sx3	169
Skull	Variable	NS		NS	
Spine	Variable	NS		NS	
Head (+c and –c)		NS	38	NS	38
Liver (−c) + A/P (+c)	20 + 50 cm	NS	88	Sx3	144
Kidney (−c) + A/P (+c)	20 + 50 cm	NS	118	Sx4	210

A/P, abdomen, pelvis; NS, nonspiral; S, spiral; Sx1, one spiral run; x2, two spiral runs, etc.

Table 23.2. Unadjusted mean room time and percentage change by examination protocol (from [1])

	Plus Classic (min)	Plus 4 (min)	Change (%)
Protocol			
Spine	46	28	40
Chest, A/P	40	24	39
Liver (−c), A/P (+c)	32	20	36
Kidney (−c), A/P (+c)	38	25	34
Chest	23	15	34
A/P	30	21	30
Head (+ or −c)	17	14	17
Head (+ and −c)	34	29	14
Simple sinus	8	9	−16
Skull or facial bones	23	28	−21

Table 23.3. Unadjusted mean scanner time and percentage change by examination protocol (from [1])

	Plus Classic (min)	Plus 4 (min)	Change (%)
Protocol			
Chest	36	26	27
Spine	48	35	27
Head (+ or −c)	22	17	22
Head (+ and −c)	36	31	15
Chest, A/P	49	43	14
Liver (−c) + A/P (+ c)	35	31	12
A/P	33	30	11
Simple sinus	9	10	− 3
Kidney (−c) + A/P (+ c)	40	43	− 7
Skull or facial bones	28	34	−24

Table 23.4. Comparison (p values) of adjusted mean room and scanner times between Plus Classic and Plus 4 scanners

Protocol	Room time	Scanner time
A/P	0.0001	0.0259
Head (+ or −c)	0.0033	0.0005
Simple sinus	0.0469	0.1600
Chest	0.0001	0.0102
Chest, A/P	0.0001	0.0102
Skull or facial bones	0.2772	0.8242
Head (+c and −c)	0.3379	0.0831
Spine	0.1113	0.0655
Liver (−c) + A/P (+c)	0.0076	0.1186
Kidneys (−c) + A/P (+c)	0.0527	0.8596

Unadjusted times should not be used in an absolute sense to compare the scanners; more outpatients were scanned on the Plus 4 scanner, and mean room and scanner time was less with outpatients. Nonetheless, when adjusted there are significant differences in overall room time and scanner time. Interestingly, there is less change with scanner time than with room time. Processing time was longer with the Plus 4; however, in many instances most if not all of the study performed on the Plus 4 reconstructed the images at half the collimation used (i.e., twice as many images reconstructed) (see differences in protocols and number of images reconstructed).

23.5
Add-Ons to the Plus 4: Does the Ceramic Detector and Turbo Reconstruction Improve Scanner and Technologist Efficiency?

One issue which radiologists face after buying a new piece of equipment is what to do the following year when a manufacturer offers them new and supposedly improved add-ons. We are often aggravated by these new add-ons as we were inevitably told that what we bought the previous year was the latest and greatest. Such is the case with the new solid detector system for the Plus 4 and the new hardware and software add-ons for rapid reconstruction (additions costing over 100–150 K in capital)

One significant advantage of the solid detector is its improved radiation absorption efficiency, an improvement of between 25% and 35% over gas detectors. With equivalent patient dose, this should improve image quality. However, in many instances this improvement in signal to noise ratio may be unnecessary. Therefore rather than scan at the same dose, we can significantly reduce the dose to achieve equivalent image quality:

- Gas detector techniques: abdomen/pelvis 120 kVp/280 or 320 mA; 0.75 s scans; 8 mm collimation
- Solid detector techniques: abdomen/pelvis 120 kVp/200 or 240 mA; 0.75 s scans; 8 mm collimation

How does this improve scanner efficiency? By using lower power settings the tube heat limits are not reached, and there is virtually no tube cooling time wasted. When multiple, back-to-back spiral runs are desired, this becomes critical. With the standard Plus 4 configuration our technologists often waited 5–10 min before the next multiple spiral examination could be performed (waiting for the tube to cool). With the solid detector addition, utilizing lower techniques, tube cooling is rarely encountered.

How does the rapid reconstruction improve patient throughput? With multiple spiral runs, often reconstructing at one-half the collimation, multiple images are now produced with extended z-axis examinations. Without rapid reconstruction it is not easy to perform an examination, remove the patient from the scanner, and have another patient on the scanner before all of the images from the prior examination are reconstructed. Again with our standard Plus 4 configuration, our technologists can wait 5–10 min before they can start scanning another patient. The rapid reconstruction virtually eliminates that problem.

Our study logs show that with the combination of the UFC detector and the turbo reconstruction 130 images can be scanned and reconstructed in 10 min. Conversely, on a Plus 4 without the detector and turbo reconstruction, the same number of images (scanned and reconstructed) take 18 min. Thus these technological improvements reduced machine time by 45%. Eight minutes does not seem substantial, but over several hours it can mean scanning many more patients (we estimate that with the Plus 4 platform we can only scan three or four patients/hour, whereas the addition of the solid detector and rapid reconstruction, we can scan five to seven patients/hour).

23.6 Interventional CT: Standard Technique vs. CARE Vision

The turbo reconstruction package also allows for CT fluoroscopy (CARE vision). Preliminary experience suggests that this will also improve efficiency.

We are currently evaluating CT fluoroscopy in a randomized, prospective fashion with each radiologist serving as his or her own control utilizing their standard technique with CT as the comparison. Unfortunately, by the present time only an insufficient number of patients have been entered into the study to have meaningful data. However, historical data is sufficient to make the following general conclusions. Overall, the total machine/room time spent for CT interventions using fluoroscopy is approximately 30%–50% less time than when using standard CT technique.

Reference

1. Herts BR, Perl J II, Seney C, Lieber ML, Davros WJ, Baker ME (1998) Comparison of examination times between CT scanners: are the newer scanners faster? AJR 170:13–18

24 Volumetric Analysis of Spiral CT Data

G. D. RUBIN

24.1 Introduction

The quality of multiplanar reformations and three-dimensional renderings is primarily influenced by the quality of the computed tomography (CT) data. A thorough understanding of spiral CT principles is required for optimal creation of multiplanar and three-dimensional renderings. No amount of sophisticated rendering and image segmentation can resurrect a poor acquisition.

Multiplanar and three-dimensional rendering techniques were applied to conventional CT data [1]; however, their accuracy and applicability have increased considerably by virtue of the contiguous volumetric data set provided by spiral CT. Three-dimensional renderings eliminate constraints of transverse tomographic imaging, allowing anatomy to be viewed from innumerable angles. Although when performing CT angiography (CTA), views can be obtained to simulate various conventional arteriographic projections, additional views that are impossible with conventional arteriography are possible. Similarly, while perspective views within tubular lumena such as the colon or bronchi can simulate fiberoptic endoscopy, the flexibility of the volume data allows substantially greater alternatives for visualization. These range from prograde and retrograde visualization along a similar axis as fiberoptic endoscopy to panoramic views of the entire internal surface of the colon. Another exciting technique for alternative analysis of spiral CT data is the quantitation of flow channels to measure luminal diameters and areas, segment lengths, and curvature independent of orientation to characterize structures in a manner that was previously unattainable.

24.2 Visualization Techniques

Current techniques for three-dimensional rendering of spiral CT data require transverse sections to be generated first and then a rendering algorithm is applied to the stack of sections. Because these algorithms enable us to view the volume of data on a two-dimensional medium, they reduce the data by eliminating information. It is impossible to reconstruct the source transverse sections from a three-dimensionally rendered image. Critical to the appropriate use of three-dimensional rendering in clinical radiology is an understanding of how the various rendering techniques are created and what information is lost in the process of rendering. To date, four rendering techniques have been employed on spiral CT scans – multi- and curved planar reformations, threshold shaded surface display (SSD), maximum-intensity projection (MIP), and volume rendering (VR).

Multiplanar reformations are coronal, sagittal, or oblique single voxel thick planes created from the stacked transverse sections. They are excellent for displaying anatomic relationships that are co-planar. Because tubular structures are not constrained to a specific plane, it is rare to visualize a vessel, airway, or bowel segment along its entire course on a single reformatted section. Curved planar reformations can be very helpful for displaying tortuous vessels that cannot be completely visualized on a flat planar section. They are prescribed from a curve drawn on either a transverse section, reformatted section, or three-dimensional projection, which is then extended through the entire data set. The resultant "curved plane" is flattened and displayed as a two-dimensional image. Multi- and curved planar reformations preserve all of the relative X-ray attenuation information and do not suffer from the limitations that overlapping vessels have on three-dimensional renderings. They are particularly valuable for visualizing the true wall of abdominal aortic aneurysms by showing mural thrombus relative to the patent arterial lumen, differentiating eccentric calcification on arterial walls from adjacent luminal patency, and evaluating the interior of metallic stents. Curved and multiplanar reformations are exceedingly operator dependent. Displays do not incorporate information from adjoining voxels, and therefore inaccurate plane selection can falsely simulate lesions which are not present or can exclude true lesions from the rendering. Curved planar reformations can be particularly misleading, because distances are referenced to the curve and not the Cartesian coordinate system of all other planar images. Measurements should never be made from curved images, and caution should be taken when assessing the relative position of structures. Therefore, curved reformations must always be interpreted in association with axial sections and three-dimensional rendering techniques.

SSD were first applied to CT data for the display of musculoskeletal system [2]. They provide an exquisite view of complex three-dimensional relationships, particularly in regions of overlapping structures and at the origins of aortic branches. Contiguous voxels at the boundary of a predefined threshold range are modeled as surfaces by the computer. The computer then generates an imaginary source of illumination to depict surface reflections which are encoded in the image gray scale [3,4]. Unfortunately, for all their pizzazz, SSD are the most reduced form of three-dimensional rendering. The majority of information regarding relative X-ray attenuation is lost in the thresholding process. In their simplest and most commonly used form, SSD are the product of binarized data, displaying the transitions between pixels within and those outside of the selected threshold range. Two main limitations of surface displays are: (1) threshold selection profoundly affects the appearance of luminal stenoses, polyps, or normal surface details such as haustra and (2) structures within the threshold range with different attenuations, e.g., calcium and luminal contrast, cannot be differentiated. SSD can be made with multiple threshold levels and colorized display to enable segmentation of structures with varying attenuation [5].

The advent of spiral CT angiography brought the first widespread application of MIP to CT [6]. A view angle is preselected along which rays are cast through the volumetric data set. The maximum value encountered by each ray is encoded in a two-dimensional projectional display [7, 8]. MIP gray scale thus reflects relative X-ray attenuation. The absence of a thresholding step, as in SSD, enable subtle variations in attenuation to be appreciated. This has tremendous importance in the differentiation of calcified atheroma and intraluminal contrast. Two main disadvantages of the MIP are that depth relationships cannot be appreciated from a single image and, in regions of vessel overlap, only one structure will be represented in any single pixel, making discrimination of structures difficult or impossible. This latter limitation is particularly germane when assessing the origins of aortic branches with CTA. The lack of depth information can in part be countered by generating multiple MIP at regular intervals around an axis of rotation. The resultant images are viewed as a cine loop to enable appreciation of depth relationships.

A further limitation of MIP and some SSD is that highly attenuating structures such as bone, metallic implants, or intensely enhancing parenchyma can mask target anatomy. Because the MIP selects only the brightest pixel along each ray, a high-attenuation structure anywhere along the path of the ray will dominate and thus mask a structure of lesser attenuation. Alternatively, SSD have the property of occlusivity. Less attenuating structures will obscure target vessels if their attenuation falls above the selected threshold and if they are closer along the selected viewing path than the target vessel.

To overcome this limitation, manual or semi-automatic techniques must be employed to remove the high-attenuating structures prior to rendering all MIP and many SSD. Editing can be divided into two basic approaches – planar and sculpted editing. Planar editing or "thin-slab" and "cut-plane" rendering is based upon the selection of a multiplanar reformation that is then broadened by a user-defined thickness to create a slab that is always viewed en fosse. Visualization of the voxels along the slab's axis of depth can be via MIP, minimum-intensity projection, SSD, or VR. The most useful and flexible implementations of thin-slab rendering allow real-time control of the slab thickness, orientation, position, and rendering options. The technique can be very effective for assessing limited regions of anatomy such as the renal or proximal mesenteric arteries and has also been suggested for assessing parenchymal abnormalities within the lung and liver. However, complex three-dimensional structures are inadequately displayed for many applications, as only a fraction of the anatomy may be displayed within the rendered subvolume.

Sculpting techniques can be characterized by varying degrees of automation. At the simplest level, manual editing involves region-of-interest drawing on individual transverse sections to isolate structures to be retained or excluded from the rendering. Manual techniques rely upon an operator who has an excellent knowledgeable of cross-sectional anatomy. Although this technique can be time-consuming (30–60 min), it allows the greatest degree of control over what structures are included or excluded in the rendering. A faster approach to manual segmentation that removes some control is to divide the imaging volume into multiple slabs or subvolumes and to perform an MIP on each slab. A region of interest is drawn on each slab MIP and then extended to all individual axial sections represented within the slab.

Semi-automated segmentation techniques employ three-dimensional connectivity or "region growing" to identify contiguous pixels within a threshold range [9]. A "seed" is manually planted on a representative section with the region to be excluded. This seed is then allowed to grow in three dimensions into neighboring pixels within the prescribed threshold range. Once identified, the pixels are assigned values of −1000 HU. Segmentation of abdominal aortic CT angiograms are the most laborious due to the need for separating the entire aneurysm (both patent and thrombosed portions) from adjacent abdominal structures. Currently, two-dimensional region-of-interest drawing appears to be the only adequate means of performing this segmentation prior to MIP. Threshold-based three-dimensional connectivity, although theoretically capable of achieving similar results, has not been adequately employed to date. Limitations of the three-dimensional connectivity include region-of-interest spread into the spine and bowel segments which contact the aneurysm.

A comparison of multiplanar reformation, MIP, and SSD rendered following sculpted editing is summarized in Table 24.1 and Fig. 24.1.

VR is the newest visualization technique to be applied to spiral CT data [10]. There are many different versions and interfaces for VR, but the general approach is that all voxel values are assigned an opacity level that varies from total transparency to total opacity (Fig. 24.2). This opacity function can be applied to the histogram of voxel values as a whole or to regions of the histogram that are classified as specific tissue types. With the latter approach, rectangular or trapezoidal regions areas are selected that correspond to the range of attenuation values for a structure [11, 12]. The "walls" of the trapezoid slope from an opacity plateau to the baseline

Table 24.1. Comparison of three-dimensional rendering techniques

	Multiplanar/curved planar reformation	Maximum intensity projection	Shaded surface display
Advantages	"Slices" through the center of the vessel to show lumen, useful with arterial stents or eccentric calcifications	Differentiates calcification or stents from contrast column and mural calcium	Displays complex anatomic relationships in regions of vessel overlap or tortuosity
Disadvantages	Inaccurate curve drawing can falsely imply lesions not present	Confusing in regions of vessel overlap, cannot image interior of metallic stent	Cannot differentiate metallic stent or mural calcium from the intra-arterial contrast column; incorrect threshold selection can falsely imply or exclude lesions
Prerendering editing	None	Minimum: removal of bones Preferred: removal of all structures other than the target vessels	Minimum: none Preferred: removal of all structures other than the target vessels
Time required	2–10 min	10–60 min	5–60 min

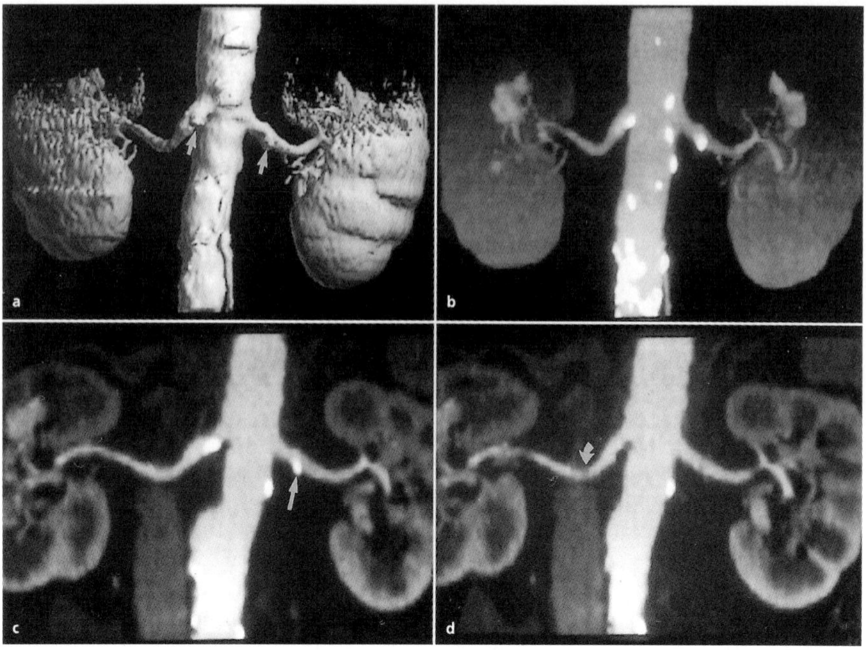

Fig. 24.1. **a** Shaded surface display (SSD) CT angiogram of the normal aorta and renal arteries. The gray scale encodes depth. All visualized pixels were above an arbitrary threshold value. Calcification at the origins of the renal arteries is seen as a contour abnormality (*arrows*). **b** Maximum-intensity projection (MIP) in the same patient. Gray scale encodes CT number. There is no depth encoding. Calcium is brighter due to its greater X-ray attenuation. Left renal arterial calcium appears to completely occlude the lumen in this view. **c** One pixel thick curved planar reformation (CPR) demonstrating eccentric mural calcification of the proximal renal arteries bilaterally. The left renal arterial origin calcification is shown to be nonocclusive (*straight arrow*). **d** CPR, reconstructed from a slightly different curve, completely eliminates the mural calcification from the arteries, attesting to the eccentricity of the calcified plaque and the absence of significant renal artery stenosis. The luminal narrowing in the right renal artery (*curved arrow*) is spurious due to inaccurate curve drawing. (Reprinted with permission from [15])

of complete transparency in an attempt to account for partial volume effects at the edges of structures. Lighting effects may be simulated in a similar fashion as with SSD. Because there is no surface definition with VR, lighting effects are applied based upon the spatial gradient (i.e., variability of attenuation within a local neighborhood of voxels). Near the edges of structures, the spatial variation in attenuation changes more rapidly (a high gradient) than in the center of structures (a low gradient). Lighting effects are most pronounced in regions of high spatial gradients. Because lighting effects and variations in transparency are simultaneously displayed, it is frequently useful to view VR in color. The color is applied to the attenuation histogram to allow differentiation of pixel values and to avoid ambiguity with lighting effects, which are encoded in gray scale. Other variables such as specular reflectivity, which models the "shininess" of a surface, may be available, but should be used with caution to avoid confounding the visualization.

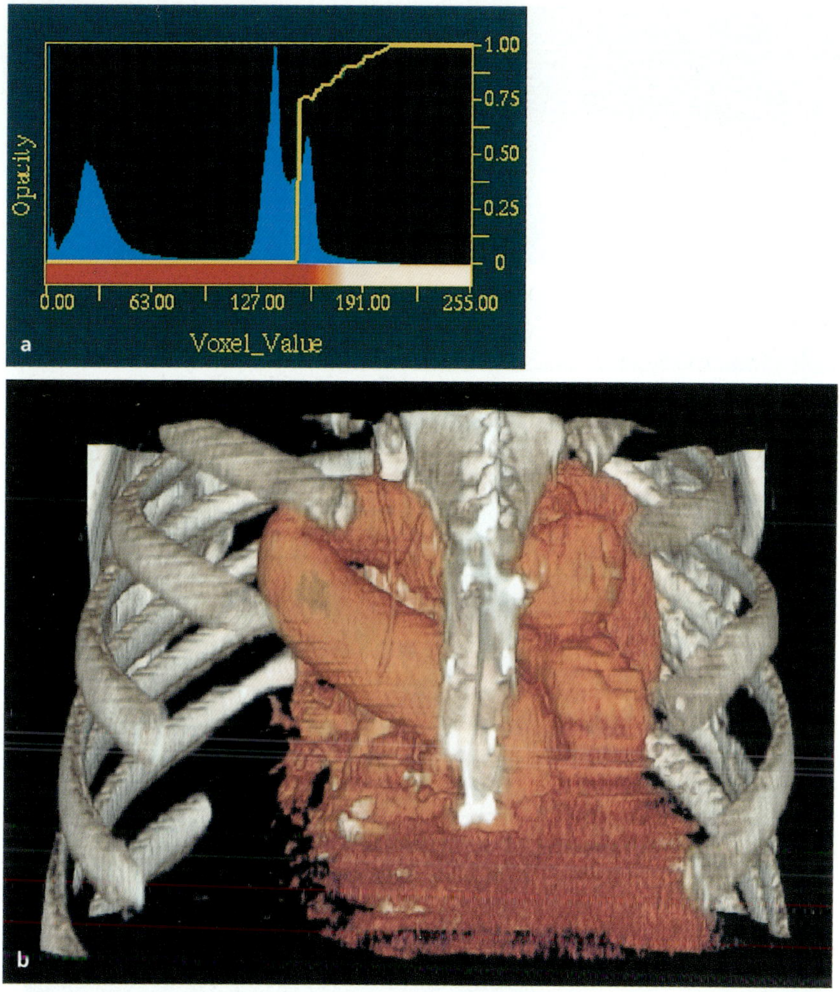

Fig. 24.2. a Histogram of voxel values within a spiral CT data set of the thorax. The *yellow line* is the opacity curve which is drawn to demonstrate the vasculature and bones. Opacity of 0 indicates complete transparency, and opacity of 1.00 indicates complete opacity. Intermediate values are semiopaque. The color scale is indicated between the x-axis and the histogram plot. The color scale enables differentiation of the blood vessels from the bones. **b** Volume rendering corresponding to opacity and color values defined in **a.** Figure continues on next page

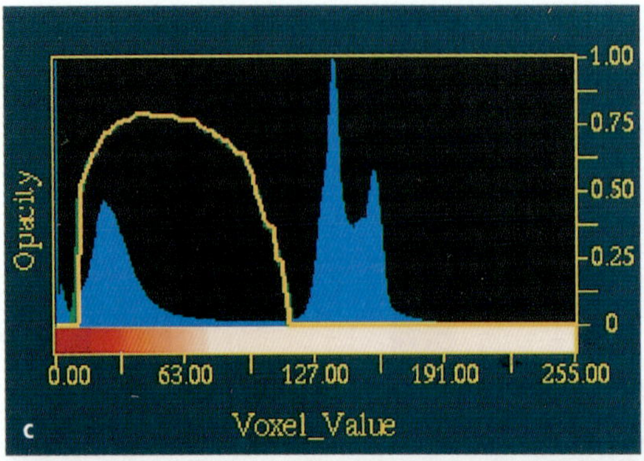

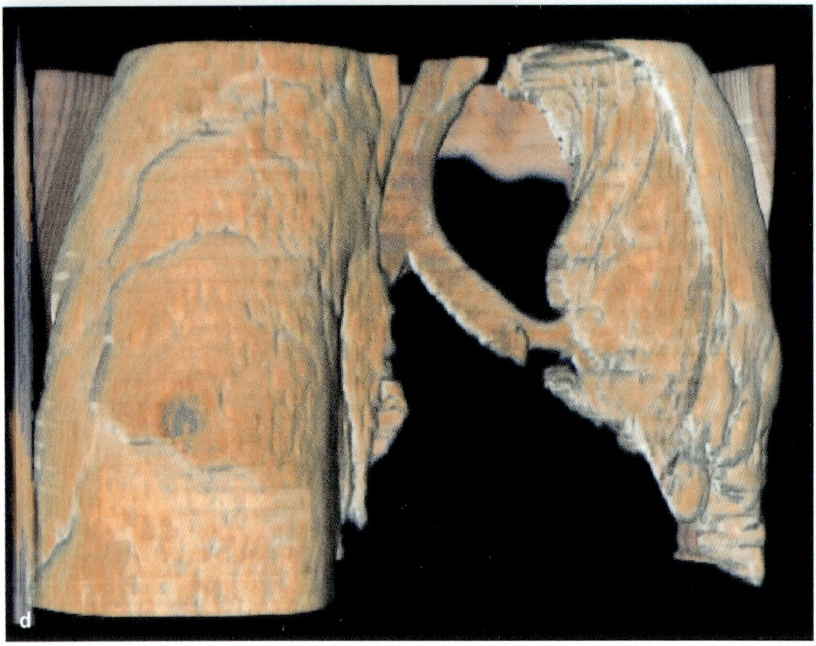

Fig. 24.2. c Same data as in **a** with opacity curve and color scale to demonstrate the pulmonary parenchyma and the central airways. **d** Volume rendering corresponding to opacity and color values defined in **c**. (Reprinted with permission from [13])

The application of VR to spiral CT data sets has been less popular than MIP and SSD because of its requirement for more powerful computer hardware and because it has required a complex software user interface with a long, steep learning curve. The recent introduction of fast computer graphics workstations has enabled VR tools to be developed that can be practically applied to CT data sets. The challenge of creating practical VR interfaces is to reduce the substantial degrees of freedom to a small feature set that is both fast and easy to use and flexible enough to provide uncompromised visualization of clinically relevant data.

MIP and SSD are both limited by substantial rendering losses. Rendering loss in MIP is by a factor equal to 1 minus the thickness of the volume, typically more than 99%. An important advantage of VR over SSD is that no information is lost by thresholding. Depth, surface, and relative X-ray attenuation are all conveyed with VR. Another advantage of volume rendering, which is shared by SSD, is that perspective views can be generated from within the data set, taking the viewer on a "fantastic voyage" into blood vessels, airways, or the gastrointestinal tract (Fig. 24.3) [13].

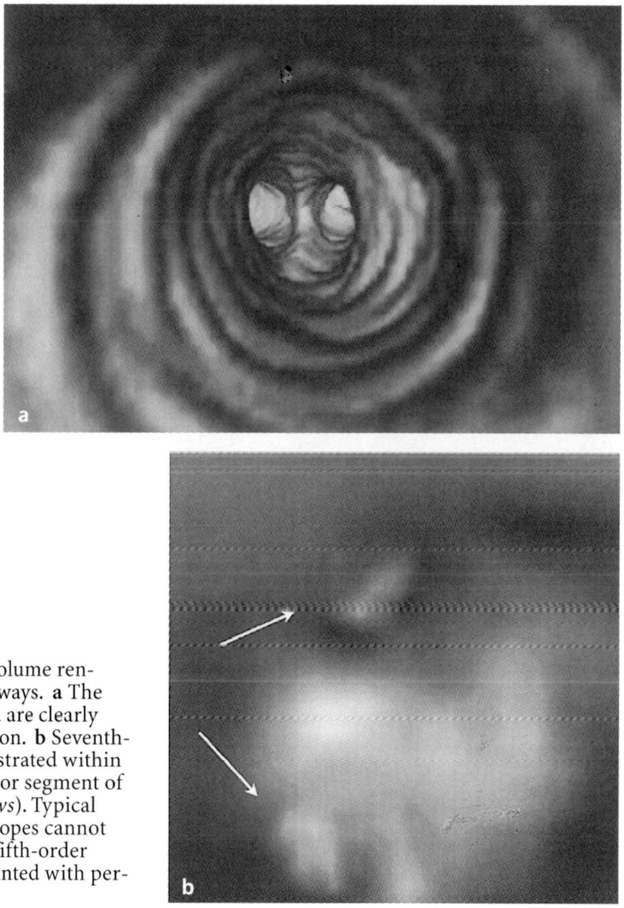

Fig. 24.3a, b. Perspective volume rendered helical CT of the airways. **a** The normal trachea and carina are clearly visualized distal to the lesion. **b** Seventh-order branching is demonstrated within a subsegment of the anterior segment of the right upper lobe (*arrows*). Typical adult fiberoptic bronchoscopes cannot pass through the ostea of fifth-order bronchial branches. (Reprinted with permission from [13])

24.3 Perspective Rendering

Currently, three-dimensional renderings are created predominantly from viewpoints external to the data set, generated using parallel rays cast through the volume or reflected off surfaces as if the model were viewed from a great distance with high-powered (telephoto) magnification. This type of visualization, termed "orthographic," results in the perceived size of structures being independent of their distance from the viewer. A more realistic technique, "perspective" visualization, renders with rays that converge at the viewer to mimic the perspective

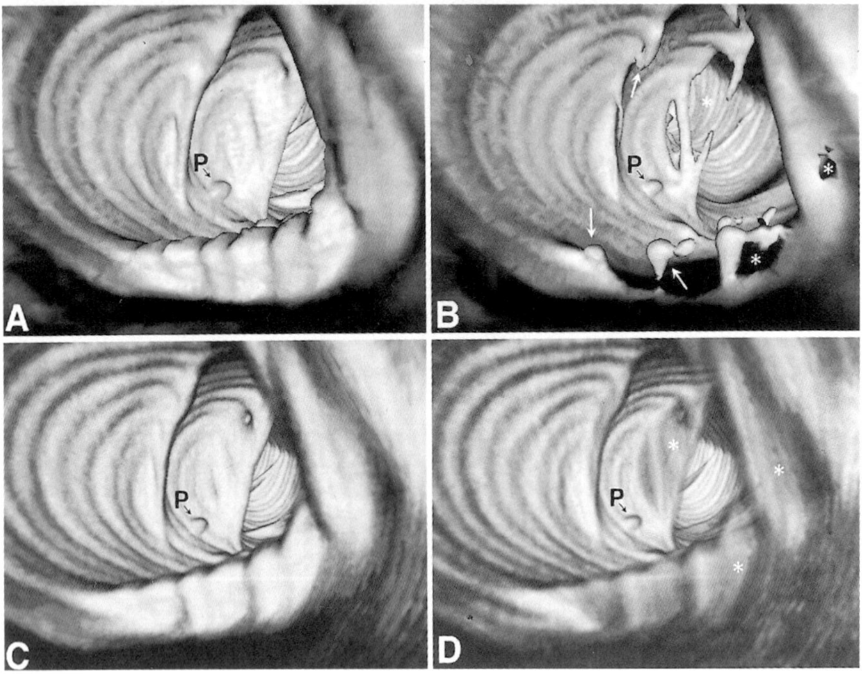

Fig. 24.4A–D. Comparison of perspective volume rendering with perspective surface display. **A** Perspective shaded surface display of colonic helical CT with threshold of –980 HU, which is optimal for displaying the interior of the colon. **B** Threshold of –930 HU, which is too high. Portions of the colonic wall are not rendered and appear as holes (*) or intraluminal juxtamural structures (arrows), which could be misinterpreted as polyps. A 5-mm polyp is visible in all views (*P*). **C** Perspective volume rendering with an opacity curve that renders all voxels above –980 as 80%–100% opaque is free from both artifactual wall discontinuities and juxtamural structures. **D** Perspective volume rendering with a different opacity curve that renders the lower densities more transparently creates a whispy appearance of the thinner structures (*). Frank discontinuities as seen with surface displays are not created. The presence of semitransparent cues on volume rendered images (**C, D**) results in easier detection of errors than on surface displays (**A, B**). Once detected, the opacity curve can be adjusted and the image rerendered in 10–20 s. Even if the error is detected on a surface display, an additional 10–15 min are required to recalculate isosurfaces based upon a new threshold value which may still be incorrect. (Reprinted with permission from [13])

provided by the human visual system, where similarly sized structures close to the viewer appear larger than those farther away [13]. While perspective rendering is not critical when viewing CT data sets from external viewpoints, it becomes critical when rendering occurs from within the data, termed "immersive" visualization. Immersive visualization enables CT renderings that simulate endoscopy. Both SSD [14] and VR [13] can be used for immersive visualization. Although SSD are less computationally intensive and thus allow near interactive rendering rates, the surface extraction process – with its inherent reduction in voxel information – ultimately limits these renderings by creating surfaces at assumed boundaries. Discontinuities in the walls of airways or blood vessels can be artifactually created, and structures typically appear irregular due to the polygonal modeling applied to the surfaces (Fig. 24.4). Thus VR is preferred, because artifacts in regions with volume averaging between luminal walls and the lumen are substantially diminished. Perspective VR has shown considerable promise for uniquely visualizing endobronchial, endovascular, and intrathoracic anatomy and disease. Immersive visualization is particularly attractive when compared to external, orthographic visualization, because editing of the data may not be required when views can be generated between structures that would overlap and obscure one another on external views.

24.4 Conclusion

Spiral CT data offer considerably greater flexibility for reconstruction than conventional CT. As a result, image quality is highly dependent on the selection of both the reconstruction parameters and the scan parameters. Because spiral CT data are volumetric, multiplanar and three-dimensional renderings are of a higher quality than when created from conventional CT data. As a result, these rendering techniques are finding increasing utility as adjuncts to transverse sections for the diagnosis and characterization of abnormalities. A thorough understanding of the benefits and limitations of these techniques is required prior to relying upon them for diagnosis.

Regardless of the three-dimensional rendering techniques employed, it is imperative to always review the unedited axial sections for unsuspected pathology or segmentation errors.

References

1. Fishman EK, Magid D, Ney DR et al (1991) Three-dimensional imaging. Radiology 181: 321–337
2. Totty WG, Vannier MW (1984) Complex musculoskeletal anatomy: analysis using three dimensional surface reconstruction. Radiology 150:173–177
3. Cline HE, Lorensen WE, Souza SP et al (1991) 3D Surface rendered MR images of the brain and its vasculature. J Comput Assist Tomogr 15:344–351
4. Magnusson M, Lenz R, Danielsson PE (1991) Evaluation of methods for shaded surface display of CT volumes. Comput Med Imaging Graph 15:247–256
5. Dillon EH, van Leeuwen MS, Fernandez MA et al (1993) Spiral CT angiography. AJR 160: 1273–1278
6. Napel S, Marks MP, Rubin GD et al (1992) CT angiography with spiral CT and maximum intensity projection. Radiology 185:607–610
7. Keller PJ, Drayer BP, Fram EK et al (1989) MR angiography with two-dimensional acquisition and three-dimensional display. Radiology 173:527–532
8. Laub GA (1988) MR angiography with gradient motion refocusing. J Comput Assist Tomogr 12:377–382
9. Cline HE, Dumoulin CL, Hart HRJ et al (1987) 3D reconstruction of the brain from magnetic resonance images using a connectivity algorithm. Magn Reson Imaging 5:345–352
10. Ney DR, Fishman EK, Niederhuber JE (1992) Three-dimensional display of hepatic venous anatomy generated from spiral computed tomography data: preliminary experience. J Digit Imaging 5:242–245
11. Johnson PT, Heath DG, Bliss DF et al (1996) Three-dimensional CT: real-time interactive volume rendering. AJR Am J Roentgenol 167:581–583
12. Kuszyk BS, Heath DG, Bliss DF et al (1996) Skeletal 3-D CT: advantages of volume rendering over surface rendering. Skeletal Radiol 25:207–14
13. Rubin GD, Beaulieu CF, Argiro V et al (1996) Perspective volume rendering of CT and MR images: applications for endoscopic imaging. Radiology 199:321–330
14. Vining DJ, Shifrin RY, Haponik EF et al (1994) Virtual bronchoscopy. Radiology 193(P):261
15. Rubin GD, Dake MD, Semba CS (1995) Current status of 3-D spiral CT for imaging the vasculature. Radiol Clin N Am 33:51–70

25 Impact of Real-Time Three-Dimensional Rendering of CT Data on Diagnostic Performance

G. P. Krestin, P. Hilfiker, P. Pelkonen, G. Verhoek

25.1 Introduction

Helical acquisition of computed tomography (CT) data enables the complete coverage of larger anatomic regions. Secondary reconstructions in additional planes out of these data volumes are therefore of better quality than reconstructions from sequentially acquired axial slices. The usefulness of such reconstructed images has been proved in several prospective and retrospective studies, particularly for planning surgical interventions and for evaluating post-traumatic alterations or in certain expansive diseases [1, 3, 4, 12, 13, 16, 19]. However, all these studies compared only the added value of data postprocessing and did not consider the diagnostic effectiveness of the reconstructed images by using them instead of those acquired in the axial plane.

Recent advances in image processing hardware and software enable more efficient data processing methods to be used. Even large data volumes can now be handled in real time, with the possibility of direct use for primary diagnostic interpretation instead of simple hard copy reading representing axial images alone.

The aim of this study was to compare the diagnostic performance of a new prototype real-time three-dimensional rendering workstation with a conventional hard copy based interpretation of CT data and with the diagnostic performance of a screen-based reading with a commercially available workstation.

25.2 Material and Methods

The study population consisted of 100 consecutive CT examinations in different parts of the body in patients with suspected disease requiring images with fairly thin (less than 5 mm) collimation. Forty women and 60 men were included in the study, with an age range of 17–84 years (mean, 50.4 years). The covered regions were the soft tissues of the neck ($n=12$), the chest ($n=7$), the upper abdomen ($n=24$), and the pelvis ($n=22$) and the musculoskeletal structures of the spine ($n=13$), the shoulder ($n=14$), the elbow ($n=1$), the wrist ($n=4$), and the foot ($n=3$).

All data were acquired with a spiral CT (Somatom Plus 4, Siemens, Erlangen, Germany) with a 2- to 5-mm collimation and a pitch of 1. Reconstruction intervals ranged from 2 to 3 mm. Each acquired data set was evaluated by three different observers using three different modalities:

- Printed hard copies
- A conventional postprocessing workstation, allowing viewing of the axial slices, and secondary reconstructions (Sunspark 20, SUN Microsystems, Mountain View California), equipped with a "Magic View" software package (Siemens, Erlangen, Germany).
- A real-time three-dimensional rendering workstation (Onyx, Silicon Graphics, Mountainview, California) equipped with a prototype software

The observers switched between the viewing modalities after every ten examinations to avoid performance bias. Each set of data was analyzed with respect to primary and secondary pathologic findings. Primary findings were considered to have a meaning for the patients' suspected disease, while secondary findings were classified as being abnormalities without implication for the actual problem. A final consensus reading by all three observers, based on all three modalities, was used as a standard of reference.

The Wilcoxon matched-pairs signed rank test was used for statistical testing.

25.3 Results

The consensus reading allowed 147 primary and 101 secondary findings to be defined. A total of 96.6% of the primary and 74.3% of the secondary findings were seen on the hard copies. The conventional workstation allowed the depiction of 96.6% and 77.2% of the diagnoses, respectively. Using the three-dimensional real-time rendering workstation, 100% of the primary and 96% of the secondary findings were detected.

The missed primary findings were the same on the hard copies and using the conventional workstation: a pulmonary metastasis, a pathologic lymph node in the abdomen, an abdominal aneurysm, and spine and rib osteolytic lesions, respectively (Fig. 25.1). Among the secondary findings, the observers particularly missed calcified alterations (calcified lymph nodes, two bone hemangiomas, two other bone lesions, and some gall stones) on the hard copies, but also some liver cysts, renal cysts, a diverticulum of the bladder, and a colon diverticulum. Using the conventional workstation, almost the same lesions were missed as in the hard copy interpretation. On the real-time three-dimensional rendering workstation, the undetected lesions were as follows: a spinal hemangioma, a cystic bone lesion, a dilated common bile duct, and a colon diverticulum.

There was no significant difference between the detection rate for primary lesions. However, the sensitivity for detection of secondary findings was significantly higher with the three-dimensional real-time rendering workstation than with the more conventional techniques.

No significant differences were described between the real-time three-dimensional rendering workstation and the standard of reference, although a couple of lesions were missed. However, the performance of reading based on hard copies and on the conventional workstation was significantly poorer than the standard of reference.

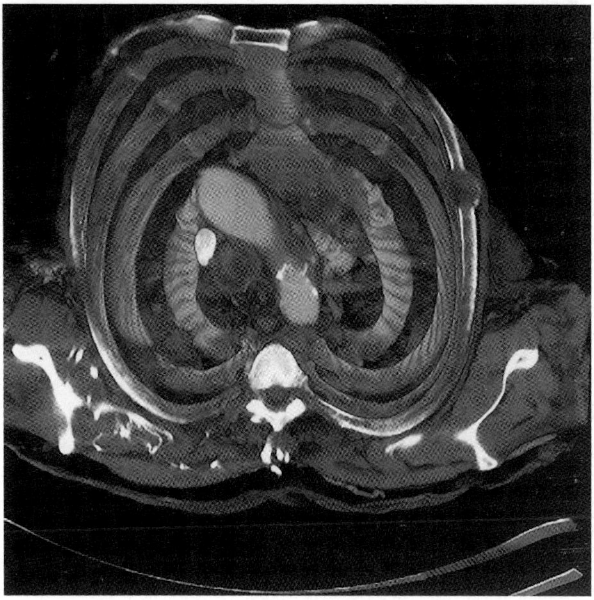

Fig. 25.1. Volumetric presentation of helical CT of the chest in a patient with a rib metastasis on the left. This finding was detected only with the real-time three-dimensional rendering workstation

The average time necessary for interpretation of an examination was shorter using the real-time three-dimensional rendering workstation than using the conventional workstation (7.3 and 8.6 min, respectively). The time requested for hard copy readings could not be registered.

25.4 Discussion

Due to the increasing number of digital archiving and communication systems, there is an increasing demand in radiology for switching from film reading to direct screen reading using workstations [2, 5, 11]. There are, however, still limitations of this kind of imaging interpretation, particularly due to the longer time periods still needed to analyze a large amount of data on screen. On the other hand, modern workstations equipped with postprocessing software capabilities allow volumetric data to be reconstructed in any desired plane. In this way, the diagnostic accuracy of CT images may be increased in some anatomic areas [6–10, 14, 15, 17, 18].

These clear advantages of image postprocessing capabilities are, however, decreased by the additional amount of time needed for reformating in additional planes. The overall efficiency of screen interpretation sessions still remained doubtful.

Use of a real-time three-dimensional rendering workstation therefore theoretically has a twofold advantage:

- Rapid scrolling through the image volume compensates for the somewhat limited capabilities of the display compared to hard copy reading.

- Real-time capabilities do not increase the time necessary for postprocessing purposes.

The data obtained in this study underscore the expected increase in efficiency offered by image interpretation on the real-time three-dimensional rendering workstation. Not only was the necessary reading time significantly decreased compared to readings based on the conventional workstation, but the number of detected lesions was also significantly higher than in the hard copy or workstation reading sessions.

One of the limitations of the present study is the lack of a golden standard for the described pathological alterations. However, the purpose of this prospective evaluation was only to compare the different modalities, and therefore some of the possible false-positive or false-negative results do not affect the outcome of this study.

There was no difference between image evaluation on hard copies and using the conventional workstation, although the workstation allowed for adjustment of level and window values as well as for reformats in additional planes. However, the time-consuming reconstructions were not regarded as necessary in all cases and therefore some of the lesions were missed.

An additional explanation for the better performance of interpretations using the real-time rendering workstation is its capability to interactively scroll through the acquired volumetric image data. This interactive viewing in any desired plane significantly facilitates the detection of even very small alterations (e.g., cysts of the liver or kidneys) [5]. The additional capability of a real-time reconstruction is helpful, especially in the detection of those lesions that are insufficiently displayed in the axial plane (aneurysms of the aorta, alterations of the spinal canal).

There are still some limitations associated with the new viewing workstation. The time-consuming loading of image data in the workstation should be automatically performed in the future. A comparison of several data volumes acquired in different phases of contrast enhancement or at different times for follow-up purposes is another drawback of the actual system. However, these are only limitations related to the prototype version of this equipment and may easily be improved in future.

In conclusion, evaluation of CT images using a real-time three-dimensional rendering workstation had no limitations compared to hard copy readings. Diagnostic accuracy was not diminished compared to the other methods. Following some further technical improvements of this technique, screen reading could become the method of choice for interpretation of CT data in the future.

References

1. Alder ME, Deahl ST, Matteson SR (1995) Clinical usefulness of two-dimensional reformatted and three-dimensionally rendered computerized tomographic images: literature review and a survey of surgeons' options. J Oral Maxillofac Surg 53:375–386
2. Fishman EK, Ney DR, Kawashima A, Scott WW jr, Robertson DD (1993) Effect of image display on the quality of multiplanar reconstruction of computed tomography data. Invest Radiol 29:146–149

3. Gandhe AJ, Hill DL, Studholm C, Hawkes DJ, Ruff CF, Cox TC, Gleeson MJ, Strong AJ (1994) Combined and three-dimensional rendered multimodal data for planning cranial base surgery: a prospective evaluation. Neurosurgery 35:463–471
4. Gregroy A, Lipczynski RT (1994) The three dimensional reconstruction and monitoring of facial surfaces. Med Eng Phys 16:249–252
5. Gur D, Good WF, Oliver JH, Thaete FL, Baron RL, Federle MP, Campbell WL, Rosenthal MS (1994) Sequential viewing of abdominal CT at varying rates. Radiology 191:119–122
6. Katz M, Konen E, Rozenman J, Szeinberg A, Itzckak Y (1995) Spiral CT and 3D image reconstruction of vascular rings and associated tracheobronchial anomalies. J Comput Assist Tomogr 19:564–568
7. Kauczcor HU, Wolcke B, Fischer B, Mildenberger P, Lorenz J, Thelen M (1996) Three-dimensional helical CT of the tracheobronchial tree. AJR 167:419–424
8. Kuhlman JE, Fishman EK, Ney DR, Magid D (1989) Two- and three-dimensional imaging of the painful shoulder. Orthop Rev 18:1201–1208
9. Lee KS, Yoon JH, Kim TK, Kim JS, Chung MP, Kwon OJ (1997) Evaluation of tracheobronchial disease with helical CT with multiplanar and three-dimensional reconstruction: correlation with bronchoscopy. Radiographics 17:555–567
10. LoCicero J III, Costello P, Campos CT, Francalancia N, Dushay KM, Silvestri RC, Zibrak JD (1996) Spiral CT with multiplanar and three-dimensional reconstructions accurately predicts tracheobronchial pathology. Ann Thorac Surg 62:811–817
11. Lohrum R, Becker G, Boesecke R, Werner T, Schlegel W, Lorenz WJ (1992) A medical workstation for the evaluation of alternative 3D radiotherapy treatment plans. Comput Med Imaging Graph 16:301–309
12. McEnery KW, Wilson AJ, Murphy WA jr (1994) Comparison of spiral computed tomography versus conventional computed tomography multiplanar reconstructions of a fracture displacement phantom. Invest Radiol 29:665–670
13. Noh HM, Scott WW jr, Fishman EK (1996) Imaging of pelvic trauma: the role of CT with multiplanar and three-dimensional reconstruction. J South Orthop Assoc 5:111–125
14. Quint LE, Francis IR, Williams D, Bass JC, Shea MJ, Frayer DL, Monaghan HM, Deeb GM (1996) Evaluation of thoracic aortic disease with the use of helical CT and multiplanar reconstructions: comparison with surgical findings. Radiology 201:37–41
15. Seltzer SE, Judy PF, Adams DF, Jacobson FL, Stark P, Kikinis R, Swensson RG, Hooton S, Head B, Feldman U (1995) Spiral CT of the chest: comparison of cine and film-based viewing. Radiology 197:73–78
16. Sutherland CJ, Bresina SJ, Gayou DE (1994) Use of general purpose mechanical computer assisted engineering software in orthopedic surgical planning: advantages and limitations. Comput Med Imaging Graph 18:435–442
17. Tarjan Z, Pozzi Muzelli F, Frezza F, Pozzi-Muzzelli R (1996) Three dimensional reconstructions of carotid bifurcation from CT images: evaluation of different rendering methods. Eur Radiol 6:326–333
18. Tecce PM, Fishman EK (1995) Spiral CT with multiplanar reconstruction in the diagnosis of sternoclavicular osteomyelitis. Skeletal Radiol 24:275–281
19. Vannier MW, Hildebolt CF, Gilula LA, Piulgram TK, Mann F, Monsees BS, Murphy WA, Totty WG, Offutt CJ (1991) Calcaneal and pelvic fractures: diagnostic evaluation by three-dimensional computed tomography scans. J Digit Imaging 4:143–152

26 Interactive 3D Volume Rendering – Vascular Applications

P. Costello, E.W. Khoo

26.1 Introduction

Spiral CT angiography (CTA) has proven valuable for the evaluation of aortic, carotid and renal vascular disease [1–6]. Combining optimal vascular opacification with motion free data acquisition creates high-quality multiplanar and 3D vascular image reconstructions. Most clinical applications of CTA to date have employed maximum-intensity projection (MIP) and shaded-surface display (SSD). These techniques, however, are limited since they use less than 10% of the entire dataset for visualisation. This chapter describes the use of a volume rendering algorithm with real-time rendering for imaging a variety of vascular abnormalities.

Volume rendering is a method of displaying a 3D dataset onto a 2D screen whilst not losing any of the spatial detail inherent to the original dataset [7, 8]. Advances in real-time volume rendering have been limited until recently by computer hardware and software constraints. The volume rendering method employed in this study is known as planar composition, which is one of the two most popular techniques in volume rendering, the other being known as ray casting. Unlike ray casting, which has similarities to ray tracing, planar composition uses hundreds of equidistant texture mapped planes that intersect the volume dataset to display it on screen. Hence the final image is the result of many overlapping planes. The texture map associated with each plane is calculated using trilinear interpolations through an OpenGL extension.

26.2 Materials and Methods

This experience results from 256 consecutively studied patients for a variety of vascular problems. All CT scans were performed on a Siemens Somatom Plus 4 scanner with a solid-state detector. CT data were acquired with 2 or 3 mm collimation and a pitch of 2 with reconstruction intervals at 1–2 mm. Non-ionic contrast 300–350 mg iodine/ml was injected at a rate of 3–4 ml/s with total volumes of 120–150 ml. A patient-specific time delay was determined by a region of interest time-density analysis over the vessel of interest during a preliminary test injection of 20 ml contrast at 4 ml/s so that optimal vascular enhancement was obtained. We used breathholds of 30– 40 s determined by the required scan length and related to table speed and collimation as detailed by Rubin [9].

26.2.1 Three-Dimensional Volumetric Rendering Methodology

A Silicon Graphics reality graphics subsystem was used to visualise the volumetric data in real time (about 3 frames/s). The machine was configured with one 180 MHz R10000 microprocessor and 128 MB of system memory. The Reality graphics subsystem consists of two geometry engines and one raster manager with 16 MB of texture memory which yields a maximum voxel (volume-rendered pixel) throughput of 160 million trilinear interpolations per second. The technique employed in visualising the volume data on the Silicon Graphics machine is based on the 3D texture mapping algorithm developed by Silicon Graphics as part of the extended OpenGL application programming interface. In 3D texture mapping multiple planes are 'cut' into the volume data, and the pixels that lie on these planes are calculated using trilinear interpolations.

The normals of these planes are parallel to the line of sight of the observer. The end result of having multiple equally spaced planes cutting through the volume data allows the whole volume to be sampled and viewed as a stack of planes. The technique just described is best known as planar composition.

Volume rendering generates a 2D image that conveys 3D spatial information inherent in the dataset. The observer can modify and rotate the volume of data on hardware accelerated OpenGL workstations in real time to visualise anatomy and pathology. The user manipulates the images through the use of transfer functions and three button mouse control for rotation, slicing, zooming and fly-throughs.

The volume-rendered images are calculated graphically using a percentage classification transfer function. In this method a graph with Hounsfield units as the x-axis and frequency of voxels as the y-axis is used. Hence the frequency of voxels are plotted according to their Hounsfield unit values.

The actual transfer function comes in the form of a trapezoid superimposed onto the graph. The position, length and slopes of the sides of the trapezoid can be manipulated under mouse control. Voxels with a particular Hounsfield unit range (e.g. to represent bone or soft tissue) can be selectively displayed by placing the origin of the upslope at the lower range and the conclusion of the downslope at the upper end of the range. It is these voxels that are drawn to screen.

Hence altering the 3D image is a simple matter of positioning the trapezoid over the appropriate range of Hounsfield units. Many trapezoids can be used to provide more spatial information. In our studies two trapezoids are used. For example, when examining a vascular stenosis, say of the carotid or renal artery, one trapezoid is used for the opacified vessel lumen and another to represent calcified plaque. The two trapezoids are positioned manually by a radiologist to best display the two entities in question. In addition, a particular colour can be associated with each trapezoid; red is used to colour the trapezoid which shows lumen and yellow to represent calcified plaque.

Modifying the slopes of the trapezoid changes the image in several ways. It is the lower density voxels and high density voxels that are affected by the slopes of the trapezoid. Decreasing the slope increases the grey scale and decreases image contrast while increasing the slope does the opposite. Manipulation of these

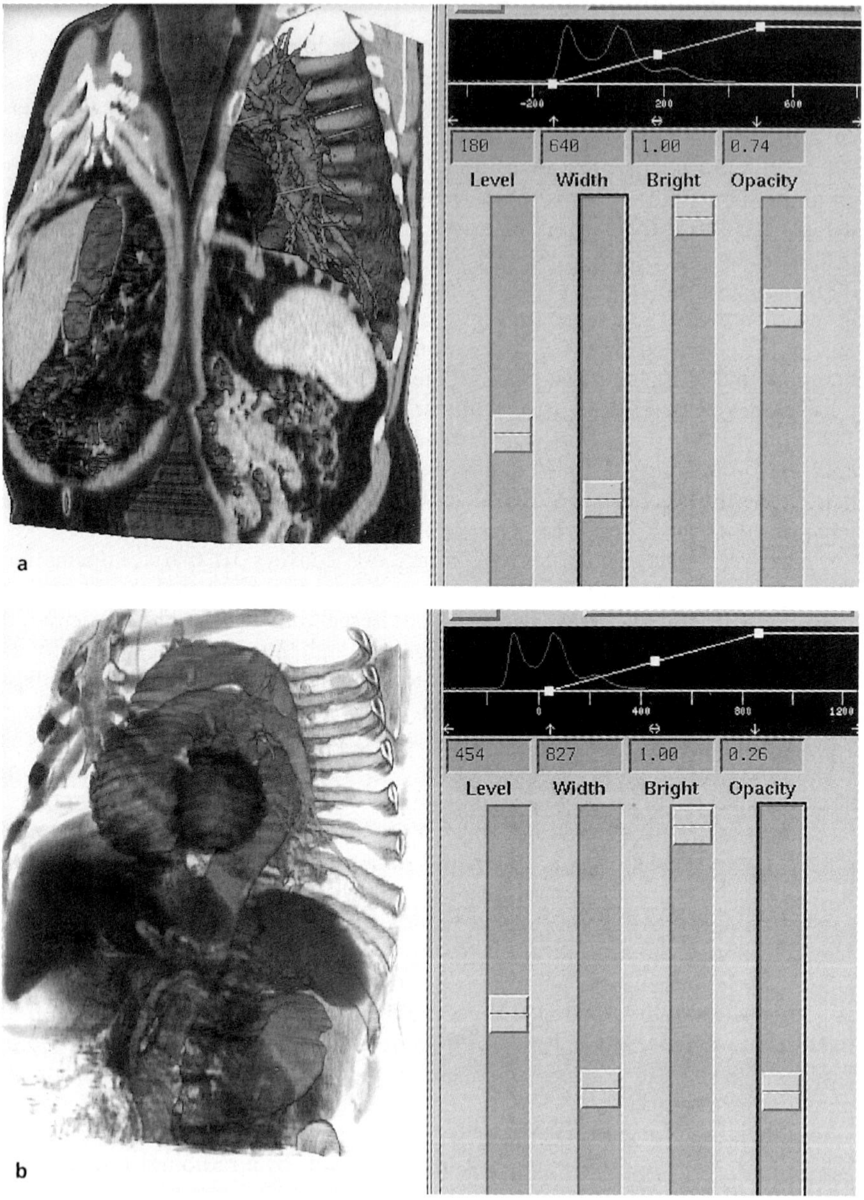

Fig. 26.1a, b.

slopes can enhance vital diagnostic information such as solid organs or mural thrombus in an aneurysm, or vascular stenoses and calcifications (Fig. 26.1).

The results of changing the position, size and shape of the trapezoid are viewed in real time and interactively changed to yield the best visual results.

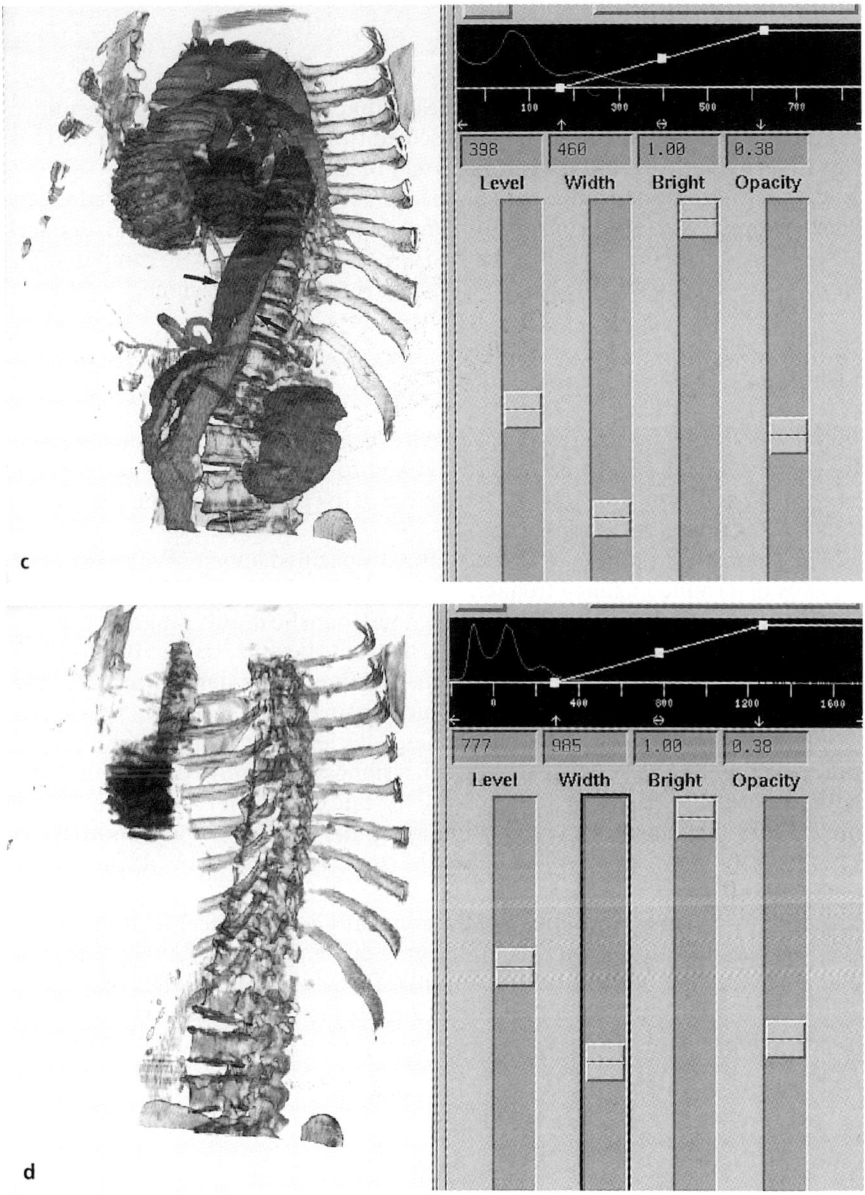

◀ **Fig. 26.1a–d.** CT volume rendering of thorax and abdomen in a patient with type B thoracic aortic dissection. Clip planes applied to the anterior and left side of the data volume. **a** Level and width set to visualise the parechymal organs including liver, spleen and thoracic vasculature. **b** By increasing the window level and width, tissues become translucent with visualisation of the pulmonary arteries and descending thoracic aorta. **c** Reducing the window width and level with an increase in opacity, it is now possible to visualise the vasculature more clearly with recognition of the lumina of the aortic dissection (*arrows*). **d** Increasing the window level and width provides exclusive visualisation of bony structure

26.2.2 Manipulating the Volume Data

Occasionally it is necessary to reduce the computational load and remove unnecessary bony structures by the standardised editing process prior to data analysis; this is particularly needed for carotid artery bifurcation visualisation.

Before the carotid arteries are volume rendered, it is necessary to reduce the computational load and remove other unwanted structures. Raw data from neck CT are first edited on a slice by slice basis by hand on a SunSparc computer. The slices are then passed to the Silicon Graphics visualisation machine.

26.2.3 Identifying and Imaging Vascular Stenoses

Initially both carotid arteries are viewed externally using the Hounsfield unit range for contrast usually above 170 HU and to help identify the external and internal branches and stenosis or occlusions. This involves rotating the volume dataset 360° about the vertical axis.

The Hounsfield unit range of the contrast-opacified lumen of the carotid arteries is determined using a frequency histogram below 166 ± 33 HU; the pixels in this range are coloured red. Similarly, the Hounsfield unit range of calcified plaques are determined using the same histogram above 425 ± 101 HU; the pixels within this range are coloured yellow. This technique provides subtraction of luminal contrast and is the basis for our "endoluminal view".

A movie scene is then produced from an anterior aspect which shows the volume rotating 180° from right to left. When a stenosis is identified, a cutting plane, with its normal oriented perpendicular to the line of sight of the observer, is then moved into the dataset, producing a longitudinal section of the carotid artery. This assists quantification of the degree of stenosis produced by plaque according to NASCET criteria.

A fly-through inside the lumen of the abnormal carotid artery is attempted for every patient to better appreciate the degree of stenosis and the relationship of plaque to the walls of the artery. The virtual fly-through starts within the lumen of the common carotid artery, heading towards the bifurcation and ends in the internal carotid artery. A movie scene is then produced based on the same flight path.

26.2.4 Common Carotid Artery Bifurcation Assessment

The North American Carotid Endarterectomy Trial and European Carotid Surgery Trial lists have proven that patients with high grade carotid artery stenosis (70%–99%) benefit from carotid endarterectomy [10, 11]. Determination of the degree of disease is therefore essential. Preliminary results have shown that CTA is superior to colour-coded duplex sonography for the evaluation of carotid disease and shows promise in determining which patients may require surgery, with the potential to replace the gold standard, digital subtraction angiography [12].

As little as 80 ml contrast can be used for assessment of the common carotid bifurcation. Using interactive volume rendering alone has in our preliminary series, shown a high degree of accuracy in assessing carotid artery disease compared to catheter angiography and transverse CT with MIP images. Using MIP display it is often impossible to discern the true residual lumen because of heavily calcified concentric plaque. The advantage of volume rendering is related to an ability to perform window and level functions and to cut through the vessel in any plane to optimally estimate the degree of luminal narrowing (Figs. 26.2, 26.3). Tortuous vessels are occasionally difficult to follow on transverse planes, particularly when they overlap, and the ability to image from multiple angles

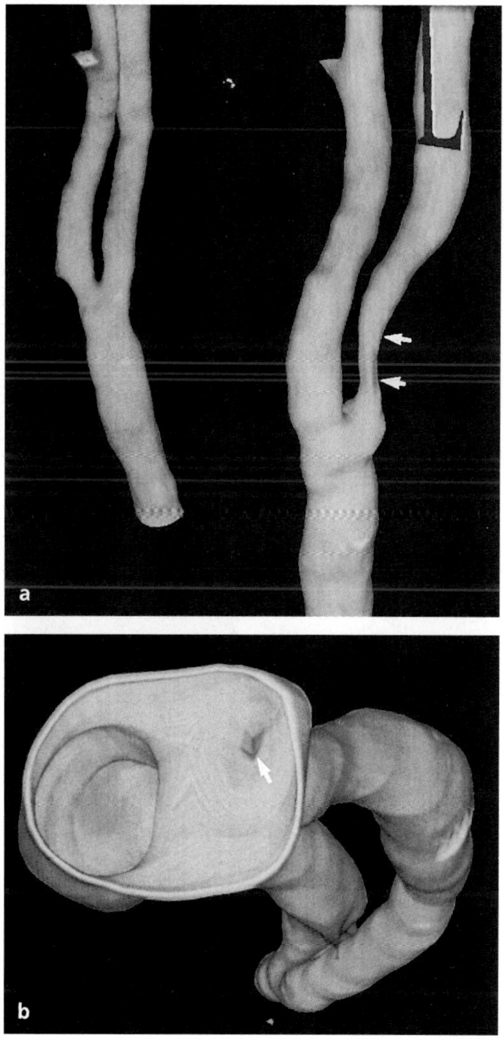

Fig. 26.2a, b. Left carotid artery stenosis. **a** Left anterior oblique projection of both carotids. Smooth stenosis of the left internal carotid artery (*arrows*). **b** Common carotid endoluminal view shows tight stenosis at the origin of the internal carotid artery (*arrow*); note widely patent external carotid origin

Fig. 26.3a, b. Carotid artery stenosis. **a** Lateral view shows multiple calcified plaques, coloured yellow, (*arrows*) surrounding a narrowed internal carotid artery (*arrowhead*). **b** Common carotid endoluminal view shows narrowed internal carotid (*curved arrow*) and calcified plaques, coloured yellow (*arrows*)

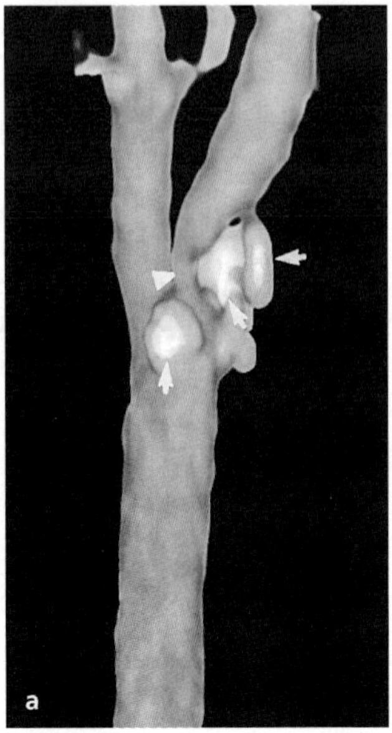

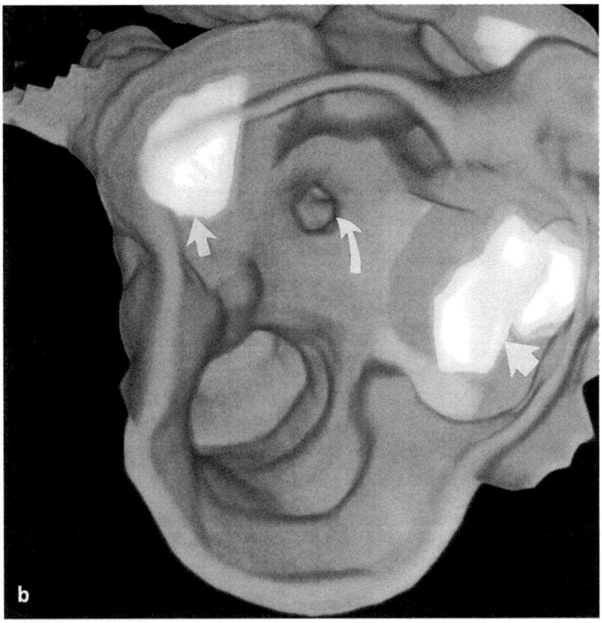

with clip plane application to remove the overlying bony structures is a distinct advantage of volume rendering. Colour coding of calcified plaque and subtraction of luminal contrast when combined with an endoluminal fly-through assists in understanding more complex vascular stenoses related to the bifurcation.

26.2.5
Intracranial Applications

The circle of Willis and vertebrobasilar system can be visualised from spiral CT datasets, enabling recognition of vascular stenoses, occlusions and aneurysms. One particular advantage of volume rendering compared to SSD and MIP displays is the ability to retain bony landmarks when visualising aneurysms or vascular stenoses (Fig. 26.4). Interactive manipulations allow visualisation of the relationship between bony landmarks in preparation for surgical intervention (Fig. 26.5). All intracranial studies are performed with 1-mm collimation and a pitch of 1.5 and overlapping reconstructions at 0.8-mm intervals.

26.2.6
Abdominal Aorta

Pre-operative assessment of abdominal aortic aneurysms require visualisation of the relationship of the aneurysm to major aortic branch vessels, accessory renal arteries, associated renal artery stenoses and inferior mesenteric artery patency [2]. This information can be achieved by spiral CTA and provides a better understanding than conventional arteriography. Spiral CTA is routinely used prior to

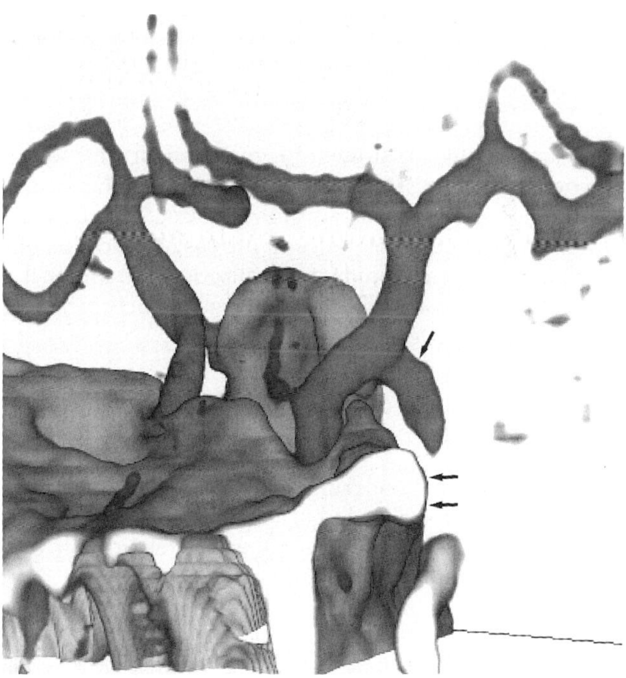

Fig. 26.4. CT angiogram of the circle of Willis with clip planes applied to remove a portion of the sella (*arrows*). There is a wide mouthed posterior communicating artery aneurysm (*arrow*) projecting from the left internal carotid artery

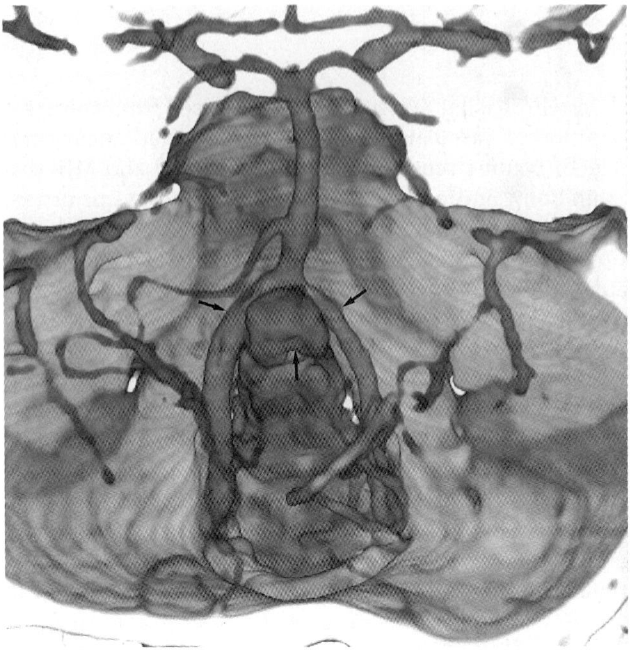

Fig. 26.5. Rheumatoid arthritis. The odontoid process (*arrow*) has migrated superiorly with impingement on both vertebral arteries (*arrows*) where they join to become the basilar artery

endoluminal stent treatment of aortic aneurysms and post-operative patients can be assessed for stent position and patency [13].

Volume rendering has advantages over SSD and MIP displays in that bony landmarks can be preserved, and the easy application of clip planes can remove overlying viscera allowing for visualisation of both renal and mesenteric branches. Real-time visualisation of relationships between clot, contrast and calcified plaque can be conveyed interactively.

26.2.7 Thoracic Aorta

Interactive volume rendering has several advantages over conventional CT with MIP display for visualisation of aortic aneurysms and aortic dissections [14]. The versatility of volume rendering allows the relationship between branching vessels and the aortic arch to be readily portrayed and in particular the relationship between thrombus and the aneurysm (Fig. 26.6). By lowering opacity the viewer can look through contrast columns, perhaps improving the diagnosis of subtle intravascular filling defects [8]. The intimal tear of aortic dissection can be viewed longitudinally by clip plane application, showing how it relates to aortic branches (Fig. 26.7). Large pulmonary emboli can be demonstrated with an angiographic-like appearance by volume rendering (Fig. 26.8).

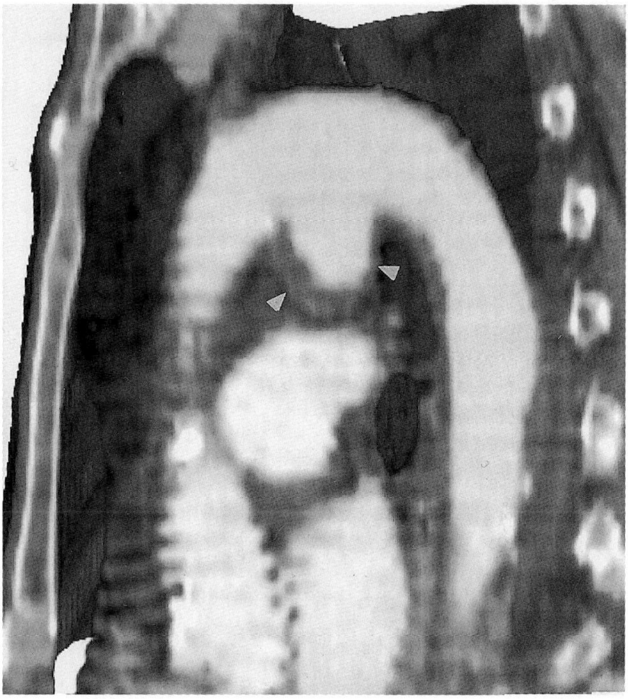

Fig. 26.6. Thoracic aortic aneurysm. Visualisation of an aneurysm projecting into the aorto-pulmonic window with associated mural thrombus (*arrowheads*)

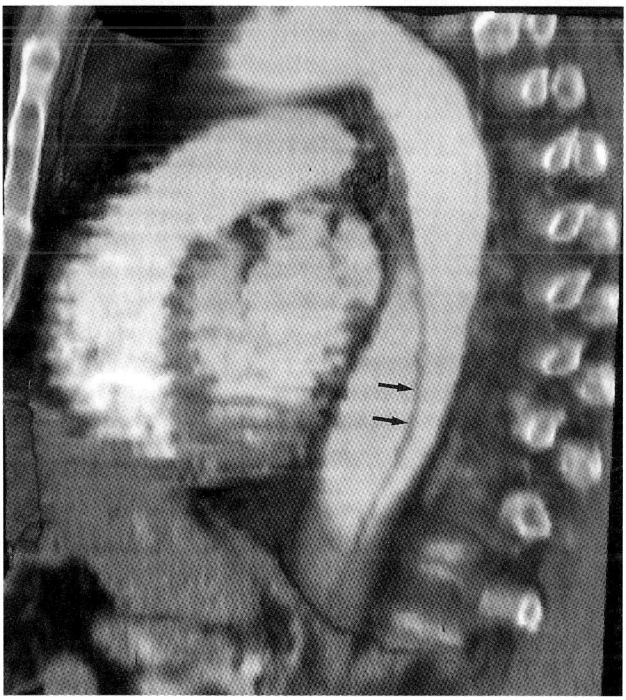

Fig. 26.7. Type B aortic dissection. Using clip planes the overlying ribs and soft tissues are removed to show the initmal tear (*arrows*). Note preservation of both high and low attenuation structures in the image (i.e. both vessels and solid organs)

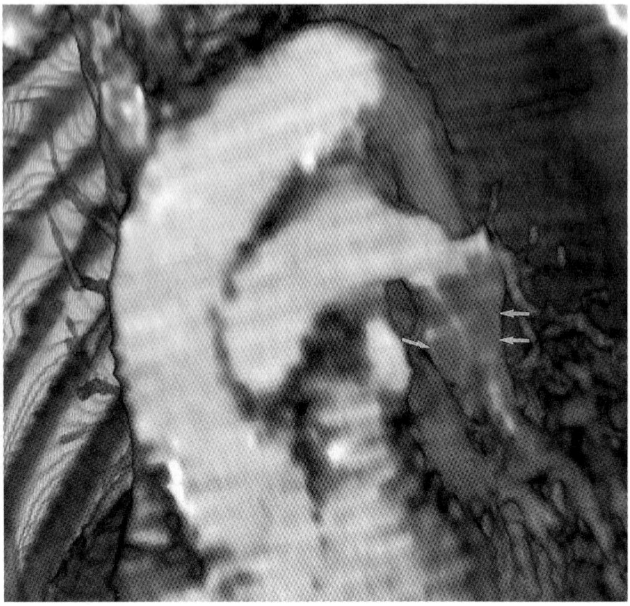

Fig. 26.8. Pulmonary embolus. Contrast-enhanced spiral CT viewed from a left anterior oblique projection. Using clip planes we can visualise a massive left lower lobe embolus (*arrows*). Contrast-filled main pulmonary artery and partially filled lower lobe vessels and thrombus are all discernible in this volume-rendered image

26.2.8 Renal Artery Assessment

Several authors have shown that CTA has the same accuracy as conventional angiography in detecting renal artery stenosis greater than 50% [4, 15, 16]. Grading of renal artery stenoses is 80% accurate with MIP CTA and only 55% accurate with SSD CTA. Volume rendering should improve our accuracy, particularly when applying clip planes and endoluminal visualisation of plaque to discriminate between calcified plaque and the enhanced lumen which can typically fall at a threshold level selected by conventional visualisation techniques. Very tortuous anatomy is more easily understood utilising volume rendering tools and has proven valuable in assessing patients who have undergone renal transplantation in whom there is a suspicion of renal artery stenosis. The tortuous complex anatomy of graft anastomoses is better visualised by volume rendering tools (Fig. 26.9).

26.3 Discussion

Unlike other rendering tools such as MIP and SSD, with volume rendering it is not essential to set single threshold parameters or routinely edit images. More importantly, since it is an interactive process, the effects of different thresholds and ranges can be explored by the user.

Unlike MIP display, true anatomical spatial relationships are better visualised with volume rendering techniques, giving a clearer understanding of three di-

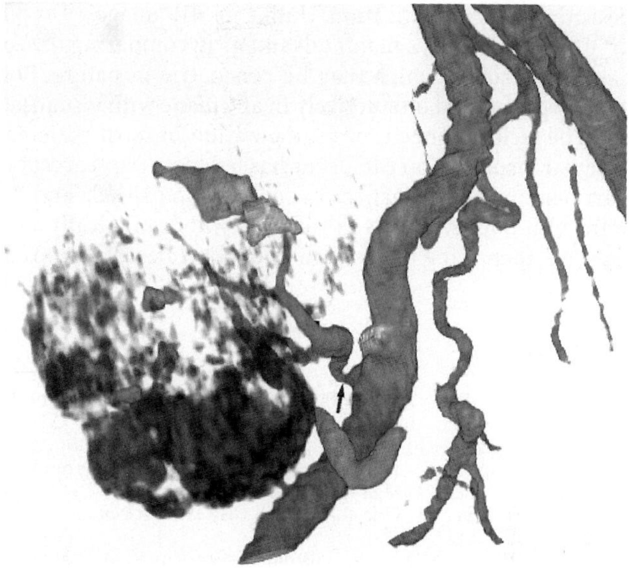

Fig. 26.9. Renal transplant artery stenosis. An end-to-side anastomoses shows severe narrowing at the origin of the transplanted vessel (*arrow*)

mensional relationships since a wide range of tissues can be explored and viewed in real time.

Volume rendering usually eliminates the need for the image editing essential to MIP images. When required, interactive editing can be performed by applying clip planes which remove slabs of data and permit centrally located structures to be visualised more readily. Clip planes can be applied to any depth level, thereby removing unnecessary or obscuring anatomy. Editing using most commercially available software tools prior to rendering is currently cumbersome and can take between 15 and 40 min. Since the volume rendering process is interactive, clip planes and parameters can be altered or restored rapidly with the advantage of immediate visualisation.

Volume rendering techniques minimise the potential to overestimate vascular stenoses because volume-averaged voxels that contribute to vascular structure are incorporated into the image with a relatively lower attenuation.

26.4 Conclusion

Refinements in computer processing with increased speeds of volume rendering have facilitated an interactive manipulation of CT data at the workstation, leading some to believe that perspective volume rendering may become an alternative to review of transverse sections for primary CT interpretation [17]. Simple manipulation of window level and width with the application of colour to voxels enables visualisation of complex vascular relationships and vascular stenoses. As the entire dataset is used during volume rendering, fewer inaccuracies in data analysis are likely. It is no longer necessary to select arbitrary thresholds stipulated with binary classification. Unlike in MIP images, it is possible to obtain proper 3D relationships, a major advantage in comparing the contrast-filled lumen to calcified plaques, which may be concentric in nature. Rotation of the image is rapidly performed interactively in any plane with visualisation of the entire dataset. The lack of a need for segmentation in most patients and the speed which vascular visualisation can occur has led to its rapid acceptance in our clinical Department. Further advances in computation speeds and the lower costs of hardware with improvements in software will dramatically alter the future use of CT datasets, increasing the versatility of clinical applications of these tools.

References

1. Rubin GD, Dake MD, Napel SA, McDonnell CH, Jeffrey RBJ (1993) Abdominal spiral CT angiography: Initial clinical experience. Radiology 186:147–152
2. Rubin GD, Walker PJ, Dake MD, Napel S, Jeffrey RB, McDonnell CH, Mitchell RS, Miller DC (1993) 3D spiral CT angiography: an alternative imaging modality for the abdominal aorta and its branches. J Vasc Surg 18:656–666
3. Costello P, Ecker CP, Tello R, Hartnell GG (1992) Assessment of the thoracic aorta by spiral CT. AJR 158:1127–1130
4. Rubin GD, Dake MD, Napel S, Brooke Jeffrey Jnr R, McDonnell CH, Sommer FG, Wexler L, Williams DM (1994) Spiral CT of renal artery stenosis: comparison of three-dimensional rendering techniques. Radiology 190:181–189
5. Marks MP, Napel S, Jordan JE, Enzmann DR (1993) diagnosis of carotid artery disease: preliminary experience with maximum-intensity-projection spiral CT angiography. AJR 160: 1267–1271
6. Cumming MJ, Morrow IM (1994) Carotid artery stenosis: a prospective comparison of CT angiography and conventional angiography. AJR 163:517–523
7. Johnson PT, Heath DG, Bliss DF, Cabral B, Fishman EK (1996) Three-Dimensional CT: Real-time interactive volume rendering. AJR 167:581–583
8. Kuszyk BS, Heath DG, Ney DR, Bluemke DA, Urban BA, Chambers TP, Fishman EK (1995) CT angiography with volume rendering: imaging findings. AJR 165:445–448
9. Rubin GD, Dake MD, Semba CP (1995) Current status of three-dimensional spiral CT scanning for imaging the vasculature. Radiol Clin North Am 33:51–70
10. North American Symptomatic Carotid Endarterectomy Trial collaborators (1991) Beneficial effect of carotid endarterectomy in symptomatic patients with high-grade carotid stenosis. N Engl J Med 325:445–453
11. European Carotid Surgery Trialists' Collaborative Group (1991) MRC European Carotid Surgery Trial: interim results for symptomatic patients with severe (70–99%) or with mild (0–29%) carotid stenosis. Lancet 337:1235–1243
12. Link J, Brossmann J, Penselin V, Gluer CC, Heller M (1997) Common Carotid Artery Bifurcation: Preliminary results of CT angiography and color-coded duplex sonography compared with digital subtraction angiography. AJR 168:361–65
13. Rubin GD, Dake MD, Napel S, Jeffrey RBJ (1993) Three-dimensional CT angiography as an alternative to conventional arteriography in planning and in vivo evaluation of aortic stent grafts. Radiology 189 (P):112
14. Johnson PT, Heath DG, Kuszyk BS, Fishman EK (1997) CT angiography: Thoracic vascular imaging with interactive volume rendering technique. J Comput Assist Tomography 21 (1): 110–114
15. Galanski M, Prokop M, Chavan A, Schaefer CM, Jandeleit K, Nischelsky JE (1993) Renal arterial stenoses: spiral CT angiography. Radiology 189:185–192
16. Olbright, CJ, Paul K, Prokop M, Chavan A, Schaefer-Prokop CM, Jandeleit K, Koch KM, Galanski M (1995) Minimally invasive diagnosis of renal artery stenosis by spiral computed tomography angiography. Kidney Int 48:1332–1337
17. Rubin GD, Beaulieu CF, Argiro V, Ringl H, Norbash AM, Feller JF, Dake MD, Brooke Jeffrey R, Napel S (1996) Perspective volume rendering of CT and MR images: applications for endoscopic imaging. Radiology 199:321–330

27 Guidance of Nonvascular Interventional Procedures with Real-Time CT-Fluoroscopy: Early Clinical Experience with C.A.R.E. Vision CT

J. J. FROELICH, K. J. KLOSE

27.1 Introduction

Nonvascular interventional radiological procedures may be guided by various imaging techniques such as ultrasonography, fluoroscopy, computed tomography (CT), and magnetic resonance imaging (MRI). Because of high spatial resolution, superior reproducibility, a wide field of view, and applicability to air-filled and bone structures, CT-guided interventional procedures have become important clinical tools in recent years. A great disadvantage with CT-guided interventions, however, has been the lack of real-time imaging capability, which is available with ultrasound and fluoroscopy. Especially in body regions where extensive respiratory movement is present, small target lesions may shift and disappear during conventional CT-guided punctures. This seems to be one of the most important reasons why CT-guided interventions are unsuccessful or must be repeated [12]. To overcome this limitation, C.A.R.E. Vision CT (Combined Applications to Reduce Exposure), a CT-fluoroscopy system, was developed and installed on a Siemens Somatom Plus 4 CT scanner providing real-time image reconstruction and display of CT images on a monitor at a frame rate of three or six images per second.

To evaluate the efficacy of this new technology, biopsy and drainage procedures were performed prospectively with either conventional CT guidance or with CT fluoroscopy. We report here our initial clinical experience in these interventions. Reduction of radiation exposure in drainage procedures, decrease in examination time, and fewer punctures promise to make CT fluoroscopy a valuable tool for future routine applications, establishing new horizons for future nonvascular radiological interventions.

27.2 Materials and Methods

27.2.1 Instruments

A continuous rotation, fan-beam geometry CT scanner (Somatom Plus 4, Siemens, Forchheim, Germany) was modified by adding a high-speed array processor to increase image reconstruction speed and image display (up to 6/s). This has resulted in virtually real-time reconstruction and display of CT images on a monitor.

CT fluoroscopic images are acquired at a gantry rotation speed of 0.75 s and generally at 50 mA and 120 kV. Three power steps up to 10.8 kW (corresponding to 50, 70, and 90 mA at 120 kV) are available. A display rate of three or six images per second with an interimage spacing of 0.17 s can be obtained while all standard collimator settings (1–10 mm) may be selected. Image reconstruction is performed on a 256 × 256 matrix with images displayed in full screen resolution of a 1024 × 1024 matrix.

Generated images are displayed on an in-room monitor next to the patient table directly facing the interventional radiologist. The field of view may be selected from 5 to 50 cm, and gantry tilt is possible. During fluoroscopy the patient table may simultaneously be moved in and out of the gantry controlled by a joystick. Duration of continuous fluoroscopy is limited to 80 s. However, after stopping radiation for only a few seconds, multiple other consecutive fluoroscopy sessions are available each without limitation in respect to 80-s intervals. Similar to conventional fluoroscopy, C.A.R.E. Vision CT is started by pressing and holding down a foot pedal. Reconstructed images are converted to standard television signals, and a video recorder interface card allows connection to a VCR for documentation of the complete set of images, acquired during CT-fluoroscopy. The last fluoroscopic image always remains displayed on the monitor (last image hold) until fluoroscopy is reactivated. Only last images are stored on hard disk (last image store). The basic configuration of the C.A.R.E. Vision CT set-up is shown in Fig. 27.1.

Patient access during the interventions is facilitated by a large 70-cm-diameter gantry aperture with a wide flared opening, a scan plane, which is located close to front of the gantry, and a table design providing improved space between table pedestal and gantry. As a control, conventional CT-guided biopsies have been performed with the same Somatom Plus 4 scanner. Depending on patient consti-

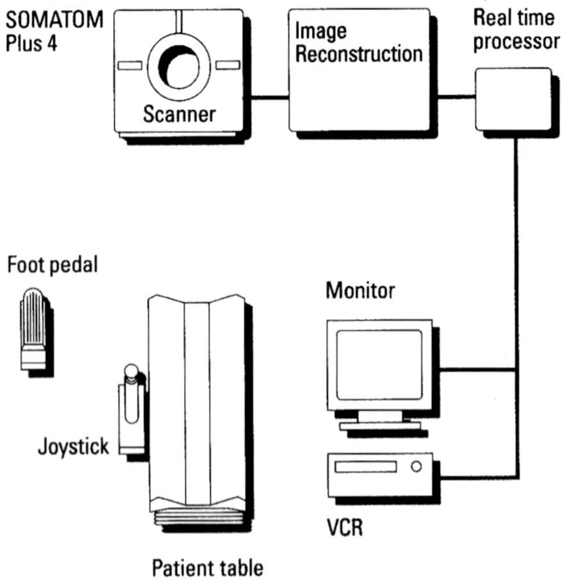

Fig. 27.1. Configuration of the CT fluoroscopy system CARE Vision

tution and target location, various single scans ranging from 150 to 250 mA at 140 kV were obtained. Gantry rotation speed generally was 1-s per slice. No targeting guides such as lasers, skin marker plates, and angulation devices were used for conventional or CT fluoroscopic interventional procedures

27.2.2 Patients

All patients receiving interventional CT-guided biopsy or drainage procedures were randomized to either conventional or fluoroscopic CT guidance while patient preparation remained identical for the two modalities. All procedures were performed by experienced interventional radiologists who were already familiar with conventional and fluoroscopic CT-guided interventions. After a target lesion had been defined by preinterventional CT and marked on the skin, a virtual access route was planned. Generally, diagnostic interventional biopsies were performed with an 18- or 20-G high-speed biopsy needle (BIP, CCC Crowne-Core-Cut Biopsy Needle, Türkenfeld, Germany). Fluid collections were initially punctured with a 22-G needle, and a 0.014-in. soft-tip guidewire was consequently introduced into the collection to be exchanged for a 0.035-in. J-tip guidewire over a coaxial catheter introducer system (Accustick, Boston Scientific, Watertown, MA, USA). Depending on the initial size and content of the fluid collection, sump drainages with diameters between 10 and 14 Fr were introduced (Van Sonnenberg Sump Drainage, Boston Scientific). Various CT single scans or CT fluoroscopy intervals were performed during the interventions whenever the operator needed to monitor the positioning of any interventional tools.

Locations and diameters of lesions, total number of punctures, procedure time, outcome, and radiation doses were evaluated separately for conventional CT guidance and for CT fluoroscopy in thoracic, abdominal, and drainage procedures.

27.3 **Results**

27.3.1 Overall

Twenty-two patients were examined between June and October 1997. Conventional CT-guided procedures were performed in half of these patients and CT fluoroscopy in the other half. Twelve interventions were performed for drainage of abdominal or pelvic fluid collections, six patients underwent pulmonary biopsy, and from four patients biopsies of abdominal lesions were obtained. Due to a problematic anatomical situation in the neighborhood of a postoperative abscess within the right upper abdomen, conventional puncture and drainage of this fluid collection was not possible in one patient. This patient had to be excluded from the study protocol to be successfully treated with CT fluoroscopic guidance. All other fluid collections and biopsy targets were completed with either conventional or CT fluoroscopic guidance according to the initial randomization protocol.

Image quality proved to be sufficient with both modalities despite the low CT fluoroscopy doses of generally 50 mA. CT fluoroscopy was able to monitor the complete biopsy and drainage procedures without requiring additional conventional CT or fluoroscopy and was performed in 11 patients. The CT fluoroscopic images sufficiently depicted important anatomical details within high- and low-contrast organ regions. Radial artifacts were occasionally observed during CT fluoroscopy. These were generally caused by moving objects within the gantry (e.g., fingers, needle holders). A characteristic shading artifact was observed in virtually all punctures at the tip of the puncture needle, indicating a correct needle position (Fig. 27.2a, 27.3b). No technical problems were observed during the interventions.

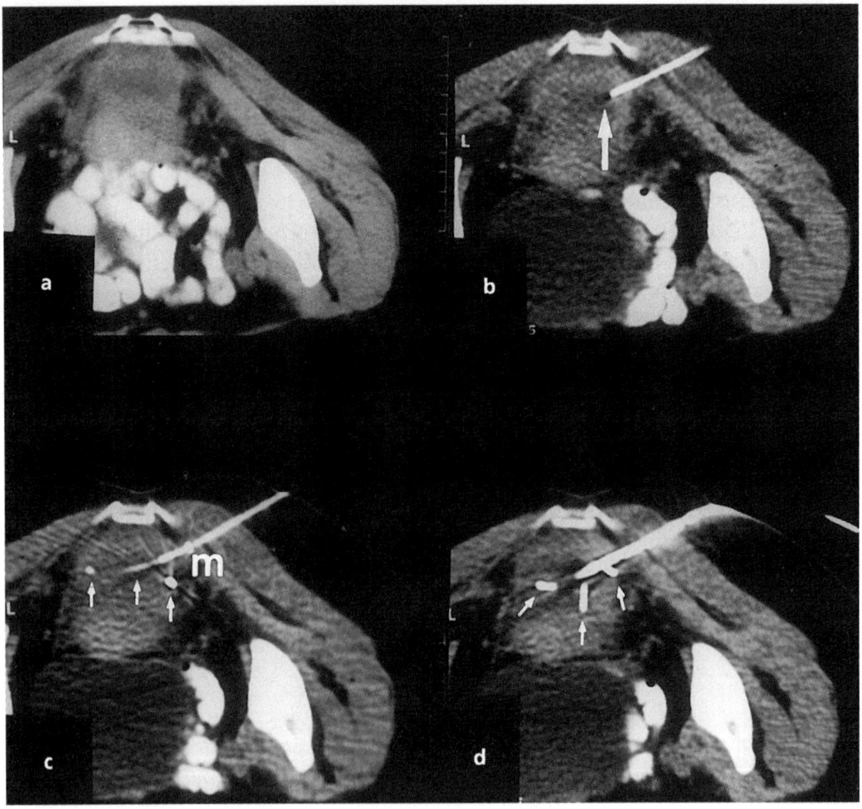

Fig. 27.2. CT fluoroscopic guidance for drainage of a presacral pelvic abscess after amputation of the rectum for carcinoma. The patient is placed in prone position. **a** Diagnostic spiral CT demonstrates fluid collection with a diameter of 4 cm and central density of 20–25 HU within the former bed of the rectum located between uterus and the sacral bone. **b** CT fluoroscopic image after puncture of the abscess with a 22-G needle from a right dorsal parasacral access route. The needle-tip sign (*arrow*) indicates correct positioning of the needle within the target area. **c** CT fluoroscopy demonstrates correct placement of a small guidewire coiled-up within the abscess (*arrows*) and the distal tip-marker of a coaxial drainage introducer system (*M*). **d** Correct positioning of a 10-Fr sump drainage within the abscess. A 0.035-in. guidewire is still left within the abscess (*arrows*)

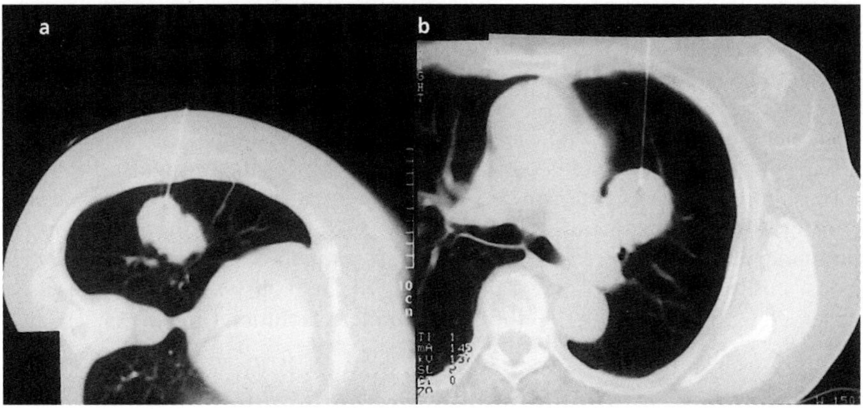

Fig. 27.3. CT-guided biopsies of pulmonary tumors with CT fluoroscopy (**a**) and conventional CT guidance (**b**) show no differences in image quality. In both modalities the needle-tip sign is located within the target lesions, again indicating correct position of the biopsy needles

27.3.2 Drainages

Mean maximum diameters of abdominal fluid collections were similar for conventional and CT fluoroscopic procedures without significant difference. Regarding depth of the fluid collections, there was also no apparent difference between the two guiding modalities. Although all target regions could be punctured easily with only one needle passage, procedure times were distinctly shorter with CT fluoroscopy than with the conventional CT-guided approach. Mean procedure time was 11.8 ± 4.4 min for CT fluoroscopic drainages and 17.6 ± 8.1 min for conventional CT guidance. A mean of 2712 ± 1362 mAs was applied with CT fluoroscopy while 4875 ± 5804 mAs was used with conventional CT guidance. Mean fluoroscopy time with C.A.R.E. Vision CT was 24.8 ± 11.5 s. No difference between CT fluoroscopy and conventional CT guidance was found regarding clinical outcome or patient recovery. After initial puncture of the target lesion introduction and coiling of guidewires, catheters, introducers, and drainages was demonstrated well with CT fluoroscopy (Fig. 27.2a–d) while additional scans within different axial levels had to be obtained during conventional CT-guided interventions.

27.3.3 Biopsies

Diameters of pulmonary and abdominal biopsy targets were also similar for CT fluoroscopy and conventional CT-guided procedures, and the depth of target lesions was almost identical in the two groups. Slightly fewer pleural/peritoneal needle passes were necessary with C.A.R.E. Vision CT than with conventional CT-guided biopsies (1 versus 1.5). The mean procedure times for biopsy of pulmonary lesions proved to be distinctly shorter for CT fluoroscopy than for conventional CT guidance (15.7 ± 4.4 versus 31.7 ± 24.7 min). Slightly higher doses, however, were applied with CT fluoroscopy (mean 5276 ± 2507 mAs) than with conventional CT guidance (mean 3692 ± 2004 mAs). Mean duration of CT fluoroscopy was 40 ± 10 s with use of C.A.R.E. Vision CT. Assessment of histologic specimens, again, showed no difference between conventional and fluoroscopic CT. CT fluoroscopy depicted pleural bulging during needle passage and in small intrapulmonary lesions; downward displacement was observed during needle contact. No procedure-related complications such as pneumothorax and intrapulmonary bleeding were observed in the six patients with intrapulmonary lesions, studied until now. Correct positioning of the biopsy needle tip was easily observed with both guiding methods at a similar resolution (Fig. 27.3).

27.3.4 Special Procedures

Generally positioning of the needle tip was found to be so precise that even slightly dilated intrahepatic bile ducts could easily be punctured with CT-fluoroscopic guidance (Fig. 27.4a). Bile fluid was aspirated continuously, and injection of diluted contrast medium confirmed correct positioning of the needle tip within the biliary tree. However, although puncture and positioning of the needle tip was managed very easily, it was not possible to perform adequate percutaneous biliary drainage in two of three patients with pancreatic tumors and intrahepatic cholestasis since guidewire advancement in the coronal plane could not be depicted sufficiently with axial CT fluoroscopy – even when using extensive joystick-controlled table feed. In one of these cases, however, a 6-Fr drainage was successfully placed within the right intrahepatic biliary tree without using additional C-arm fluoroscopy (Fig. 27.4b).

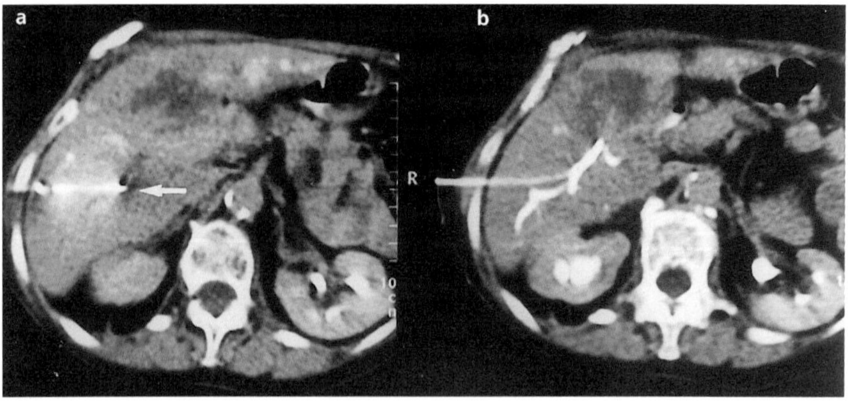

Fig. 27.4. a Percutaneous CT fluoroscopic puncture of a bile duct within the 6th segment of the right hepatic lobe. The needle tip is positioned precisely within the dilated bile duct (*arrow*). **b** Consequent introduction of a 6-Fr drainage and application of contrast material finally demonstrates correct intraductal positioning

27.4 Discussion

Nonvascular interventional radiological procedures such as biopsies and drainages may be guided by various imaging modalities such as ultrasonography [4–6, 8, 9, 11, 15, 16, 20], fluoroscopy [14, 17, 23, 25], CT [2, 3, 22, 24], combined CT and fluoroscopy [7], and magnetic resonance imaging [1, 10, 18, 19, 21]. Especially CT guidance has distinct advantages over other imaging modalities since it can be used simultaneously in soft tissue, fluid, air-filled, and bone structures. CT also offers superior reproducibility, a wide and variable field of view, easy patient access, and high spatial resolution and precision.

Disadvantages in CT-guided punctures, however, are procedure-related radiation exposure and the lack of real-time imaging capability because a few seconds of postprocessing time are required for generation of a single CT image. Patient motion due to the inability of the patient to remain still and respiratory motion of target lesions especially within the base of the lung and the upper abdomen may therefore cause the target to disappear during the procedures. This problem becomes more aggravated with small-sized lesions. Such limitations may require repeat punctures, resulting in a decrease of the primary success rate and accuracy. Additionally, complication rates are increased and procedure times become prolonged. As observed by Katada et al. [12], it would be more appropriate to refer to such conventional CT approaches as "CT-assisted" rather than "CT-guided" procedures.

To overcome the constant lack of real-time imaging during CT interventions, a CT fluoroscopy system was developed, providing real-time image reconstruction and display of CT images on a monitor at a frame rate of three or six images per second. Our initial experience comparing conventional CT assistance and fluoroscopic CT guidance in biopsy and drainage procedures shows distinct advantages for the new CT fluoroscopy system. Targeting and advancement of needles, guidewires, catheters, and drainages was clearly monitored with CT fluoroscopy. Procedure times proved to be shorter for drainages and for diagnostic biopsies. Fewer punctures were generally necessary for biopsy of pulmonary target lesions with CT fluoroscopic guidance. As observed in one case, a conventional CT-guided access may become critical in problematic anatomical situations and cannot be performed safely without risk to the patient. Especially in such situations, C.A.R.E. Vision CT allows safe puncture of the target because the advancement of puncture needles is monitored in real-time CT fluoroscopy.

Since positioning of needles, guidewires, catheters, and drainages is easily visible in real-time mode, the operator's skill, which is essential for CT-guided biopsies and drainages, might be a less important factor for future interventions guided by C.A.R.E. Vision CT. CT fluoroscopy therefore offers high success rates to even less experienced operator's. Also, the precise placement of biopsy needles within special areas of a target lesion can be monitored to ensure positive biopsy of a tumor area rather than obtaining only tumor necrosis for the definite histologic report.

With the introduction of CT fluoroscopy we have observed modifications in puncture technique compared with conventional CT-guided procedures. Especially in pulmonary lesions located within the base of the lung and close to the diaphragm or in subphrenically located liver lesions respirational shift often causes targets to disappear from the puncture plane during conventional CT-guided procedures. As reported by Katada et al. [12], CT fluoroscopic puncture of such lesions may be performed during respiration while the target is shifting along. Especially in uncooperative patients a target lesion may suddenly be punctured whenever it appears within the axial CT plane after correct needle angulation has been established within the subcutaneous tissue. Also, obstruction of the needle access during conventional CT-guided procedures due to bone structures (e.g., ribs) often requires repeated punctures and additional confirmation of correct needle placement.

With C.A.R.E. Vision CT the puncture needle however, may easily be guided across obstacles, retargeted and safely placed within the target area during a single CT fluoroscopic interval – repeat punctures and pleural passages may therefore be avoided in most cases. Target shifting due to needle contact in hard tumors and needle pull-back due to rebound of subcutaneous tissue can clearly be observed with C.A.R.E. Vision CT [12]. The needle-tip sign which is observed in conventional and fluoroscopic CT-guided procedures helps to ensure correct positioning of a needle tip within the target, especially when punctures must be performed from the axial plane. This sign is described as a shading artifact resulting from a sudden change in Hounsfield units between the needle tip and the surrounding tissue. Correct positioning within the target is indicated by the needle-tip sign [12]. Whenever the shading artifact at the needle-tip sign is absent, the needle is likely to be positioned outside from the axial plane and must be relocated by sliding the patient couch in or out of the gantry by means of joystick control.

Persistent concerns exist regarding radiation exposure to patient and surgeon during CT fluoroscopy. As reported previously, the dose to the patient's skin and the operator's hands has been found to be as high as 1.14 ± 0.02 mGy/s [13]. The dose to the physician's hand, however, may be reduced by using needle holders or special radiation protection gloves (Boston Scientific). As with C-arm fluoroscopy, radiation exposure remains a general disadvantage associated with CT-guided procedures, although only low doses are applied during CT fluoroscopy [8, 10]. While the radiation dose in terms of total mAs may be slightly less with C.A.R.E. Vision CT than with conventional CT procedures for drainages, it is distinctly higher in biopsy procedures. The observed decrease in total mAs during drainages probably reflects the problematic situation in conventional CT-guided interventions, where repeated punctures, introductions and relocations of various needles, guidewires, and coaxial exchanges are necessary for different drainages and multiple confirmations of correct positioning in single CT scans. With CT fluoroscopy the positioning of interventional instruments, however, can be monitored in real-time by simply sliding the patient table in and out of the gantry. The advantage of reducing total mAs as observed in drainage procedures, however, did not become apparent with CT-guided biopsies since target lesions generally had to be punctured only once to obtain sufficient biopsy samples with either modality. Extensive needle manipulations or replacements have not been necessary during our preliminary biopsy experience.

We have found that CT fluoroscopy generally facilitates nonvascular interventional procedures. By providing real-time monitoring a major disadvantage of CT-guided procedures has finally been overcome. Our initial clinical experience well demonstrates the apparent advantages of CT fluoroscopy over conventional CT-guidance in drainage and biopsy procedures of the abdomen and the chest. CT fluoroscopy has proven to be an efficient method for real-time monitoring of various interventional procedures at a reasonably high resolution. We believe that this innovative technology is generally applicable for true guidance of nonvascular interventions. A possible combination of CT fluoroscopy with C-arm fluoroscopy may offer even further horizons for challenging future interventional radiological procedures such as instant and precise placement of percutaneous biliary drainages, TIPSS, and neurosurgical and embolization procedures.

References

1. Adam G, Neuerburg J, Bucker A, Glowinski A, Vorwerk D, Stargardt A, Van Vaals JJ, Günther RW (1997) Interventional magnetic resonance. Initial clinical experience with a 1.5-tesla magnetic resonance system combined with C-arm fluoroscopy. Invest Radiol 32:191–197
2. Aideyan OA, Schmidt AJ, Trenkner SW, Hakim NS, Gruessner RW, Walsh JW (1992) CT-guided percutaneous biopsy of pancreas transplants. Radiology 201:825–828 (1996)
3. Barton P, Schurawitzki H, Karnel F, Klepetko W (1927) Percutaneous CT-guided catheter drainage of intrathoracic fluid accumulations. Rofo 156:47–52
4. Bazzocchi M, Zuiani C, Degano GP, Dalpiaz G, Anania G, di Loreto C (1993) The use of automatic devices for ultrasonography-guided histologic biopsy of breast lesions. Radiol Med 86:599–602
5. Bret PM, Guibaud L, Atri M, Gillett P, Seymour RJ, Senterman MK (1992) Transvaginal US-guided aspiration of ovarian cysts and solid pelvic masses. Radiology 185:377– 380
6. Bunk A, Unger W, Friedberg R, Hildebrandt E (1990) Results of sonographically-guided percutaneous procedures for therapy of liquid-filled space-occupying lesions in acute abdomen. Zentralbl Chir 115:1101–1111
7. Damascelli B, Porcelli G, Spreafico C, Marchiano A, Milella M, Garbagnati F, Frigerio LF, Salvetti M, Bonalumi MG, Cozzi G (1990) CT-fluoroscopy link-up (CTF) potential for special procedures. Eur J Radiol 11:81–86
8. Dodd GD 3rd, Esola CC, Memel DS, Ghiatas AA, Chintapalli KN, Paulson EK, Nelson RC, Ferris JV, Baron RL (1996) Sonography: the undiscovered jewel of interventional radiology. Radiographics 16:1271–1288
9. Flament JB, Delattre JF, Palot JP, Avisse C, Burde A (1991) Ultrasound-guided percutaneous drainage of intraperitoneal fluid collections. An experience of a surgical team with 205 patients. Chirurgie 117:298–310
10. Frahm C, Gehl HB, Weiss HD, Rossberg WA (1996) Technique of MRT-guided core biopsy in the abdomen using an open low-field scanner: feasibility and initial clinical results. Rofo 164:62–67
11. Holm HH, Skjoldbye B (1996) Interventional ultrasound. Ultrasound Med Biol 22:773– 789
12. Katada K, Kato R, Anno H, Ogura Y, Koga S, Ida Y, Sato M, Nonomura K (1996) Guidance with real-time CT fluoroscopy: early clinical experience. Radiology 200:851–856
13. Kato R, Katada K, Anno H, Suzuki S, Ida Y, Koga S (1996) Radiation dosimetry at CT fluoroscopy: physician's hand dose and development of needle holders. Radiology 201:576–578
14. Lemmi A, Lupattelli L, Barzi F, Malaspina C, Rizzo F (1992) The advantages of combined US-fluoroscopic guidance in the drainage of abdominal abscesses. Radiol Med 83:81–84
15. Memel DS, Dodd GD 3rd, Esola CC (1996) Efficacy of sonography as a guidance technique for biopsy of abdominal, pelvic, and retroperitoneal lymph nodes. AJR Am J Roentgenol 167:957–962
16. Mueller PR, Simeone JF, Butch RJ, Saini S, Stafford SA, Vici LG, Soto-Rivera C, Ferrucci JT Jr (1986) Percutaneous drainage of subphrenic abscess: a review of 62 patients. AJR Am J Roentenol 147:1237–1240
17. Nakamura K, Ooe T, Matsushita T, Nakagawa K, Aoki K, Mamada K, Ono M, Kurokawa T (1997) Stereo fluoroscopy-assisted percutaneous needle puncture of the vertebral body. J Spinal Disord 10:102–105

18. Schoenenberger AW, Steiner P, Debatin JF, Pfammatter T, Kacl GM (1996) Puncture with an open-sided, interventional MRI system. Illustration with a case report. Radiologe 36: 705–708
19. Steiner P, Schoenenberger AW, Penner EA, Erhardt P, Debatin JF, von Schulthess GK, Kacl GM (1996) Interactive stereotaxic interventions in superconducting, open 0.5-tesla MRI tomography. Rofo 165:276–280
20. Tsatalis JT, Rifkin M (1989) Abdominal abscesses: ultrasound guided percutaneous therapy. Del Med J 61:413–416
21. Vosshenrich R, Fischer U, Grabbe E (1996) MRI-controlled intervention in suspected lesions of the breast. Geburtshilfe Frauenheilkd 56:173–176
22. Waddill W 3rd, Wright W Jr, Unger E, Stopeck A, Akporiaye E, Harris D, Grogan T, Schluter S, Hersh E, Stahl S (1997) Human gene therapy for melanoma: CT-guided interstitial injection. AJR Am J Roentgenol 169:63–67
23. Westcott JL (1980) Direct percutaneous needle aspiration of localized pulmonary lesions: results in 422 patients. Radiology 137:31–35
24. Westcott JL, Rao N, Colley DP (1997) Transthoracic needle biopsy of small pulmonary nodules. Radiology 202:97–103
25. Zornoza J, Snow J Jr, Lukeman JM, Libshitz HI (1977) Aspiration biopsy of discrete pulmonary lesions using a new thin needle: results in the first 100 cases. Radiology 123:519–520

Subject Index

A
abdomen / abdominal 147 ff.
- aneurysm 208
- aorta, abdominal 151, 219
- - fly-around view 151
- diagnostic puncture, contribution of fast and SCT 171–174
- perimeter 4
abscess 176, 180
- intramuscular 180
absorption efficiency 10
ACA (anterior cerebral artery) 59
acetabulum, trauma 175
- fracture 178, 179
acquisition time 3
afterglow 9, 10
AIDS 175
air-trapping 121
airway disease 120
ALARA principle 3, 32
allergic reaction 107
amplitude, maxiumum modulation amplitude 28
anatomically adapted tube, dose reduction in CT 27 ff., 35 ff.
aneurysms
- abdominal 208
- cerebral 59–69
- - diagnosis with CTA 60
- - infraclinoidal 61–63
- - intracavernous 59
- thoracic aortic 221
angiography
- CTA (computed tomography angiography) 45, 59 ff., 84 ff., 149, 150
- DSA (digital subtraction angiography) 59, 61, 107
- MRA (magnetic resonance angiography) 59, 61
anticoagulant therapy 106
aortic
- arch 87
- coarctation 124
- dissection 86, 101
- root 87
apex fractures, orbital 77
arterial
- encasement 165
- inflow 50
- rise time 52
arteriovenous malformations 118
arthritis, rheumatoid 220
artifacts 3, 36, 37, 44, 71, 85, 93, 94, 126
- clipping artifacts 93
- motion artifacts 44
- pulsation 94
- radial artifacts 228
- rotation / stair-step 3
- SCT vs. CCT, breath and motion artifacts 71
- shading artifacts 93, 228
- - shaded three-dimensional surface displays 93
- stepping artifacts 142
- streak artifacts 85, 94, 126
aspiration, fine-needle 171
atheroma 132

B
BA (basilar artery) 59
basal ganglia 51
beam hardening 5, 37
- effect 37
biliary drainge 230
biopsies 144, 145, 171, 172, 229, 230
- anaesthetics and preparation 172
- biopsy gun 171
- bone biopsy 172
- chest, CT-guided punctures 144, 145
- coaxial puncture 172
- complications 173
- end notch 171
- fine-needle aspiration 171
- hybrid needles 171
- pulmonary tumors 229
- side-notch biopsy 171
- tissue biopsy needles 171
biphasic examinations 16, 70, 154
- contrast-enhanced CT 154
- SCT 70, 154
bladder, diverticulum 208
blood
- blood-brain barrier 49
- blood gas analysis 107
- flow tracers 49
blurring 126
bolus 45, 49, 154 ff.
- kinetics 49
- saline Chaser bolus 90
- tracking, liver 154–164
- triggering (CARE bolus) 90, 91, 96, 154, 156

bone
- biopsy 172
- hemangiomas 208
- marrow transplants 175
brachiocephalic veins 85
brain
- blood-brain barrier 49
- ischemia 49
- perfusion 49–58
breakthrough, CT 171
breast carcinoma 102
breath-hold scanning 3
bronchiectasis 120, 132
bronchiolitis obliterans 121
bronchus / bronchi
- absent 121
- cardiac 121
- dehiscence, bronchial 121
- ectopic 120
- hypoplastic 121
- supernumerary 121

C
calcification, coronary 132, 137–140
calcium score 132
cardiac / cardio
- bronchus 121
- cardio-delta 137
- cardio-interpolation 137, 139
- - linear 139
- CT with prospective cardic gating 126–136
- cycle 138
- insufficiency 51
- perforation 107
CARE
- bolus (bolus triggering) 90, 91, 96, 154, 156
- vision CT 195, 225–234
carotid artery
- bifurcation 216
- internal carotid artery (ICA) 56, 59
- stenosis 217, 218
Catphan phantom 13
cavernous sinus 63
- intracavernous aneurysms 59
CBF (cerebral blood flow) 49, 50, 53
- calculation of 50
CBV (cerebral blood volume) 50, 52
- calculation of 52–54
- fractional 52
ceramics scintillator 9
cerebral
- aneurysms (see there) 59–69
- arteries
- - ACA (anterior cerebral artery) 59
- - BA (basilar artery) 59
- - choiroidal arteries, anterior 63
- - communicating arteries 63, 66
- - - anterior 66
- - - posterior 63
- - MCA (middle cerebral artery) 56, 59
- - VA (vertebral artery) 59
- blood flow (CBF) 49
- blood volume (CBV) 50
- infarcts 55
cerebrospinal fluid (CSF) 54
Chaser bolus 90
chest
- CTA 83–97
- CT-guided diagnostic punctures of the chest 144, 145
- helical CT in pediatric chest 115–125
- pain 101
chloral hydrate 115
choroidal arteries, anterior 63
circle of Willis 45, 69, 219
circular cross-section 28
circumflex branch 88
clip planes 222
clipping 61
- artifacts 93
CM (contrast material) 70
coaxial puncture 172
collaterals 55
collimation 3
colon
- cancer 150
- diverticulum 208
colonoscopy, virtual 150
common duct stones 150
communicating arteries 63, 66
- anterior 66
- posterior 63
- - hypoplastic 63
compression ultrasonography 108
computed tomography angiography (see CTA) 45, 59 ff., 84 ff., 149, 150
condylar fractures 80
congenital lesions 118
conspicuity 4
contour finding 54
contrast 3
- administrations, intravenous 90
- biphasic contrast-enhanced CT 154
- enhancement threshold, liver 158
- high contrast resolution 11, 23, 117
- intravenous contrast medium 116, 154
- - chest 116
- - liver 154
- low contrast
- - detectability 14
- - phantom 3
- material (CM) 70
- in-plane contrast resolution 3
- resolution 36, 37
conventional CT (CCT) 70
- SCT vs. CCT, breath and motion artifacts 71
coronary artery diseases (see also cardiac) 137–140
- calcification 132, 137–140
- right coronary artery (RCA) 88
cortex, insular 56
cost-effectiveness analysis in diagnostic management of pulmonary embolism 106–114

cross-section 28
- circular 28
- non-circular 28
CSF (cerebrospinal fluid) 54
CTA (computed tomography angiography) 45, 59 ff., 84 ff., 149, 150
- accuracy in detection and characterization 60
- chest CTA 84–97
- comparison of diagnostic usefulness betwwen CTA, DSA and MRA 61
- 3D CTA 149
- diagnosis of cerebral aneurysms with CTA 60, 61
- disadvantages of CTA 61
- role of CTA in surgical planning 65, 66
- thoracic aorta, applications of CTA 92
CTDI measurements 17–19
- in air 19
CT-guided intervention 225
CT-scopy 173
curved planar reformations 149
cut-plane 198

D
3DI (three-dimensional imaging) 44 ff., 59 ff., 93, 149 ff., 176, 199, 207 ff.
- comparison of 3D rendering techniques 199
- CTA (computed tomography angiography) 45, 59–69, 149, 150, 212–224
- interactive 3D volume rendering, vascular applications 212–224
- postprocessing 3DI 44, 207 ff.
- radiosurgery planning 48
- real-time 45
- - 3D rendering 45
- - impact of, rendering of CT data on diagnostic performance 207–211
- - modeling 45
- - volume rendering 45, 46
- shaded three-dimensional surface displays 93, 149
- skeletal trauma with 3DI 176
- virtual applications of SCT 149–153
data interpolation 17
D-dimer 112
detector
- array 10
- multirow detector systems 143
- photodetectors 9
- solid-state detectors 9
- UFC detector technology 9–15
- xenon detectors 9
dextrocardia 123
diagonal branch 88
digital subtraction angiography (DSA) 59, 61, 107
diseases (see syndromes)
display noise 18
diverticulum
- bladder 208
- colon 208
documentations 190–193
dose
- efficiency 10, 11
- helical CT, relationship between time, dose and quality 3–8
- modulation 15
- reduction in CT 3 ff., 16 ff., 27 ff., 35 ff.
- - by anatomically adapted tube current modulation 27 ff., 35 ff.
- - - first patient studies 35–40
- - - principles and first results 27–34
- - automated reduction 5
- - vs. image quality in spiral CT 16–26
- reference dose 27
drainages 229, 230
- biliary drainge 230
DSA (digital subtraction angiography) 59, 61, 107
- comparison of diagnostic usefulness between CTA, DSA and MRA 61
dual-phase SCT 155
- liver 155
- pancreatic neoplasms 165–170
duct / ductal
- adenocarcinoma 167
- common duct stones 150
- interrupted duct 168
dye dilution theory 133
dynamic CT 50
dyspnoe 101

E
EBCT (electron beam CT) 126
ECG-oriented reconstruction from subsecond SCT scans 137–143
ECG-triggered interpolation / ECG triggering 94, 126 135
- applications 131–135
- methods 128, 129
- monitoring 129
- principles 128
- prospective 129, 130
- retrospective 130
echocardiography, M mode 126, 127
electron beam CT (EBCT) 126
electronic noise 19
embolism, pulmonary (see there) 85, 98–105, 222
endoluminal visualisation 222
endoscopic
- movies 150, 151
- virtual imaging 149
epiglottis, infrahyoid 74
equilibrium phase 162
ERCP 169
European Carotid Surgery Trial 216
extraocular muscles 76

F
facial fracturs, examination protocol in midfacial fractures 77

false channel 92
fast and SCT, contribution to diagnostic puncture of abdominal lesions 171–174
film reading 209
fine-needle aspiration 171
first pass of tracer 50
fistulisation 173
flow channels 196
fluoroscopy, CT 195, 225–234
fly / flying
- fly-around view, abdominal aorta 151
- fly-through view, abdominal aorta 150, 151
- flying focal spot 15
foramen, pseudoforamina 80
Fourier transformation 17
fractures 76 ff., 176
- acetabular 178, 179
- condylar 80
- frontobasis 79
- heminasoethmoidal 79
- hip joint 180
- midfacial 77, 79
- orbital 76, 77, 80
- symphyisis pubis 179
- tripod 79
frontobasis 79
functional
- imaging 49
- maps 50

G
gall stones 208
gammaknife 48
gastrointestinal invasion, pancreatic carcinoma 168
geometric / geometry
- efficiency 10
- engines 213, 225
glottis 71
grid-controlled X-ray 33

H
half-value layers 16
hard copies 208
head and neck malignancies, spiral CT vs. subsecond conventional CT 70–75
heart, imaging by ECG-oriented reconstruction from subsecond SCT scans 137–143
helical
- pediatric chest 115–125
- - applications 117, 118
- relationship between time, dose and quality 3–8
- volumetric presentation, chest 209
hemangiomas
- bone 208
- spine 208
hematopericardium 144
hematothorax 144
heminasoethmoidal fracture 79
hemoptysis 101
hepatic (see also liver)
- adenoma 159
- carcinoma, hepatocellular 160
- hepatic-arterial phase 154
hip / hip joint
- phantom 29
- trauma / fractures 175, 180
hybrid needles 171
hypopharynx 71
hypoplastic
- lung 120
- posterior communicating arteries 63

I
ICA (internal carotid artery) 56, 59
image
- noise 16, 20, 24, 28
- quality 3 ff., 16 ff.
- - dose reduction vs. image quality in spiral CT 16–26
- - helical CT, relationship between time, dose and quality 3–8
indicator-dilution theory 49
infection / inflammatory diseases 175
inflow, arterial 50
infrahyoid epiglottis 74
insular cortex 56
interpolation 128
- algorithm 22
- linear 139
- trilinear 212
intimal flap 89
ionization chamber 13
islet cell tumors 170

J
jaundice 165
jugular veins 72, 89
- internal 72

K
Kernel 16

L
LAD (left anterior descending) 88
Lefort level I 79
lipoma 183
liver (see also hepatic)
- automatic bolus tracking for SCT 154–164
- biphasic contrast-enhanced CT 154
- contrast enhancement threshold 158
- - intravenous contrast medium 116
- cysts 208
- dual-phase SCT 155
- monophasic SCT 162
- parenchymal disease 162

lung
- hypoplastic 120, 123
- metastatic lung cancer to paraspinal muscle 184
- scintigraphy 107, 108
lymph nodes 71
lymphadenopathy 150
lymphoma suspicion 173

M
magnetic resonance angiography (MRA) 59, 61, 149
maps, functional 50
mAs settings 14
mass characterization 118
maxillary sinuses 80
maxillofacial trauma, SCT 76–82
maximum
- MIP (maximum intensity projection) 55, 93, 149, 198, 212
- slope model 50
MCA (middle cerebral artery) 56, 59
mean transit time 50
mediastinal
- survey 124
- tumors 117
mesenteric artery, inferior 219
metastasis 173
microangiopathy 55
MIP (maximum intensity projection) 55, 93, 149, 198, 212
misregistration 126
modulation
- amplitude 28, 30
- - maximum modulation amplitude 28
- dose modulation 15
- functions 28
- MTF (modulation transfer function) 11
monophasic SCT, liver 162
MPR (multiplanar reformatted reconstructions) 77, 93, 177, 196
MRA (magnetic resonance angiography) 59, 61, 149
- comparison of diagnostic usefulness betwwen CTA, DSA and MRA 61
MRI (magnetic resonance imaging) 225
MTF (modulation transfer function) 11
multiplanar reformatted reconstructions (MPR) 77, 93, 177, 196
mural thrombus 197
muscle
- infection 176
- mass 131
musculoskeletal
- inflammation 177–181
- system, SCT 175 ff.
- tumors 181–184
myocardial
- infarction 107
- perfusion 126
- scintigraphy 133

N
NASCET criteria 216
nasopharynx 71
neck, head and neck (see there)
neuroendocrine tumors 165
neuronavigation
- real-time 43–48
- surgical 44, 45
neuroradiology, spiral CT 43–48
noise
- display noise 18
- electronic noise 19
- image noise 16, 20, 24, 28
- pixel noise 36
- propagation in CT imaging 28
- quantum noise 19
- signal-to-noise ratio 3
non-circular cross-section 28
North American Carotid Endarterectomy Trial 216

O
object
- conspicuity 4
- translucency 45
ocular, extraocular muscles 76
odontoid process 220
optic / optical
- coupling 10
- nerve canal 77, 79
orbital
- floor 77, 80
- fractures 76, 80
- - apex fractures 77
- wall 80
oropharynx 71
osteochondroma, scapula 183
osteolytic lesions 208
osteomyelitis, thoracic spine 181
osteosarcoma 119
outflow, venous 50

P
pancreatic
- carcinoma 165
- neoplasms, dual-phase SCT 165–170
- parenchyma 165
pancreatitis
- chronic 169
- puncture induced 173
parenchymal disease 117, 118, 162
- liver 162
- pancreatic 165
- pulmonary 117, 118
patient throughput 14
peak time 50
pediatric chest, helical CT 115–125
pentobarbital sodium 115
perforating arteries 63
perfusion / ventilation, lung 107, 108
pericardial constriction 131

perisplenic vesicles 165
peritonitis 173
PET (photon emission tomography) 54
pharynx 71
photodetectors 9
photodiodes 9
photomultipliers 9
PIOPED study 101, 107
piriform sinus 72
pitch / pitch factor 3, 86
planar
- compositions 213
- editing 198
- reformations 77, 93, 149
- - curved 149
- - MPR (multiplanar reformatted reconstructions) 77, 93, 177, 196
planum sphenoidale 66
plaque rupture 132
pleurisy 101
pneumonia 101, 107
pneumothorax 107, 144, 173
- biopsy 173
polyps 150
portal-venous phase 154, 155
- monophasic 155
postprocessing 207 ff.
power injector 54
productivity, scanner 189
projection angle 28
protocols 190–193
pseudoforamina 80
pterygoid processes 79
pulmonary
- acquired pulmonary hypoplasia (Swyer-James syndrome) 122
- embolism 85, 98 ff., 106 ff., 222
- - cost-effectiveness analysis in diagnostic management of 106–114
- - mortality 111
- - SCT 98–105
- - subsegmental emboli 100
- metastasis 208
- nodules 118
- parenchymal disease 117, 118
- sequestrations 118
- tumors, biopsy 229
pulsation / pulsed
- artifacts / effects 85, 94
- radiation 9
punctures (see also biopsies) 144, 145, 171, 172
- of the chest, CT-guided 144, 145
- coaxial puncture 172

Q
quality phantom 29
quantum noise 19

R
R wave 129
radial artifacts 228
radiation drift 9
radiolabeled microspheres 50
radiology 21
radiosurgery 45
raster manager 213
ray
- ray sum 150
- ray-tracing projectional techniques 150
- rays cast 204
- X-ray (see there) 14, 33
- VRT (volume ray tracing) 91, 93
Rayleigh criterion 11
RCA (right coronary artery) 88
real-time
- CT fluoroscopy 225–234
- intraoperative surgical navigation 47, 48
- neuronavigation 43–48
- three-dimensional modeling 45, 207–211
- volume rendering (see also there) 43–48
recirculation 50
reconstruction algorithm 16, 22
refractory period 130
region(s) of interest (ROIs) 17, 154, 155
renal
- artery stenosis 167, 222, 223
- cell carcinoma 150
- cysts 208
- transplantation 222, 223
rendering
- comparison of 3D rendering techniques 199
- perspective 204, 205
- surface rendering 77
- impact of real-time 3D rendering of CT data on diagnostic performance 207–211
- volume rendering (see also there) 43–48, 59, 77, 149–153, 212–224
residual flow 55
rheumatoid arthritis 220
ROIs (regions of interest) 17, 154, 155
room time 190
rotation
- angle 28, 29
- - abdomen phantom 29
- - hip phantom 29
- - quality phantom 29
- - shoulder phantom 29, 30
- artifacts 3
- partial 128
R-R interval 129

S
saline Chaser bolus 90
scanner productivity 189
scheduling 191
Scimitar syndrome 123
scintigraphy
- lung 107, 108
- myocardial 133
- VQ 98, 100, 103
scintillators 9
- UFC 9
screen reading 209

SCT (spiral CT) 16 ff., 43 ff., 70 ff., 76 ff., 98 ff., 137 ff., 149 ff., 154 ff., 165 ff., 171 ff., 175 ff., 189 ff.
- artifacts (breath and motion), SCT vs. CCT 71
- biphasic 70, 154
- contribution of fast and SCT to diagnostic puncture of abdominal lesions 171–174
- dose reduction vs. image quality in spiral CT 16–26
- dual-phase SCT 155, 165–170
- - liver 155
- - pancreatic neoplasms 165–170
- heart, imaging by ECG-oriented reconstruction from subsecond SCT scans 137–143
- liver, automatic bolus tracking for SCT 154–164
- maxillofacial trauma 76–82
- monophasic 162
- musculoskeletal system 175 ff.
- new technologies 189–195
- pulmonary embolism (see there) 98–105
- scan times 14
- spiral CT vs. subsecond conventional CT in head and neck malignancies 70–75
- three-dimensional imaging and virtual applications of SCT 149–153
- use in neuroradiology 43
- volumetric analysis of SCT data 196–206
sculpted editing 198
sedation 115
segmentation 54
shaded surface
- displays (SSD) 93, 149, 196, 197, 200, 201
- reconstruction (SSR) 59
shoulder
- region in patients, dose reduction 36, 37
- phantom 29, 30
side-notch biopsy 171
sigmoid colon 151
signal-to-noise ratio 3
single photon emission computed tomography (SPECT) 49
skeletal trauma with 3DI 176
slice
- collimation (SC) 17, 19–21, 86
- sensitivity profile 17
- thickness 4
slim-2 16
slip-ring
- gantry 43
- technology 9
slope model, maximum 50
smartscan 33
solid-state detectors 9
spatial resolution 3, 16
SPECT (single photon emission computed tomography) 49
spine / spinal
- hemangiomas 208
- osteomyelitis, thoracic spine 181
spiral CT (see SCT) 16 ff., 43 ff., 70 ff., 76 ff., 98 ff., 137 ff., 149 ff., 154 ff., 165 ff., 171 ff., 175 ff., 189 ff.
splanchnic vessels 150
splenic artery 167
SSD (shaded surface displays) 93, 149, 196, 197, 200, 201
- 3D 93, 149
SSR (shaded surface reconstruction) 59
stair-step artifacts 3
stent grafts 149
stereolithographic models 80
sterno-cleidomastoid muscle 73
streak artifacts 85, 94, 126
stroke 49
subarachnoid hemorrhage 61
subsecond scanning 15, 88
supraglottis 71
surface rendering 77
surgery / surgical
- neuronavigation 44, 45
- radiosurgery 45
- real-time intraoperative surgical navigation 47, 48
- role of CTA in surgical planning 65, 66
- three-dimensional radiosurgery planning 48
Swyer-James syndrome 122
sylvian veins 67
symphysis pubis, fracture 179
syndromes / diseases (names only)
- Scimitar 123
- Swyer-James 122

T

T wave 129
table feed 3
tachypnea 107
technical developments 187 ff.
thin-slab 198
thoracic
- aorta 220, 221
- - aneurysm 221
- - applications of CTA 92
- - CTA, perspective volume rendering 152
- helical CT, applications 117, 118
- spine, osteomyelitis 181
three-dimensional imaging (see 3DI) 44 ff., 59 ff., 93, 149 ff., 176, 199, 207 ff.
thrombosis
- deep vein thrombosis 106, 108
- mural thrombus 197
thyroid cartilage 72
TIA 55
time
- helical, relationship between time, dose and quality 3–8
- savings 190
TIPSS 233
tissue biopsy needles 171
tongue, base of 74

tracer, fist pass of 50
tracheal collapse 121
tracheobronchial tree assessment 119, 120
tracheomalacia 121
track a bolus 45, 154 ff.
tract metastasis 173
transit time 50
transplantation, post-transplantation complications 120
trigger / triggering
- CARE bolus (bolus triggering) 90, 91, 96, 154, 156
- ECG-triggered interpolation / ECG triggering 94, 126, 128, 130
- trigger delay 129
trilinear interpolations 212
triphasic examinations 16
tripod fracture 79
tube
- currents 4, 27
- - dose reduction in CT by anatomically adapted tube current modulation 27 ff., 35 ff.
- grid-controlled X-ray tubes 33
- load 13
turbo reconstruction 195

U
UFC (ultrafast ceramics)
- design goal 9–11
- - CT number stability 12
- - dose efficiency 10, 11
- - high contrast resolution 11, 23
- detector technology 9–15
- practical considerations 12–14
- scintillator 9
ultrasonography (US) 108, 225
- compression 108
uncinate process 166

V
vascular
- anomalies, mediastinum and lungs 117
- applications, interactive 3D volume rendering 212–224
- disease, chronic occlusive 49
- stenosis, identifying and imaging 216
vein / venous (vena)
- outflow, venous 50
- sampling, venous 170
- thrombosis 106, 108
- - tests of deep vein thrombosis 108
- v. cava superior 89
venography 108
ventilation / perfusion, lung 107, 108
ventricular function 131
vertebrobasilar system 219
virtual
- colonoscopy 150
- 3DI applications of SCT 149–153
- endoscopic imaging 149
- virtual-reality prosthesis 80
voltage 4
volume
- averaging 118
- manipulating volume data 216
- partial volume averaging 44
- ray tracing (VRT) 91, 93
- real-time volume rendering 43–48
- rendering 43–48, 59, 77, 149–153, 212–224
- - interactive 3D volume rendering, vascular applications 212–224
- - perspective 149–153
- - real-time 59
- volumetric analysis of SCT data 196–206
VQ scintigraphy 98, 100, 103
VRT (volume ray tracing) 91, 93

W
watershed 57
wave
- R wave 129
- T wave 129
Willis, circle of 45, 69, 219
window setting 4
workstation 208
wrist 176

X
xenon
- computed tomography 49
- detectors 9
X-ray
- grid-controlled X-ray tubes 33
- power 14

Z
zygomatic buttress 79